OXFORD MEDICAL PUBLICATIONS

Stroke Medicine

Published and forthcoming Oxford Specialist Handbooks

General Oxford Specialist Handbooks
A Resuscitation Room Guide
Addiction Medicine
Hypertension
Perioperative Medicine, Second Edition
Post-Operative Complications, Second Edition
Pulmonary Hypertension
Renal Transplantation

Oxford Specialist Handbooks in Anaesthesia
Cardiac Anaesthesia
Day Case Surgery
General Thoracic Anaesthesia
Neuroanaethesia
Obstetric Anaesthesia
Paediatric Anaesthesia
Regional Anaesthesia, Stimulation and Ultrasound Techniques

Oxford Specialist Handbooks in Cardiology
Adult Congenital Heart Disease
Cardiac Catheterization and Coronary Intervention
Cardiac Electrophysiology
Cardiovascular Magnetic Resonance
Echocardiography
Fetal Cardiology
Heart Failure
Nuclear Cardiology
Pacemakers and ICDs
Valvular Heart Disease

Oxford Specialist Handbooks in Critical Care
Advanced Respiratory Critical Care

Oxford Specialist Handbooks in End of Life Care
End of Life Care in Dementia
End of Life Care in Nephrology
End of Life in the Intensive Care Unit

Oxford Specialist Handbooks in Neurology
Epilepsy
Parkinson's Disease and Other Movement Disorders
Stroke Medicine

Oxford Specialist Handbooks in Paediatrics
Paediatric Dermatology
Paediatric Endocrinology and Diabetes
Paediatric Gastroenterology, Hepatology, and Nutrition
Paediatric Haematology and Oncology
Paediatric Intensive Care
Paediatric Nephrology
Paediatric Neurology
Paediatric Palliative Care
Paediatric Radiology
Paediatric Respiratory Medicine

Oxford Specialist Handbooks in Psychiatry
Child and Adolescent Psychiatry
Old Age Psychiatry

Oxford Specialist Handbooks in Radiology
Interventional Radiology
Musculoskeletal Imaging
Pulmonary Imaging

Oxford Specialist Handbooks in Surgery
Cardiothoracic Surgery
Colorectal Surgery
Hand Surgery
Liver and Pancreatobiliary Surgery
Operative Surgery, Second Edition
Oral Maxillofacial Surgery
Otolaryngology and Head and Neck Surgery
Paediatric Surgery
Plastic and Reconstructive Surgery
Surgical Oncology
Urological Surgery
Vascular Surgery

Oxford Specialist Handbooks in Neurology

Stroke Medicine

Hugh Markus

Professor of Neurology,
St George's University of London and
Consultant Neurologist,
St George's Hospital, London, UK

Anthony Pereira

Consultant Neurologist,
Department of Neurology,
St George's Hospital, London, UK

Geoffrey Cloud

Consultant Stroke Physician,
Department of Neurology,
St George's Hospital, London, UK

OXFORD
UNIVERSITY PRESS

OXFORD
UNIVERSITY PRESS

Great Clarendon Street, Oxford OX2 6DP

Oxford University Press is a department of the University of Oxford.
It furthers the University's objective of excellence in research, scholarship, and education by publishing worldwide in

Oxford New York

Auckland Cape Town Dar es Salaam Hong Kong Karachi
Kuala Lumpur Madrid Melbourne Mexico City Nairobi
New Delhi Shanghai Taipei Toronto

With offices in

Argentina Austria Brazil Chile Czech Republic France Greece
Guatemala Hungary Italy Japan Poland Portugal Singapore
South Korea Switzerland Thailand Turkey Ukraine Vietnam

Published in the United States
by Oxford University Press Inc., New York

First published 2010

British Library Cataloguing in Publication Data
Data available

Library of Congress Cataloging in Publication Data
Markus, Hugh.
Stroke medicine / Hugh Markus, Anthony Pereira, Geoffrey Cloud.—1st ed.
p. ; cm.—(Oxford specialist handbooks in neurology)
Includes bibliographical references and index.
ISBN 978–0–19–921877–6 (alk. paper)
1. Cerebrovascular disease—Handbooks, manuals, etc. I. Pereira, Anthony.
II. Cloud, Geoffrey. III. Title. IV. Series: Oxford specialist handbooks in neurology.
[DNLM: 1. Stroke. L 355 M3463s 2009]
RC388.5.M247 2009
616.8'1—dc22

Typeset by Cepha Imaging Private Ltd., Bangalore, India
Printed in China
on acid-free paper through
Asia Pacific Offset Limited

ISBN 978–0–19–921877–6

10 9 8 7 6 5 4 3 2 1

Preface

Introduction

Recent years have seen a revolution in the profile of stroke. Often thought of as an untreatable disease we now realise that, not only can many strokes be prevented, but acute treatment can have a major impact on outcome. Organised care within stroke units markedly reduces mortality. Thrombolysis is transforming the way in which acute stroke services are organised. It is encouraging both the medical profession and the general public to think of stroke as a potentially treatable "brain attack" requiring urgent diagnosis, transfer to hospital, and treatment. Recent data has shown that minor stroke and TIA is followed by a high risk of early recurrent stroke, much higher than previously appreciated. Preventing this early recurrence prevents major challenges in how we reconfigure services, and determine which early secondary prevention strategies are most effective.

These advances in stroke present many challenges in delivering services. In many countries stroke has been a 'Cinderella' specialty and there have been few senior doctors specifically trained in stroke care. Specialists from geriatric medicine, neurology and other disciplines are having to train themselves in hyperacute stroke management, and familiarise themselves with the many other advances in management which are required to deliver comprehensive stroke care. We will need many more stroke specialists in the future and this has led to the establishment of dedicated stroke training programmes, such as the UK Stroke Specialty training programme, and similar schemes in other countries.

Clinicians looking after stroke patients need rapid access to up to date practical information on how to look after stroke patients. We hope this text book of stroke medicine will provide such a source. It is written by two neurologists and a stroke physician, who together run a busy district and regional stroke service. It is aimed to provide a ready source of information for both stroke trainees and consultants. It is written to cover the syllabus of the UK stroke specialist training programme and other similar programmes worldwide.

Hugh Markus
Anthony Pereira
Geoff Cloud

Contents

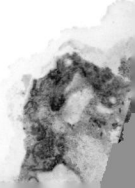

Abbreviations

ACA	anterior cerebral artery
ADC	apparent diffusion coefficient
ADL	activities of daily living
AF	atrial fibrillation
AHA	American Heart Association
AICA	anterior inferior cerebellar artery
aMTS	abbreviated mental test score
ALD	advanced life directive
ANH	artificial nutrition and hydration
APTT	activated partial thromboplastin time
ASA	atrial septal aneurysm
BMI	body mass index
BP	blood pressure
CADASIL	cerebral autosomal dominant arteriopathy with subcortical infarcts and leukoencephalopathy
CBF	cerebral blood flow
CBV	cerebral blood volume
CCD	cognitive communication disorder
CEA	carotid endarterectomy
COC	combined oral contraceptive
CPR	cardiopulmonary resuscitation
CRP	C-reactive protein
CSF	cerebrospinal fluid
CTA	computed tomography angiography
CVD	cardiovascular disease
CVP	central venous pressure
CVT	cerebral venous thrombosis
DNAR	do not attempt resuscitation
DTI	diffusion tensor imaging
DVT	deep venous thrombosis
DWI	diffusion-weighted imaging
ECG	electrocardiogram
EC–IC	extracranial–intracranial
EDV	end-diastolic velocity
ESR	erythrocyte sedimentation rate
FES	functional electrical stimulation

FLAIR	fluid-attenuated inversion recovery
GCS	Glasgow Coma Score
GDP	gross domestic product
GI	gastrointestinal
GOM	granular osmiophilic material
GRE	gradient spin echo
HbA1c	haemoglobin A1c
HDL	high density lipoproteins
HMPAO	^{99m}Tc-hexamethyl propyleneamine oxime
HRT	hormone replacement therapy
hs-CRP	highly sensitive CRP
HSP	hemiplegic shoulder pain
ICA	internal carotid artery
ICH	intracranial haemorrhage
ICP	intracranial pressure
IEED	involuntary emotional expression disorder
IMCA	Independent Mental Capacity Advocate
IMT	intima–media thickness
INR	international normalized ratio
LACI	lacunar anterior circulation infarct
LDL	low density lipoprotein
LPA	lasting Power of Attorney
LVH	left ventricular hypertrophy
MCA	middle cerebral artery
MCI	mild cognitive impairment
MELAS	mitochondrial encephalopathy with lactic acidosis and stroke-like episodes
MI	myocardial infarction
MIT	melodic intervention therapy
MMSE	mini mental state examination
MRA	magnetic resonance angiography
MRI	magnetic resonance imaging
MRS	magnetic resonance spectroscopy
MTHFR	methylene tetrahydrofolate reductase
MTT	mean transit time
NINDS	National Institute of Neurological Disorders and Stroke
NNT	number needed to treat
NSF	nephrogenic systemic fibrosis
OCSP	Oxfordshire Community Stroke Project Classification
OR	odds ratio
OSA	obstructive sleep apnoea

OT	occupational therapist
PACI	partial anterior circulation infarct
PCA	posterior cerebral artery
Pcom	posterior communicating artery
PCWP	pulmonary capillary wedge pressure
PE	pulmonary embolism
PEG	percutaneous endoscopic gastrostomy
PET	positron emission tomography
PFO	patent foramen ovale
PICA	posterior inferior cerebellar artery
POCI	posterior circulation infarct
PSV	peak systolic velocity
PVR	post-voiding residual volume
PWI	perfusion-weighted MRI
rtPA	recombinant tissue plasminogen activator
SAH	subarachnoid haemorrhage
SALT	speech and language therapist
SBP	systolic blood pressure
SCA	superior cerebellar artery
SIADH	syndrome of inappropriate ADH secretion
SLE	systemic lupus erythematosus
SNP	single nucleotide polymorphism
SPECT	single photon emission computed tomography
TACI	total anterior circulation infarct
TCD	transcranial Doppler
TED	thromboembolus deterrent
TIA	transient ischaemic attack
TOAST	Trial of Organon in Acute STroke
TOE	transoesophageal echocardiography
TOF	time of flight
TTE	transthoracic echocardiography
TTP	time to peak
VTE	venous thromboembolism
WHO	World Health Organization

Chapter 1

Epidemiology

Introduction

- Stroke is common. Someone suffers a stroke every 5 minutes in England and every 40 seconds in the USA
- Every year over 15 million people throughout the world suffer a stroke and 5 million are left significantly disabled
- In the UK and the USA, stroke is the third commonest cause of death (more than 60 000 and 160 000 deaths per annum, respectively) and is the leading cause of adult disability. There are nearly 5 million stroke survivors in the USA today
- Stroke is similarly devastating throughout western Europe
- Stroke is thought to be the second biggest killer worldwide, and is responsible for over 5 million deaths per annum
- Over half of stroke deaths are in women
- The lifetime risk of suffering stroke is approximately 1 in 4 for men and 1 in 5 for women (the latter being 2-3 times higher than the lifetime risk of breast cancer)
- In developed countries, about 15% of all strokes are haemorrhagic and 85% ischaemic
- One quarter of strokes are recurrent events
- Because stroke is such a common disease, prevention interventions which have only a small benefit to individual patients can have a large population benefit
- In the UK NHS, stroke patients have a typical hospital length of stay of 28 days and occupy over 2.6 million acute hospital bed days per year. The total economic burden of stroke is of the order of £7 billion per annum in England and Wales.

Definitions for epidemiological studies

Stroke

- A standardized definition of stroke is vital for epidemiological studies
- The World Health Organization (WHO) definition of stroke has been used for most studies and defines stroke as:
  Rapidly developing clinical signs of focal (or global) disturbance of cerebral function, with symptoms lasting 24 hours or longer, or leading to death, with no apparent cause other than of vascular origin
- This definition *includes* ischaemic stroke, intracerebral haemorrhage and subarachnoid haemorrhage. It *excludes* transient ischaemic attack, subdural haematoma and haemorrhage or infarction secondary to tumour or infection.

Transient ischaemic attack

- Stroke symptoms which last less than 24 hours are termed transient ischaemic attack (TIA)
- One should not think of TIA as an independent entity but rather a very short-lived stroke
- About 15% of strokes are preceded by a TIA
- MRI of patients who have suffered a TIA lasting longer than 1 hour shows that over 50% have visible areas of infarction. Technically, they have not suffered a 'stroke' but they have suffered cerebral infarction. This emphasizes that TIA and stroke are a continuum
- A revised definition of TIA has been proposed which excludes patients with cerebral infarction on imaging but it has not yet been widely adopted:
  A brief episode of neurological dysfunction caused by focal brain or retinal ischaemia, with clinical symptoms typically lasting less than 1 hour, and without evidence of acute infarction.

Reversible ischaemic neurological deficit (RIND)

- This term is now rarely used and is not terribly useful
- It defines a type of minor stroke caused by cerebral infarction whose clinical course lasts between 24 and 72 hours
- RIND is used in some countries to describe a minor stroke with complete recovery
- It is probably better to think of RIND as 'minor stroke'.

Most stroke physicians now accept that the terms TIA and RIND are artificial and think of these clinical syndromes as merely identifying different durations of symptoms from the same underlying disease process.

Stroke subtyping

- The definition of stroke does not differentiate between haemorrhagic and ischaemic stroke or between subtypes of ischaemic stroke
- Stroke subtyping attempts to address this
- Stroke subtyping has been attempted using the following classifications.

Clinical classifications

These rely on clinical features and were introduced before the widespread availability of brain and cerebral vascular imaging. The most used is the Oxfordshire Community Stroke Project Classification (OCSP, Table 1.1). The OCSP:

- Is simple and easy to apply
- Relates to prognosis and is useful to look at case-mix between populations
- Does not differentiate pathophysiological subtypes well (e.g. the OCSP stroke syndrome may not match the identified infarct; (for example an expected LACI may turn out to be a PACI on MRI and not the expected LACI)
- Is less suited to look at the pathological process causing the stroke, and the risk factor profiles for different stroke subtypes.

Pathophysiological classifications

Here the results of additional investigations are taken into account before identifying a subtype of stroke. For example, brain imaging may show a cortical infarct; the Doppler may show 80% stenosis due to atherosclerotic plaque and the echocardiogram (Echo) and ECG may be normal. This stroke is classified as a large artery atherosclerotic infarct.

Pathophysiological classifications:

- Are aimed at identifying the causes of individual subtypes
- Need intensive investigation (e.g. extracranial and ideally intracranial cerebral artery imaging, echo, etc. if they are to provide useful data)
- May not identify a mechanism even if the patient is fully investigated (approximately 25% of strokes remain of unknown cause).

The most used is the Trial of Organon in Acute STroke (TOAST).

The Trial of Org 10172 in Acute Stroke Treatment (TOAST) study, was a 7-year, randomized, double-blind, placebo-controlled, multicentre study of 1281 acute stroke patients in 36 centres across the USA. Sponsored by the National Institute of Neurological Disorders and Stroke (NINDS), it was the largest trial of an intravenously administered anticoagulant drug for treatment of acute ischaemic stroke.

Table 1.1 Oxfordshire Community Stroke Project Classification

Stroke type	Symptoms/presentation
LACI (lacunar infarct) Outcome = sometimes good	Pure motor *or* pure sensory stroke *or* a combination of motor and sensory (sensorimotor) *or* ataxic hemiparesis
TACI (total anterior circulation infarct) Outcome = usually poor	Motor and/or sensory deficits which affect the arm, leg and face in at least two areas *and* hemianopia (visual problems) *and* higher cerebral dysfunction such as dysphasia
PACI (partial anterior circulation infarct) Outcome = varied	Any two components of a TACI *or* isolated cerebral dysfunction, which are more restrictive than in a LACI classification
POCI (posterior circulation infarct) Outcome = varied	Symptoms of brainstem dysfunction *or* hemianopia (isolated)

Reproduced from Bamford J, Sandercock P *et al.* (1991). Classification and natural history of clinically identifiable subtypes of cerebral infarction. *Lancet* **337**, 1521, with permission of Elsevier.

Trial of organon in acute stroke (TOAST) classification

The TOAST classification denotes five subtypes of ischaemic stroke (Table 1.2):

1) Large-artery atherosclerosis
2) Cardioembolism
3) Small-vessel occlusion
4) Stroke of other determined aetiology
5) Stroke of undetermined aetiology
6) Stroke caused by more than one potential cause

The original TOAST classification:

- Divided most causes into probable and possible. However, many clinicians use only one category for both probable and possible when using it clinically or for research
- Used risk factors in the definition of subtype: e.g. hypertension for lacunar stroke. This is often not applied, particularly in studies looking at risk factor profiles as it will, of course, exaggerate the role of hypertension as a risk factor for lacunar stroke.

Table 1.2 TOAST Diagnostic Classification

Diagnostic Group	Case Description	Collapsed Group	
1	Atherosclerosis, probable	Atherosclerosis	New onset left hemiparesis with sensory deficit affecting face and arm more than leg. Left homonymous hemianopsia. Left hemispatial neglect. CT shows loss area of ill-defined loss of gray–white junction in right parietotemporal region. Doppler shows >95% stenosis in right ICA. Angiogram shows 80% stenosis right ICA with branch occlusion in right MCA. Patient in normal sinus rhythm. ECG normal. Echocardiogram normal. No coagulopathy.
2	Atherosclerosis, possible		New onset left hemiparesis with sensory deficit affecting face and arm more than leg. Left homonymous hemianopsia. Left hemispatial neglect. CT shows loss area of ill-defined loss of gray–white junction in right parietotemporal region. Doppler shows >60% stenosis in right ICA. Angiogram shows <50% stenosis right ICA with branch occlusion in right MCA. Patient in normal sinus rhythm. ECG normal. Echocardiogram normal. No coagulopathy.
3	Cardioembolic, probable	Cardioembolic	New onset left hemiparesis with sensory deficit affecting face and arm more than leg. Left homonymous hemianopsia. Left hemispatial neglect. CT shows loss area of ill-defined loss of gray–white junction in right parietotemporal region. Doppler shows <50% stenosis in ICAs. Patient in atrial fibrillation. Echocardiogram dilated left atrium without clot. No coagulopathy.
4	Cardioembolic, possible		New onset left hemiparesis with sensory deficit affecting face and arm more than leg. Left homonymous hemianopsia. Left hemispatial neglect. CT shows loss area of ill-defined loss of gray–white junction in right parietotemporal region. Patient in atrial fibrillation. Echocardiogram dilated left atrium without clot. No coagulopathy.
5	Lacunar, probable	Lacunar	History of hypertension. New onset left hemiparesis affecting face, arm, and leg to same extent. No cognitive, visual, or sensory deficits. CT shows loss area of ill-defined decreased attenuation in right internal capsule. Doppler shows <50% stenosis in ICAs. Patient in normal sinus rhythm. ECG normal. Echocardiogram normal. No coagulopathy.
6	Lacunar, possible		History of hypertension. New onset left hemiparesis affecting face, arm, and leg to same extent. No cognitive, visual, or sensory deficits. CT shows loss area of ill-defined decreased attenuation in right internal capsule. Doppler shows <50% stenosis in ICAs. Patient in normal sinus rhythm. ECG normal. Echocardiogram patent foramen ovale. No coagulopathy.

7	Other determined aetiology, possible	Other determined aetiology	History of DVT and spontaneous abortion. New onset left hemiparesis affecting face, arm, and leg to same extent. No cognitive, visual, or sensory deficits. CT shows loss area of ill-defined decreased attenuation in right internal capsule. Doppler shows <50% stenosis in ICAs. Patient in normal sinus rhythm. ECG normal. Echocardiogram normal. PTT prolonged without anticoagulants.
8	Other determined aetiology, probable		History of DVT and spontaneous abortion. Prior workup showed protein C deficiency. New onset left hemiparesis affecting face, arm, and leg to same extent. No cognitive, visual, or sensory deficits. CT shows loss area of ill-defined decreased attenuation in right internal capsule. Doppler shows <50% stenosis in ICAs. Patient in normal sinus rhythm. ECG normal. Echocardiogram normal.
9	Undetermined aetiology, complete evaluation	Undetermined aetiology	New onset left hemiparesis with sensory deficit affecting face and arm more than leg. Left homonymous hemianopsia. Left hemispatial neglect. CT shows loss area of ill-defined loss of gray–white junction in right parietotemporal region. Doppler shows <50% stenosis in ICAs. Angiogram normal. Patient in normal sinus rhythm. ECG normal. Echocardiogram normal. No coagulopathy.
10	Undetermined aetiology, incomplete evaluation		New onset left hemiparesis with sensory deficit affecting face and arm more than leg. Left homonymous hemianopsia. Left hemispatial neglect. CT shows loss area of ill-defined loss of gray–white junction in right parietotemporal region. Patient in normal sinus rhythm. No coagulopathy.
11	Multiple possible aetiologies		New onset left hemiparesis with sensory deficit affecting face and arm more than leg. Left homonymous hemianopsia. Left hemispatial neglect. CT shows loss area of ill-defined loss of gray–white junction in right parietotemporal region. Doppler shows >70% stenosis in right ICA. Angiogram shows 80% stenosis in right ICA with branch occlusion in right MCA. Patient in atrial fibrillation. Echocardiogram dilated left atrium without clot. No coagulopathy.

ICA indicates internal carotid artery; MCA, middle cerebral artery; DVT, deep vein thrombosis; and PTT, partial thromboplastin time.
Criteria reprinted with permission.
Data from Adams HP, Bendixen BH, Kappelle LJ, Biller J, Love BB, Gordon DL, Marsh E (1993). Classification of subtype of acute ischemic stroke. Definitions for use in a multicenter clinical trial. TOAST. Trial of Org 10172 in Acute Stroke Treatment. *Stroke* **24**: 35–41, and Goldstein LB, Jones MR, Matchar DB, Edwards LJ, Hoff J, Chilukuri V, Armstrong SB, Horner RD (2001). Improving the reliability of stroke subgroup classification using the Trial of ORG 10172 in Acute Stroke Treatment (TOAST) criteria. *Stroke* **32**:1091–8.

Incidence and prevalence

Incidence is the number of new cases of stroke per annum in a population. ***Prevalence*** is the total number of patients who have had stroke at any time within a population.

Stroke incidence (Fig 1.1)

Stroke incidence is probably under-reported for several reasons:

- Owing to the limitations of epidemiological studies using the WHO clinical definition alone
- The fact that not all stroke patients go to hospital
- Stroke diagnosis may not be recorded in those individuals who die shortly after stroke onset (brain imaging is required to confirm a diagnosis of stroke)
- There are no reliable estimates of incidence in developing countries.

The incidence of stroke varies geographically but in the UK is typically 2–3/1000 per annum.

This would mean a family doctor (general practitioner) in a practice of 5000 would have more than 10 patients a year with new stroke and a typical general hospital serving a population of 250 000 may admit over 500 stroke cases a year.

Stroke incidence has been falling in many westernized countries. For example, over 20 years or more of prospective study in Oxford (UK), incorporating both OCSP and OXVASC studies, incidence seems to have fallen by about a third. This is thought to be due principally to a reduction in levels of hypertension and smoking within the population, and the introduction of statin and antiplatelet therapy for primary prevention of those with vascular risk factors. However, there are at least 110 000 new strokes per annum in England and 780 000 in the USA.

Interestingly, although stroke incidence has fallen in Oxfordshire, case fatality has remained at about 17%, emphasizing the importance of prevention rather than cure.

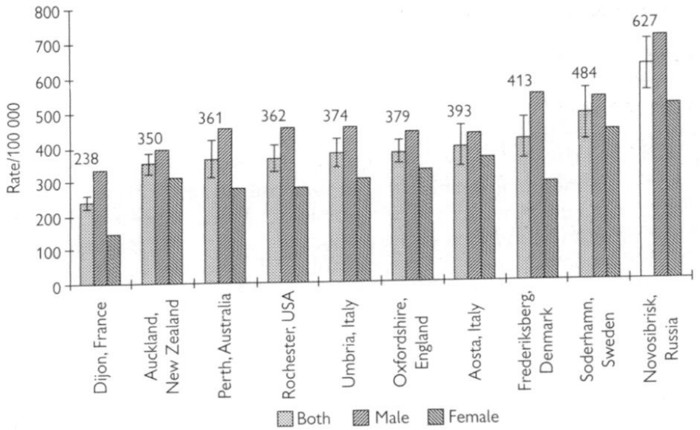

Fig. 1.1 Incidence of stroke (ischaemic and haemorrhagic) amongst 10 different communities according to age groups 45 years and older. Adapted from Sudlow CL, Warlow CP (1997) Comparable studies of the incidence of stroke and its pathological types: results from an international collaboration. *Stroke* **28**, 491–9, with permission.

Stroke prevalence (Fig. 1.2)

- In England there are nearly 1 million stroke survivors and over half are dependent on others for everyday activities, with 300 000 living with significant disability from their stroke
- In the USA there are over 4.8 million survivors (approximately 2.6% of the total population).

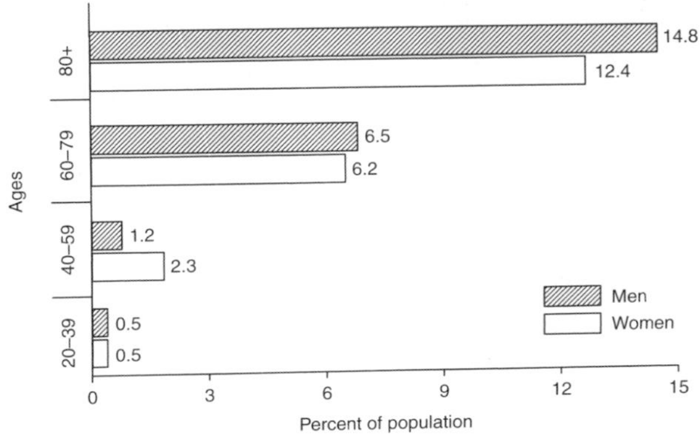

Fig. 1.2 Stroke prevalence in the USA by age and gender. Data from the National Health and Nutrition Examination Survey (NHANES) 1999–2005.

Stroke mortality

- Estimates of stroke mortality are more robust than those of incidence as minor (almost all non-fatal) strokes are more easily missed than major ones
- Within Europe, there is a fivefold gradient of increased stroke mortality, from France and Switzerland with the lowest mortality rates to Russia and the former Soviet bloc with the highest. This difference is mainly determined by socioeconomic factors. About 66% of the variance can be ascribed to the amount of gross domestic product (GDP) countries spend on stroke care. GDP is not the whole story, however, as countries such as Norway with high GDP spent on stroke care still have relative increased stroke mortality rates in comparison to other countries such as France
- Overall, rates of stroke mortality are:
  - decreasing in western Europe
  - increasing in eastern Europe
  - seem to have 'bottomed out' in both the USA and Japan
- Within western European countries, comparative studies have shown high mortality rates in the UK compared with other countries, such as France, despite overall resources consumed being similar. The reasons for this are uncertain but it has been suggested that it is due to less intensive therapy early during the acute phase. The poorer outcome is then associated with greater disability which increases costs
- Stroke mortality is falling in the UK but still 20–30% of people die within 28 days of stroke—with case fatality twice as high in patients aged over 85 as those below 65 years
- Stroke mortality is highest for haemorrhagic subtypes.

Table 1.3 Thirty-day case-fatality rates for stroke in the USA in 1999. Figures are for first-ever stroke, by ethnicity and stroke subtype

	% Case-fatality rates (95% CI)		
	All†	**Black***	**White***
All stroke subtypes	14.7	12.8	16.9
Ischaemic	10.2	9.1	11.5
Intracerebral haemorrhage	37.6	36.2	39.0
Subarachnoid haemorrhage	31.3	28.2	34.7

*Adjusted for age and gender. †Adjusted for age, gender and race. Adapted from Kleindorfer D, Broderick J, Khoury J *et al.* (2006) The unchanging incidence and case-fatality of stroke in the 1990s: a population-based study. *Stroke* **37**, 2473–8.

Economic cost of stroke care

- Acute stroke care in England is responsible for 6% of all NHS expenditure – around £2.8 billion (see Table 1.4). Stroke patients have a typical hospital length of stay of 28 days and occupy over 2.6 million acute hospital bed days per year
- With the cost of lost productivity and disability estimated at £1.8 billion and the cost of informal carers at £2.4 billion, the total annual cost of UK stroke care is estimated at £7 billion, comparable to coronary heart disease
- The cost of stroke (indirect and direct) in the USA was estimated in 2004 to be \$53.6 billion, with a mean lifetime cost of \$140 048 per stroke
- Over one-quarter of strokes occur in people of working age
- Cerebrovascular disease is also the second commonest cause of dementia, is the commonest cause of late onset epilepsy and a major cause of depression, compounding the healthcare economic burden of stroke disease.

Costs (in pounds sterling) of stroke in England (total population of 50 million) from the National Audit Office report

Table 1.4 Total cost of stroke in England (in pounds sterling)

Cost items	Cost
Diagnostic costs	9,600,000
Inpatient care costs	530,000,000
Outpatient care cots	46,200,000
Outpatient drug costs	507,200,000
Community care costs	1,741,100,000
Total annual direct care cost	**2,834,100,000**
Informal care costs	**2,406,400,000**
Income lost due to mortality	483,700,000
Income lost due to morbidity	604,100,000
Benefit payments	686,600,000
Total annual indirect costs	**1,774,400,000**
Total	**7,014,900,000**

- In an ageing population, the incidence, prevalence and cost are all set to rise
- The number of people in England aged 65 years and over increased by nearly 4 million between 1952 and 2002. The proportion of older people is predicted to rise from 16% in 2003 to 23% in 2031. The total cost of stroke care is predicted to rise in real terms by 30% between 1991 and 2010.

Table 1.5 Interim life table for England. This shows the main number of years of remaining life at different ages.

	0	1	2	3	4	5	6	7	8	9	10	11	12	13	14	15	16	17	18	19	20	Age now
Male	76.52	75.95	74.98	74.00	73.02	72.03	71.04	70.05	69.05	68.06	67.07	66.07	65.08	64.09	63.10	62.12	61.13	60.15	59.19	58.23	57.26	Life added years
Female	80.93	80.30	79.33	78.35	77.36	76.37	75.38	74.39	73.39	72.40	71.40	70.41	69.42	68.43	67.44	66.44	65.45	64.47	63.49	62.50	61.52	
	21	22	23	24	25	26	27	28	29	30	31	32	33	34	35	36	37	38	39	40	41	Age now
Male	56.31	55.35	54.39	53.44	52.48	51.52	50.56	49.60	48.65	47.69	46.74	45.78	44.83	43.88	42.93	41.98	41.04	40.09	39.15	38.21	37.27	Life added years
Female	60.54	59.56	58.58	57.59	56.61	55.63	54.65	53.67	52.69	51.71	50.73	49.75	48.78	47.80	46.83	45.86	44.89	43.93	42.96	42.00	41.04	
	42	43	44	45	46	47	48	49	50	51	52	53	54	55	56	57	58	59	60	61	62	Age now
Male	36.33	35.40	34.48	33.55	32.63	31.72	30.81	29.91	29.02	28.13	27.25	26.38	25.51	24.65	23.80	22.95	22.11	21.28	20.47	19.67	18.88	Life added years
Female	40.08	39.13	38.18	37.23	36.29	35.35	34.42	33.50	32.57	31.66	30.75	29.84	28.93	28.04	27.14	26.26	25.38	24.50	23.64	22.78	21.93	

	63	64	65	66	67	68	69	70	71	72	73	74	75	76	77	78	79	80	81	82	83	Age now
Male	18.12	17.35	16.61	15.87	15.15	14.44	13.75	13.07	12.40	11.76	11.14	10.54	9.96	9.40	8.86	8.35	7.85	7.38	6.93	6.51	6.11	Life added years
Female	21.09	20.26	19.44	18.63	17.84	17.05	16.27	15.51	14.75	14.02	13.30	12.60	11.92	11.26	10.63	10.01	9.41	8.83	8.28	7.75	7.24	

	84	85	86	87	88	89	90	91	92	93	94	95	96	97	98	99	100	Age now
Male	5.72	5.33	4.96	4.62	4.33	4.06	3.82	3.56	3.32	3.10	2.91	2.70	2.53	2.37	2.22	2.10	1.96	Life added years
Female	6.75	6.28	5.83	5.40	5.03	4.67	4.34	4.02	3.73	3.46	3.22	3.01	2.81	2.62	2.46	2.31	2.15	

Determining risk

Definition of a risk factor and causality

A risk factor for stroke is a characteristic which, when possessed by an individual, increases their liability to suffer a stroke.

Such an association does not necessarily imply causality. Causality depends upon a number of factors, including:

- Biological and epidemiological plausibility
- A temporal sequence between risk factor and stroke
- The strength of the association
- The reproducibility and consistency of the association in different studies and populations
- Independence from confounding factors
- The demonstration that reduction or treatment of that risk factor reduces stroke risk.

Absolute and relative risk

Absolute risk is the risk of developing a disease in a given population in a given time. For example, in the population of patients aged over 60 who have atrial fibrillation, their risk of suffering a stroke is 5% per year. Therefore, their absolute annual risk of stroke is 5%.

The absolute risk will be affected by treatment. In the population of atrial fibrillation patients aged over 60 years treated with warfarin, the risk of stroke is about 2% per annum. Therefore, treating the person with warfarin reduces their absolute risk to approximately 2%.

The absolute risk reduction is simply 5% minus 2%, making 3%. Therefore, warfarin reduces the absolute risk of stroke by 3% per annum. The patient on warfarin now has a 2% risk of stroke compared to the 5% they would have had untreated, i.e. 40% of the original risk. This is their relative risk. Their risk has gone down from 100% of the absolute risk to 40% of the absolute risk, i.e. a relative risk reduction of 60%.

Therefore, relative risk can be thought of as the ratio of the absolute risk in the population with the risk factor to the absolute risk in the control population without the risk factor.

Relative risk = absolute risk in risk population/absolute risk in control population

If the relative risk is greater than 1, then the risk factor increases stroke risk. If the relative risk is less than one then the 'risk factor' is protective.

Population-attributable risk

This describes the overall contribution a risk factor makes to stroke disease burden. The population-attributable or absolute risk is the proportion of disease for which the risk factor accounts.

This greatly depends on the prevalence of the risk factor in the population. This can be illustrated with hypertension. For example, elevation of systolic blood pressure to greater than 180 mmHg confirms a greatly increased relative risk of stroke, which is much greater than the relative risk of stroke owing to a blood pressure in the range 160–180 mmHg. However, such marked elevations of blood pressure are rare while more modest elevations are much more common. Therefore the population absolute risk associated with a blood pressure elevation in the range 160–180 is greater than that due to blood pressure elevation of greater than 180 mmHg.

Number needed to treat

The absolute risk allows a calculation for the number needed to treat. This is the number of patients needed to treat to prevent one additional bad outcome. It is calculated from the absolute risk reduction. It gives a good idea of the benefit of a treatment and is a simple and honest way to present the potential benefit of a treatment to a patient.

In the example above, treating patients aged over 60 years old who are in atrial fibrillation with warfarin reduces their risk of stroke by 3% per year.

- Therefore treating 100 patients per year would save three from having a stroke
- Therefore treating 33 patients per year would save one from having a stroke
- Therefore the number needed to treat per year is 33 to prevent one stroke.

Alternatively:

- The absolute risk reduction is 3% per year
- Therefore, the absolute risk reduction would be 30% after 10 years
- Now, treating 100 people for 10 years would save 30 strokes
- Therefore, treating 3.3 people for 10 years would save 1 stroke
- Therefore, the number needed to save 1 stroke is 3.3 (for 10 years).

Odds ratio versus relative risk

Relative risk is used in prospective cohort studies, or prospective clinical trials to indicate the increased risk associated with a specific risk factor.

Odds ratio (OR) is used instead to indicate the increased risk associated with a risk factor in cross-sectional (non-prospective) studies.

The difference is illustrated by the following example.

Consider the question: Does smoking cause stroke?

This can be answered in two ways:

1. It could be done by prospectively following up a whole population of people and identifying the smokers and non-smokers and see who develops stroke during follow up. The absolute risk of having a stroke if you smoked and the absolute risk if you didn't could be calculated, and then the relative risk could be worked out. An easy concept but the downside of this is that it would take a long time (many years) to perform the study. This is because the population incidence of stroke is fairly low and a large number of patients and/or many years of follow up are required to obtain sufficient endpoints (strokes)

2. Alternatively, a cohort of stroke patients could be collected who have been seen over a shorter period and how many of them smoked could be determined. This calculation would give the risk of being a smoker in an individual stroke population; it would not give the absolute risk of having a stroke from smoking. This sort of study is called a cross-sectional case-controlled study. It is relatively easy to do but does not allow relative risk calculation. Instead, it provides the OR.

Therefore the OR is used because:

- It can be used in case-controlled studies
- It is relatively easy to manipulate mathematically
- It can be corrected for confounding variables in logistic regression models.

It may be possible to look at several other risk factors which produce different ORs. You could then look at the particular risk factor of interest and correct for all the others (logistic regression analysis) to see which risk factors are independent risk factors.

Example of how to calculate an odds ratio
Let us use the table below:

		The outcome (e.g. stroke event)	
		+	–
Risk factor exposure	+	*a*	*b*
	–	*c*	*d*
		a/c Odds of being exposed in cases	*b/d* Odds of being exposed in controls
			OR = a/c ---- b/d

	Stroke	
	Yes	**No**
Risk factor	20	10
No risk factor	30	40

- The odds of having the risk factor if the patient suffered a stroke are 20:30, i.e. 2/3 (0.66)
- The odds of having the risk factor if the person didn't suffer a stroke are 10:40, i.e. 1/4 (0.25)
- The OR is 0.66/0.25, i.e. 2.64. An OR of greater than 1 suggests the risk factor plays a part in causing the stroke. Note this is *not* a relative risk of 2.64.

Stroke risk factors

Risk factors for stroke: general considerations

Population-based prospective studies

- The most reliable identification of stroke risk factors comes from prospective cohort studies such as the Framingham study
- These give true population-based estimates and avoid referral bias
- Stroke subtyping and characterization is often suboptimal because stroke cannot all be investigated in one hospital but may occur in the community or present to remote hospitals
- Even in large prospective studies, the number of strokes during the follow-up period may be small.

Case-control studies

- Allow much more detailed evaluation of each individual stroke in a standardized fashion than population-based studies
- Allow better differentiation between different stroke subtypes
- However, they are subject to potential bias, both in patient and control-case selection.

In many studies, particularly population-based ones, there has been little or no division of stroke into cerebral haemorrhage and ischaemia, let alone any division of ischaemia into its different pathogenic subtypes. Because most strokes are due to infarction, most of these studies primarily tell us the risk factors for infarction rather than haemorrhage.

Because a large number of ischaemic strokes are related to the complications of atherosclerosis (e.g. carotid stenosis, embolism secondary to myocardial infarction, atrial fibrillation secondary to coronary heart disease), these studies have similar risk factor profiles to those of coronary heart disease. However, there do seem to be some differences, particularly in the importance of different risk factors for coronary heart disease and stroke.

More recent studies have included imaging, allowing differentiation of different stroke subtypes; this suggests that the risk factor profile of the different subtypes may vary.

A further problem with the population studies is that frequently the diagnosis of stroke is obtained from hospital records or death certification. Both may be unreliable.

Specific stroke risk factors

Many have been proposed and they are best thought of in terms of *modifiable* and *non-modifiable* risk factors for stroke. See Table 1.6.

Table 1.6 Risk factors for stroke

Non-modifiable	Modifiable
Older age	**Major—well described and/or most important**
Male sex	Socioeconomic class
Ethnicity	Obesity
Genetic predisposition	Physical inactivity
	Smoking
	Alcohol
	Hypertension
	Diabetes and metabolic syndrome
	Cholesterol
	Previous stroke or TIA
	Atherosclerosis
	Atrial fibrillation
	Structural cardiac abnormalities
	Minor—less well described and/or less important
	Diet
	Homocysteine
	Recreational drug use
	Sleep disordered breathing
	Thrombophilia
	Inflammation
	Infection
	Migraine
	Oral contraceptive pill use
	Hormone replacement therapy
	Other drugs

Non-modifiable stroke risk factors

Age

- Stroke incidence increases exponentially with age
- Each decade above 55 years leads to a doubling of stroke risk
- Under the age of 50, incidence of stroke is evenly represented between haemorrhagic and ischaemic subtypes, but the former declines with age, leaving an overall majority of 85% of all strokes being ischaemic in origin
- The lifetime risk of suffering stroke if a person lives to 85 years is approximately 1 in 4 for a man and 1 in 5 for a woman.

Gender

- Male sex confers an increased risk of ischaemic stroke (relative risk about 1.3 compared to female)
- Although stroke risk is higher in men than in women, more women die from stroke owing to their greater life expectancy
- Overall, women have more severe stroke, more significant stroke disability and more post-stroke depression and dementia
- There is no clear genetic basis to explain the gender difference and the excess risk in men is less than that seen in ischaemic heart disease.

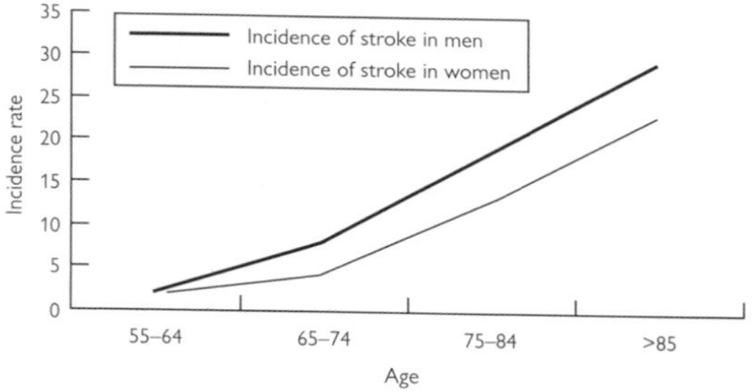

Fig. 1.3 Graph showing incidence rate per 1000 person-years for stroke in relation to age and gender. Adapted from Hollander M *et al.* (2003) Incidence, risk, and case fatality of first ever stroke in the elderly population. The Rotterdam Study. *Journal of Neurology, Neurosurgery and Psychiatry* **74**, 317–21, with permission from BMJ Publishing Group Ltd.

Ethnicity

There are ethnic differences in both stroke incidence and the relative frequency of stroke subtypes.

Blacks

In the USA, relative risk of stroke is highest in blacks, who also have increased stroke mortality compared to Mexican Americans and white Americans. The American Heart Association estimated prevalence of stroke in males in the US is:

- 4.1% black Americans
- 3.1% Mexican Americans
- 2.4% white Americans

In the UK, data from the South London Stroke register has suggested that:

- Incidence rates of first ever stroke adjusted for age and sex are twice as high in black compared to white people
- This excess incidence cannot be accounted for by differences in social class in the age group 35–64 years
- Black people tend to have their first stroke at a younger age than white people
- Small-vessel cerebrovascular disease (lacunar stroke) and intracranial atherosclerosis are more common in black than white patients
- In contrast, extracranial larger artery disease is less common in black people
- Hypertension is common and often severe and this contributes to the small-vessel disease risk but does not explain it fully
- However, in general, black patients in a south London population with first ever stroke were more likely to survive than white patients (the exceptions being in those aged <65 years and those with a prior Barthel score <15). This is likely to be related to their ischaemic stroke subtype which is mainly subcortical small volume stroke—as opposed to large-vessel atherosclerotic or cardioembolic stroke—associated with generally larger volume, cortical infarcts.

Far Eastern Asian

- Stroke is reportedly more common in Far East countries although with marked geographical variation within the region
- Northern China has increased incidence of stroke of the order of 80% compared to white America, Japan (39%) and Taiwan (23%). Stroke is the second leading cause of death in China, Korea and Taiwan, third in Japan and Singapore, sixth in the Philippines and tenth in Thailand
- Stroke in patients of Chinese ethnic origin often has a different aetiological subtype, with a greater incidence of intracranial stenoses and primary haemorrhage (especially subarachnoid haemorrhage) compared to white European populations. A similar increase in these subtypes is found in Japan
- Multivariate analysis has suggested that hypertension is a more important risk factor in Far Eastern populations compared to white Americans but does not explain the variation in stroke incidence within the geographical region.

South Asian

- South Asians (from India, Pakistan and Bangladesh) also have increased incidence of stroke
- In the UK, South Asian immigrants have particularly high levels of diabetes (sixfold greater than the rest of the population) and seem to have a predominantly small-vessel form of cerebrovascular disease
- Interestingly, South Asians studied in Singapore have predominantly intracranial large-vessel stenoses as a cause of stroke.

Genetic predisposition

- Twin and family studies suggest that genetic factors contribute to the risk of stroke, although the degree of risk they contribute is uncertain
- Having a first degree family member with a history of stroke before the age of 65 is associated with a twofold increased risk of ischaemic stroke. The genetic basis for this is not clear. Genetic predisposition to stroke may act either directly through vascular risk factors with their own genetic basis (e.g. hypertension and diabetes), independently of such factors or by modulating the effect of risk factors
- Genetic factors are believed to be primarily polygenic (multiple genes having small effects) with interaction with environmental and other risk factors
- The genes causing polygenic stroke are poorly understood. Many studies have looked at genetic variants (polymorphisms) in candidate genes as risk factors. Results have been conflicting. New chip technology allows screening of as many as 1 million single nucleotide polymorphisms (SNPs) spanning the whole chromosome in a genome- wide association scan. This technology has been applied successfully to other complex diseases (e.g. diabetes) and is being applied to stroke. Gene loci discovered using this approach as risk factors for atrial fibrillation and for ischaemic heart disease have also been shown to be risk factors for cardioembolic and larger artery ischaemic stroke, respectively
- The differences in stroke mortality rates between, for example, eastern and western Europe suggest that potentially modifiable factors may be more important than genetic differences for stroke susceptibility
- The results of migrant studies also support this view. Japanese populations in the USA experience rates of stroke similar to the American white host population rather than to the indigenous Japanese population in Japan. However, it is likely that there are complex interactions between genetic and environmental influences, and environmental influences may only increase the risk of stroke in those with pre-existing genetic susceptibility
- A number of monogenic (single gene) disorders cause stroke but these are rare on a population basis (see 🕮 Chapter 11 for details).

Major modifiable stroke risk factors

Socioeconomic class

- Low socioeconomic class is associated with increased stroke risk
- Stroke mortality across Europe significantly correlates with GDP (a surrogate for the economic status of the country).

Obesity

- Obesity is associated with increased stroke risk, but much of this may be via other risk factors such as hypertension and diabetes
- There has been no trial data to demonstrate weight reduction reduces stroke risk, but weight reduction has been shown to reduce systolic blood pressure by about 4 mmHg for every 5 kg reduction. Obesity also closely relates to type 2 diabetes

Evidence for obesity to be a risk factor is divided:

For:

- The Whitehall study showed that body mass index (BMI) was predictive of stroke in both smokers and non-smokers
- Increased weight seems to be associated with an increased stroke risk in a dose–response fashion. In the Korean Medical Insurance Corporation Study, adjusted RR for all stroke was approximately 1.04.

Against:

- Much of the association between BMI and stroke is reduced when confounding variables such as hypertension, diabetes, smoking, and exercise are taken into account. Therefore obesity may not be an independent risk factor but be increasing via these risk factors
- In multivariate analysis that controls for other vascular risk factors, the relationship between obesity and stroke is attenuated but persists.

Physical inactivity

Sedentary or inactive lifestyle is an independent risk factor for stroke. At least 30 minutes of moderate exercise—such as continuous walking three times a week—has been shown to reduce risk of recurrent stroke.

The mechanisms for this may include:

- Improved risk factor (e.g. hypertension, diabetes) control
- Increase in plasma tissue plasminogen activator activity
- Increase in HDL concentrations
- Decrease in fibrinogen levels and platelet activity.

Smoking

- The risk of ischaemic stroke in smokers is twice that of non-smokers
- The risk of haemorrhagic stroke in smokers is between two and four times higher than that of non-smokers
- Increased stroke risk is halved by 2 years of cessation and almost back to baseline within 5 years of smoking cessation (Framingham data)
- In the USA, 12–14% of all stroke deaths are attributable to smoking.

The mechanisms by which smoking increases stroke risk include:

- Increased fibrinogen levels
- Increased platelet aggregation
- Increased haematocrit
- Increased homocysteine levels
- Decreased HDL levels
- Decreased blood vessel compliance
- Increased inflammation, promoting atherosclerosis.

Alcohol

- Alcohol excess can increase stroke risk in a number of ways:
  - Increasing hypertension
  - Increasing large-vessel atherosclerotic cerebrovascular disease through dyslipidaemia
  - Causing atrial fibrillation and cardiomyopathy which may produce cardioembolic ischaemic stroke
  - Causing a pro-atherogenic low grade inflammatory response
- Binge drinking causes surges in blood pressure and is particularly associated with increased haemorrhagic stroke risk
- There is a U-shaped relationship between alcohol and cardiovascular disease, including stroke
  - Alcohol in moderation (20–30 g per day) appears protective—the relative risk reduction for stroke is in the order of 25–30%
  - Alcohol intake of >60 g per day causes an increased relative risk of all stroke of about 1.6 but is over 2 for haemorrhagic stroke
- In the UK, the recommended alcohol intake is 21 international units for a man and 14 for a woman per week.

Hypertension

Hypertension is the strongest risk factor for all stroke. The relationship between risk of stroke and degree of hypertension is approximately linear (Fig. 1.4). There is a similar association with high blood pressure and recurrent stroke (Fig. 1.5).

- Increasing blood pressure is strongly and independently associated with both ischaemic and haemorrhagic stroke
- There appears to be no threshold blood pressure below which the stroke risk plateaus, at least not over the normal range of blood pressures studied from 70 to 100 mmHg diastolic
- The proportional increase in stroke risk associated with a given increase in blood pressure is similar in both sexes and almost doubles with each 7.5 mmHg increase in diastolic blood pressure
- Although there is less data on the relationship between stroke and systolic blood pressure, the association may be even stronger than for diastolic blood pressure. Even 'isolated' systolic hypertension, with a normal diastolic blood pressure, is associated with increased stroke risk
- Approximately 40% of strokes can be attributed to a systolic blood pressure of more than 140 mmHg

- The causal nature of the relationship is strongly supported by the results of randomized controlled trials demonstrating that stroke can be prevented by treating blood pressure—this was seen most dramatically in the PROGRESS study where lowering blood pressure in patients with conventionally 'normal' blood pressure after stroke produced an almost 30% reduction in recurrent stroke incidence over 5 years
- Hypertension increases the risk of ischaemic stroke, both by promoting large-vessel atherosclerosis and intracranial small-vessel disease. It has been shown to be strongly associated with carotid stenosis, carotid plaque, and carotid intima-media thickness demonstrated using carotid ultrasound
- Hypertension is a particularly strong risk factor for small-vessel disease with leukoaraiosis. About 80–90% of patients with lacunar stroke and leukoaraiosis have hypertension. It is also strongly related to white matter MRI hyperintensities in community populations
- Hypertension is the major risk factor for cerebral haemorrhage and is most often associated with subcortical haemorrhage.

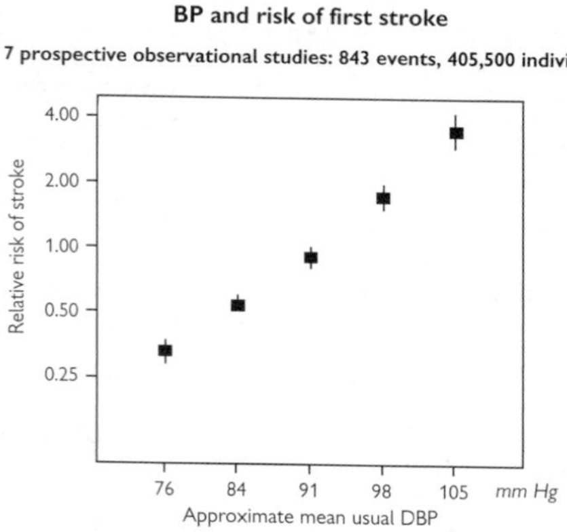

Fig. 1.4 Blood pressure and risk of first stroke. Reproduced from MacMahon S, Peto R, Cutler J *et al.* (1990) *Lancet* **335**, 765–74, with permission from Elsevier.

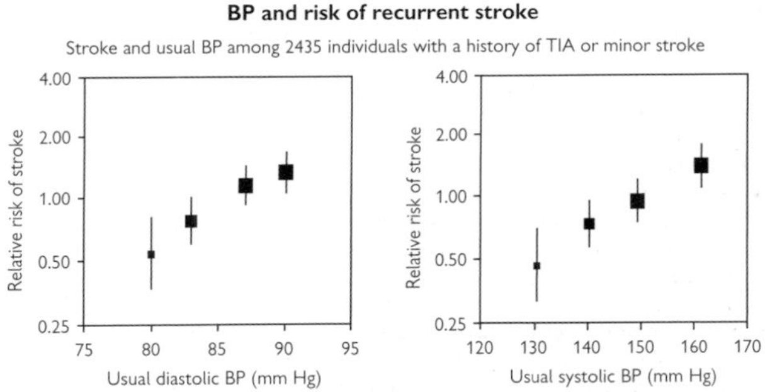

Fig. 1.5 Graph showing linear relationship between recurrent stroke risk and hypertension. Reproduced from Rogers A *et al.* (1996) Blood pressure and risk of stroke in patients with cerebrovascular disease. *BMJ* **313**, 147, with permission from BMJ Publishing Group Ltd.

Diabetes

- Type 2 diabetes is associated with a relative risk of stroke in the order of 2–2.5 (and up to six times increase in some populations)
- Diabetes is a risk factor for carotid atherosclerosis and small-vessel cerebrovascular disease
- Aggressive blood pressure control reduces stroke risk in diabetics
- The role of tight glycaemic control is still unproven in hyperacute stroke. In secondary prevention, glycosylated haemoglobin (HbA1c) levels of 7% or less are associated with reduced microvascular complications but no clear reduction in stroke.

Metabolic syndrome

- This is defined by the American Heart Association (AHA) as the presence of three or more of the following:
  - Elevated waist circumference:
    Men ≥102 cm (40 inches)
    Women ≥88 cm (35 inches)
  - Elevated triglycerides:
  - ≥150 mg/dL (1.7 mmol/L)
  - Reduced HDL ('good') cholesterol:
  - Men <40 mg/dL (1.0 mmol/L)
    Women <50 mg/dL (1.3 mmol/L)
  - Elevated blood pressure:
    >130/85 mmHg
  - Elevated fasting glucose:
    ≥100 mg/dL(5.6 mmol/L).
- The WHO modified the definition to include hyperinsulinaemia

- Metabolic syndrome is highly prevalent in the USA: it is estimated that over 23% (47 million) of Americans have it. It is present in almost one in three Mexican Americans
- Metabolic syndrome is a well described risk factor for coronary and cardiovascular disease, but the relationship to stroke is as yet unclear.

Hypercholesterolaemia

- Increased total cholesterol and LDL cholesterol are strong risk factors for ischaemic heart disease, while high levels of HDL cholesterol appear to be protective. The relationship to stroke appears to be weaker
- This may be partly due to most studies including both haemorrhagic and ischaemic stroke. Those studies looking at ischaemic stroke separately have shown a similar relationship to that seen for ischaemic heart disease. In contrast, some studies have suggested low cholesterol levels increase cerebral haemorrhage risk
- Reducing cholesterol with statin therapy reduces stroke in patients with coronary disease (LIPID, WOSCOPS), patients at risk of stroke (ASCOT, HPS) and those with symptomatic stroke disease (SPARCL)
- The HPS study showed a reduction in stroke even in those individuals with conventionally 'normal' cholesterol levels
- SPARCL is the only randomized controlled trial to date which has taken a treatment group of stroke patients to assess the effect of statin treatment; it showed a 2.2% absolute risk reduction in all stroke with atorvastatin (see 📖 p. 288)
- Statin therapy has been shown to reduce carotid intimal-media thickness and plaque in prospective studies and therefore could be expected to be more effective in preventing stroke in large artery stroke—a subgroup analysis from the SPARCL trial suggest this may be the case
- No statin therapy trial has shown a definite increase in intracerebral bleeding as a side effect, but the benefit of statin therapy in reducing recurrent haemorrhagic stroke is uncertain
- There is still doubt around the role of cholesterol reduction in the very elderly to reduce stroke risk alone.

Previous TIA/stroke

The recurrent stroke risk after TIA is highest in the first few days after TIA, making TIA a powerful predictor/risk factor for future stroke.

A recent risk stratification tool to identify individuals at high early risk of stroke after transient ischaemic attack has been developed between groups in California and Oxford. It is called the ABCD2 score.

- **A** (Age); 1 point for age ≥60 years
- **B** (Blood pressure ≥140/90 mmHg); 1 point for hypertension at the acute evaluation
- **C** (Clinical features); 2 points for unilateral weakness, 1 for speech disturbance without weakness
- **D** (Symptom duration); 1 point for 10–59 minutes, 2 points for ≥60 minutes
- **D** (Diabetes); 1 point

Total scores ranged from 0 (lowest risk) to 7 (highest risk).
Stroke risk at 2 days, 7 days, and 90 days:

- Scores 0–3: low risk
- Scores 4–5: moderate risk
- Scores 6–7: high risk.

Early (3–7-day) risk of stroke stratified according to ABCD score at first assessment in the OXVASC TIA patient cohort

Table 1.6 7-day risk of stroke stratified according to ABCD score at first assessment in the OXVASC validation cohort of patients with probable of definite TIA

	Patients (%)	Strokes (%)	% risk (95% CI)
ABCD score			
≤ 1	2(1%)	0	0
2	28(15%)	0	0
3	32(17%)	0	0
4	46(24%)	1(5%)	2.2(0–6.4)
5	49(26%)	8(40%)	16–3(6.0–26.7)
6	31(16%)	11(55%)	35.5(18.6–52.3)
Total	188(100%)	20(100%)	10.5(6.2–14.9)

Reproduced with permission from Johnston SC, Rothwell PM, Nguyen-Huynh MN *et al.* (2007) Validation and refinement of scores to predict very early stroke risk after transient ischaemic attack. *Lancet* **369**, 283–92.

Atherosclerosis

- Atherosclerosis is associated with stroke because:
  - It may be the cause of the stroke itself, usually by artery to artery embolism
  - It is a marker of systemic atherosclerosis
- Therefore, risk factors for stroke are:
  - Cardiac atherosclerosis (myocardial infarction, angina or other ischaemic heart disease)
  - Peripheral vascular atherosclerosis (e.g. intermittent claudication)
  - Aortic atherosclerosis.

Results published from the REACH registry (multicentred international database of 68 000 patients with either three or more risk factors for atherothrombosis or established coronary disease or stroke) suggest that stroke patients with concomitant peripheral vascular disease have twice the absolute risk of vascular death, myocardial infarction or recurrent stroke at 1 year—emphasizing the need to consider global vascular risk in stroke patients.

Asymptomatic internal carotid artery stenosis

- The annual risk of stroke from an asymptomatic atherosclerotic internal carotid (ICA) stenosis of >50% is between between 1.5 and 2.0%
- The risk of major complications (stroke/death) from carotid endarterectomy (CEA) in asymptomatic patients is about 3% in good units
- Two large prospective trials (ACAS and ACST) have shown a significant approximately 40% relative risk reduction in stroke. However, due to the lower risk of stroke, the absolute risk reduction and the overall population benefit is small (see 📖 Chapter 10 for more details)
- Sometimes to make operations more palatable, the statistics can be presented in a different way. Therefore:
  - 50 patients need to be treated to prevent one stroke over 2 years
  - 20 patients need to be treated to prevent one stroke over 5 years
  - 10 patients need to be treated to prevent one stroke over 10 years
  - 5 patients need to be treated to prevent one stroke over 20 years
  - The numbers needed to treat are approximately doubled when only disabling stroke is considered, which is probably most relevant for the patient
- Subgroup analysis suggests younger men benefit most and there is little or no benefit in women.

Atrial fibrillation (AF)

- Atrial fibrillation is the commonest cause of cardioembolic stroke
- Present in 5–6% of the population, it increases exponentially with age
- The risk of first stroke in a patient aged >60 with AF is 5% per year
- In a patient with stroke and AF the future stroke risk is 12% per year
- AF causes over one-third of strokes in the over 80s—mainly large intracranial artery occlusions or striatocapsular infarcts
- Consequently, patients with stroke due to AF tend to have severe neurological deficits and high associated mortality
- Anticoagulation with warfarin to an INR target 2.5 (range 2.0–3.0) has been shown to be superior in preventing stroke in comparison to aspirin, with a 60–70% relative risk reduction compared to 21% for aspirin alone
- In people aged <60 years with non-valvular or 'lone' AF and no other vascular risk factors, aspirin alone is recommended as primary prevention
- The risk of stroke in newly diagnosed AF can be estimated from the Framingham Score (Fig. 1.6) or by using the CHADS2 (📖 p. 31)
- Anticoagulation is recommended with a CHADS2 score of 2 or more (i.e. all patients with previous ischaemic stroke).

CHADS2 item	Points
Congestive heart failure	1
Hypertension (systolic >160 mmHg)	1
Age greater than 75 years	1
Diabetes	1
Prior cerebral ischaemia	2

Table 1.7 CHADS2 scoring and adjusted annual stroke rate for patients with newly diagnosed AF

CHADS2 score	Adjusted annual stroke rate (95%CI)
0	1.9 (1.2–3.0)
1	2.8 (2.0–3.8)
2	4.0 (3.1–5.1)
3	5.9 (4.6–7.3)
4	8.5 (6.3–11.1)
5	12.5 (8.2–17.5)
6	18.2 (10.5–27.4)

Adapted from Gage BF *et al.* (2001) Validation of clinical classification schemes for predicting stroke. Results from the national registry of atrial fibrillation. *JAMA* **285**, 2864–70.

Framingham stroke risk prediction for new AF

Not valid for those already taking warfarin.

Step 1

Age (years)	Points
55 to 59	0
60 to 62	1
63 to 66	2
67 to 71	3
72 to 74	4
75 to 77	5
78 to 81	6
82 to 85	7
86 to 90	8
91 to 93	9
>93	10

Step 2

Sex	Points
Men	0
Women	6

Step 3

Systolic blood pressure (mm Hg)	Points
<120	0
120 to 139	1
140 to 159	2
160 to 179	3
>179	4

Step 4

Diabetes	Points
No	0
Yes	5

Step 5

Prior stroke or TIA	Points
No	0
Yes	6

Step 6

Add up points from steps 1 through 5.

Look up predicted five-year risk of stroke in table.

Predicted five-year risk of stroke

Total points	Five-year risk (%)
0 to 1	5
2 to 3	6
4	7
5	8
6 to 7	9
8	11
9	12
10	13
11	14
12	16
13	18
14	19
15	21
16	24
17	26
18	28
19	31
20	34
21	37
22	41
23	44
24	48
25	51
26	55
27	59
28	63
29	67
30	71
31	75

Fig. 1.6 Predicted 5-year risk of stroke. A precise equation-based risk function provided as a spreadsheet is available at http://www.nhlbi.nih.gov/about/framingham/stroke.htm. The point-based risk estimate may differ from the equation-based one, particularly in patients with uncommon combinations of characteristics.
Adapted with permission from Wang TJ, Massaro JM, Levy D *et al.* (2003) A risk score for predicting stroke or death for individuals with new-onset atrial fibrillation in the community: The Framingham Heart Study. *JAMA* **290**, 1049–56.

Structural cardiac abnormalities

Cardiomyopathy and ventricular thrombus

- Ischaemic or other forms of dilated cardiomyopathy can lead to mural thrombus within the left ventricle and cardioembolic stroke
- Following anterior myocardial infarction, mural thrombus should be treated with anticoagulation to prevent cardiac embolism. Where there is poor ventricular remodelling, a large akinetic segment or persistent reduced ejection fraction, long-term anticoagulation should be considered
- The incidence of stroke in heart failure patients seems to be inversely proportional to cardiac ejection fraction. There is, however, no randomized controlled trial evidence to date to support long-term anticoagulation over antiplatelet treatment in those patients in sinus rhythm with <30% ejection fraction.

Patent foramen ovale (PFO)

- PFO is caused by a failure of opposition of the two halves the interatrial septum, resulting in more of a patent tract or tunnel than a 'hole in the heart'. This creates a potential communication between the left and right heart. Owing to high left-sided pressure this usually has no physiological effect. However, if the defect is sizeable during a procedure such as 'valsalva', where the right-sided atrial pressure increases above that of the left, venous blood from the right heart can mix with arterial blood on the left
- PFO is a common normal variant usually of no clinical significance. It is present in 'utero', allowing blood from the right side of the heart to cross to the left side. This allows oxygenated blood to pass from the mother's placenta to the arterial tree. In most cases it closes at birth but fails to do so in between 17% and 35% of the general population
- Evidence suggests it is a risk factor for stroke but only of minor significance on its own. PFO is present in about 22% of the population but in about 44% of an age-matched population with cryptogenic stroke. However, where the inferior interatrial septum is hypokinetic or floppy and tends to 'bow' or 'balloon' (so called atrial septal aneurysm or ASA), clot may form in the right atrium and the presence of PFO then leads to left-sided cardiac arterial embolism of the thrombus resulting in stroke
- Although PFO and septal defects were originally only thought to be an issue in younger patients with apparent cryptogenic stroke, a recent study has identified that there is an increased prevalence in older (over 55 years) cryptogenic stroke patients, and cardiac embolism may in fact be the cause of stroke in this patient group too.

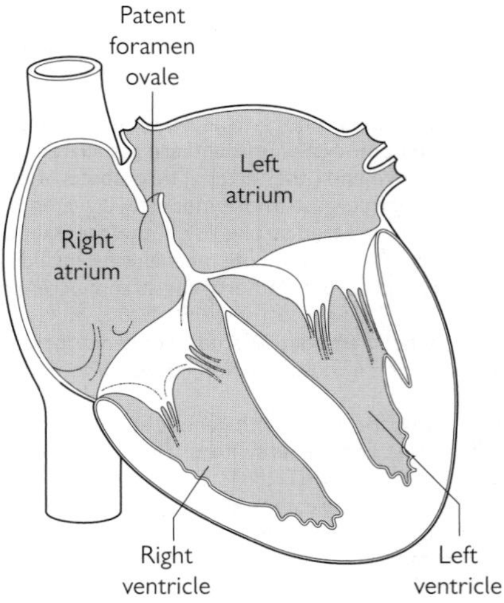

Fig. 1.7 Anatomy of a patent foramen ovale (PFO).

Minor modifiable stroke risk factors

Diet

- Numerous cohort studies have confirmed an inverse association between fruit/vegetable intake and stroke incidence and mortality
- Other studies have found that low potassium intake and low serum potassium are associated with increased stroke mortality. Potassium and magnesium supplementation and diets high in fibre may reduce stroke risk. In an 8-year study of 44 000 men, these factors were found to reduce risk of stroke by 38%
- Cross-sectional and case-control studies have generally shown an inverse association between consumption of fish and fish oils and stroke risk. In the Nurses Health Study, a significant decrease in the risk of thrombotic stroke (relative risk, 0.49; 95% confidence interval, 0.26–0.93) was observed among women who ate fish at least twice a week compared to women who ate fish less than once per month, after adjustment for age, smoking, and other cardiovascular risk factors. No association was observed between consumption of fish or fish oil and haemorrhagic stroke
- Salt ingestion is related to high blood pressure, and restriction of dietary salt intake can produce falls in blood pressure in the region of 10 mmHg or more.

Current 'healthy eating recommendations' for stroke risk prevention include:

- At least five portions of fruit and vegetables daily
- Six servings of grains daily
- Limited salt
- Limited saturated fats and cholesterol
- Twice-weekly servings of oily fish, such as tuna or salmon

Hyperhomocysteinaemia

- Very high levels of serum homocysteine occur in the autosomal recessive condition homocysteinuria, and are associated with an increased risk of stroke and other arterial thrombosis at an early age
- Considerable evidence suggests more modestly elevated homocysteine is associated with an increased stroke risk in the general population
- This association could act via multiple mechanisms, including impaired endothelial function, promoting atherogenesis and increasing thrombosis
- Meta-analysis of genetic association studies of genes increasing homocysteine supports a causal relation between homocysteine and stroke
- Homocysteine levels are under both genetic and dietary control
- A number of enzymes control its synthesis, including methylene tetrahydrofolate reductase (MTHFR)
- Low vitamin B12 and, to a greater extent, low folate levels are associated with high homocysteine levels
- Folate supplementation reduces homocysteine levels
- Raised homocysteine can be treated. Once B12 deficiency has been excluded, oral vitamin B complex (incorporating vitamins B6 and B12) and folic acid 5 mg are given

- Although there is evidence that high homocysteine contributes to stroke risk, there are no randomized controlled trial data to confirm that reduction of homocysteine actually reduces the risk of stroke
- Elevated homocysteine appears to be a particularly strong risk factor for small-vessel disease stroke with leukoaraiosis.

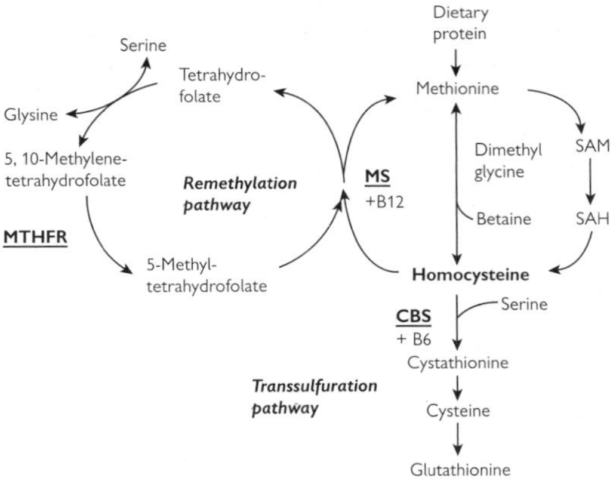

Fig. 1.8 Schematic diagram of homocysteine synthesis.

Sleep-disordered breathing/obstructive sleep apnoea (OSA)

- OSA probably has a small effect in increasing the risk of stroke
- Stroke often occurs during sleep (up to one in three strokes) and there is controversy over whether snoring and OSA have a causative association with stroke
- OSA has been associated with hypertension and increased cardiovascular events
- OSA can also cause reduced cerebral autoregulation and hypercoagulability and arrhythmias can occur during periods of oxygen desaturation
- A recent observational study suggested that independent of age, sex, and established stroke risk factors, patients with established OSA have an increased relative risk of stroke of 2 compared to controls
- Successful treatment of OSA can reduce blood pressure but there is no evidence to suggest that stroke risk is also reduced.

Inflammation and CRP

- Highly sensitive C-reactive protein (hs-CRP) is an assay of one of the acute phase proteins released by the liver that increase during systemic inflammation
- Raised CRP has been associated with atherosclerosis in both coronary and carotid arteries, although much of this association disappears after conventional risk factors are accounted for

- A level of hs-CRP of 3 mg/L or above is thought to be high risk for atherosclerotic disease. Levels of >10 mg/L usually have non-cardiovascular causes excluded (autoimmune, cancer, infection and other causes of inflammation)
- It has been suggested that testing CRP levels in the blood may be an additional way to assess cardiovascular and stroke risk, although there is currently no evidence to support this as a screening test
- CRP may be predictive of recurrent stroke and survival after stroke. However, the prognostic significance of a CRP rise after stroke is not clear
- Atherosclerosis can be thought of as a chronic inflammatory process, which may be accelerated by systemic inflammation of which hs-CRP is a marker. Increasing evidence suggests that some conventional risk factors may increase atherosclerosis via inducing a chronic pro-inflammatory state. These include smoking, alcohol excess, and obesity (adipose tissue secretes cytokines).

Infections

(HIV infection is covered in 📖 p. 354.)
Infections may cause stroke in two possible ways.

1. Acute infection precipitating acute stroke

- Case-control studies have found that recent infections (within 7 days) are more common in stroke patients. They may induce a hypercoagulable state and/or endothelial dysfunction.

2. Chronic infection and inflammation and atherosclerosis

- Cytomegalovirus (CMV), *Chlamydia pneumoniae*, *Helicobacter pylori*, and Gram-negative bacteria associated with periodontal infection have all been isolated in atherosclerotic plaque. It may well be that chronic inflammation associated with such low grade infection—rather than the bacteria itself—is responsible for inducing atherosclerotic disease.

Migraine

- Migraine can be associated with stroke in two ways:
  1. Stroke occurs during a migraine attack
  2. As a risk factor for stroke
- Stroke during a migraine attack (migrainous stroke) is very rare and more common in migraine with aura
- Epidemiological studies have shown migraine is a risk factor for stroke
- The stroke risk is highest for migraine with aura. The relative risk of migraine causing stroke is 1.5–2.0 whilst migraine with aura is up to 6
- There is an interaction between smoking, migraine (particularly with aura), and the combined oral contraceptive (COC) pill. Women who smoke, take the COC pill, and suffer migraine with aura have an increased stroke risk of up to tenfold
- Recent onset migraine with aura is thought to be associated with the greatest stroke risk
- In terms of primary prevention, there is no evidence to suggest that migraine prophylaxis reduces stroke risk.

Contraceptive use/pregnancy

- The relative risk of stroke is approximately doubled in users of the COC pill
- However, the absolute risk remains very low. This is because the incidence of ischaemic stroke in women aged under 35 is very low: three in 100 000
- More recent studies with low-dose oestrogen (<50 μg) suggest the risk is even less with modern COC
- There is no increased risk in haemorrhagic stroke and no increase in stroke mortality in COC users. COCs should not generally be prescribed to young women with established vascular risk and a family history of venous thromboembolism (VTE)
- There is no, or a much smaller increased, risk in women who take the progestagen-only contraceptive pill.

Hormone replacement therapy (HRT)

- HRT also increases the relative risk of stroke by about 2. However, it is taken by older women and their absolute risk of stroke is higher. Therefore, the potential population-attribitable risk is higher
- Therefore, current advice is to use HRT for 5 years only and to continue only in women where the unpleasant menopausal symptoms outweigh their risk of stroke
- Prior to recent trial data, it was thought that HRT may protect against cardiovascular risk and stroke, and this led to trials assessing this hypothesis which, to many people's surprise, demonstrated that they actually increased risk. The Heart & Estrogen-progestin Replacement Study (HERS) showed no effect of HRT on stroke primary prevention. HRT in the secondary prevention Women's Estrogen for Stroke Trial (WEST), however, increased the risk of recurrent fatal stroke and worsened the neurological and functional deficit of recurrent stroke in a stroke population
- HRT should not be used in primary stroke prevention for women with other vascular risk factors.

Recreational drug use

A number of commonly used recreational drugs increase the risk of stroke; these include amphetamines and cocaine. They are covered in detail in 📖 p. 350.

Other drugs

Several recently introduced classes of drugs have produced concern over increasing stroke risk. These include the following.

COX-2 inhibitors

- The selective COX-2 inhibitor, non-steroidal inflammatory drug Vioxx was withdrawn from the market in 2004 by the manufacturing company, after a post-licence trial had suggested the drug increased coronary and stroke events (but mainly myocardial infarction). The effect was small but equated to a relative risk of about 2.
The mechanism for this is possibly through inhibition of endothelial COX-2-derived prostacyclin (PG12) as well as a deleterious effect on

cellular mediators that have neuroprotective and cardioprotective actions

- Subsequently, other COX-2 drugs have similarly been suspected of increasing cardiovascular and stroke risk, and consequently those that remain on the market are heavily cautioned in patients with vascular risk factors
- For the same reason the traditional NSAIDs such as ibuprofen and diclofenac should also be used with caution.

Atypical antipsychotic medication

- Evidence from randomized trials shows a small increased risk of stroke in patients with dementia and agitation treated with the atypical antipsychotics risperidone and olanzapine. However, this is based on a small number of events, and a small increase in relative risk with wide confidence intervals. A large observational study failed to find any increased risk and probably limits the size of the effect to no more than two extra strokes per 1000 person-years of treatment. The mechanism for this small increase in stroke risk is unclear
- Nevertheless, atypical neuroleptic drugs are not recommended for treatment of behavioural problems in dementia, although they may be used under supervision for short periods of time. The licence has not been affected outside their use in dementia patients
- A recent case-controlled study argued in fact that the risk is similar in all antipsychotic medication and highest in patients on treatment with dementia.

Relative contribution of different stroke risk factors

The relative risks associated with different risk factors for stroke are shown in Table 1.8. These are representative figures derived from different studies of each risk factor.

Table 1.8 Relative contribution of different stroke risk factors

	Relative risk for stroke
Age (55–64 years versus >75 years)	5
Male sex	1.3
Afro-Caribbean	2
Social class (I versus V)	1.6
Physical activity (little or none versus some)	2.5
Smoking (current status)	2
Alcohol (>60 g per day)	1.6
Blood pressure 160/95 versus 120/80	7
Diabetes mellitus	2
Previous TIA (symptomatic ICA stenosis>70%)	5 (10)
Ischaemic heart disease	3
Heart failure	5
Atrial fibrillation	5
Oral contraceptives	2

It is important to remember that risk factors frequently coexist and often have more than summative effects on stroke risk, e.g. diabetes, hypertension, and the presence of peripheral vascular disease is associated with a more than 12-fold increase in stroke risk.

The Framingham stroke risk profile (📖 see p. 42) estimates 10-year predicted stroke risk according to common risk factors.

Framingham stroke risk

The Framingham stroke risk tables can be used to calculate stroke risk in an individual person. The tables shown apply to individuals not in atrial fibrillation.

The risk score is calculated from the first table; there are separate tables for men (Table 1.9) and women (Table 1.10). This risk score is than converted into a stroke risk over the next 10 years using the conversion table (Table 1.11).

Table 1.9 Table for calculating Framingham risk score in men, not in atrial fibrillation

Risk score	Points 0	+1	+2	+3	+4	+5	+6	+7	+8	+9	+10
Risk score for men aged 55–85 years											
Age (years)	54–56	57–59	60–62	63–65	66–68	69–72	73–75	76–78	79–81	82–84	85
Untreated SBP	97–105	106–115	116–125	126–135	136–145	146–155	156–165	166–175	176–185	186–195	196–205
Treated SBP	97–105	106–112	113–117	118–123	124–129	130–135	136–142	143–150	151–161	162–176	177–205
Diabetes	No		Yes								
Current smoker	No			Yes							
CVD	No				Yes						
ECG LVH	No					Yes					

Reproduced with permission from D'Agostino RB, Wolf PA, Belanger AJ, Kannel WB (1994) Stroke risk profile: The Framingham Study. *Stroke* 1994; **25**, 40–3.
SBP = Systolic blood pressure (mmHg); CVD = history of MI, angina, intermittent claudication or heart failure; LVH = left ventricular hypertrophy

Table 1.10 Table for calculating Framingham risk score in women, not in atrial fibrillation

Risk score	Points 0	+1	+2	+3	+4	+5	+6	+7	+8	+9	+10
Risk score for women aged 55–85 years											
Age (years)	54–56	57–59	60–62	63–64	65–67	68–70	71–73	74–76	77–78	79–81	82–84
Untreated SBP	95–106	107–118	119–130	131–143	144–155	156–167	168–180	181–192	193–204	205–216	
Treated SBP	95–106	107–113	114–119	120–125	136–131	132–139	140–148	149–160	161–204	205–216	
Diabetes	No			Yes							
Cigarettes	No			Yes							
CVD	No		Yes								
ECG LVH	No				Yes						

Reproduced with permission from D'Agostino RB, Wolf PA, Belanger AJ, Kannel WB (1994) Stroke risk profile: The Framingham Study. *Stroke* 1994; **25**, 40–3.
SBP = Systolic blood pressure (mmHg); CVD = history of MI, angina, intermittent claudication or heart failure; LVH = left ventricular hypertrophy

Table 1.11 Table for converting Framingham risk scores to 10 year probability of stroke

Conversion of points from risk factor profiles to probability of stroke over 10 years

Points	10-year probability (%), men	10-year probability (%), women	Points	10-year probability (%), men	10-year probability (%), women	Points	10-year probability (%), men	10-year probability (%), women
1	3	1	11	11	8	21	42	43
2	3	1	12	13	9	22	47	50
34	2	13	15	11	23	52	57	
44	2	14	14	13	24	57	64	
55	2	15	20	16	25	63	71	
65	3	16	22	19	26	68	78	
76	4	17	26	23	27	74	84	
87	4	18	29	27	28	79		
98	5	19	33	32	29	84		
10	10	6	20	37	37	30	88	

Reproduced with permission from D'Agostino RB, Wolf PA, Belanger AJ, Kannel WB (1994) Stroke risk profile: The Framingham Study. *Stroke* 1994; **25**, 40–3.

Further reading

Introduction

WHO Atlas of Heart Disease and Stroke. http://www.who.int/cardiovascular_diseases/resources/atlas/en/

UK National Audit Office report looking at the cost of stroke. http://www.nao.org.uk/publications/nao_reports/05-06/0506452.pdf

Definitions for epidemiological studies

Albers GW, Caplan LR, Easton JD *et al.* (2002) Transient ischemic attack—proposal for a new definition. *New England Journal of Medicine* **347**, 1713–16.

Stroke subtyping

Adams HP, Bendixen BH, Kappelle LJ (1993) Classification of subtype of acute ischemic stroke. Definitions for use in a multicenter clinical trial. TOAST. Trial of Org 10172 in Acute Stroke Treatment. *Stroke* **24**, 35–41.

Goldstein LB, Jones MR, Matchar DB *et al.* (2001) Improving the reliability of stroke subgroup classification using the Trial of ORG 10172 in Acute Stroke Treatment (TOAST) criteria. *Stroke* **32**, 1091–8.

Incidence and prevalence

Rothwell P, Coull A, Giles M *et al.* (2004) Change in stroke incidence, mortality, case-fatality, severity, and risk factors in Oxfordshire, UK from 1981 to 2004 (Oxford Vascular Study). *Lancet* **363**, 1925–33.

Non-modifiable stroke risk factors

Ethnicity

De Silva DA, Woon FP, Lee MP *et al.* (2007) South Asian patients with ischemic stroke: intracranial large arteries are the predominant site of disease. *Stroke* **38**, 2592–4.

Markus HS, Khan U, Birns B *et al.* (2007) Differences in stroke subtypes between black and white patients with stroke—The South London Ethnicity and Stroke Study. *Circulation* **116**, 2157–64.

Wolfe CD, Rudd AG, Howard R *et al.* (2002) Incidence and case fatality rates of stroke subtypes in a multiethnic population: the South London Stroke Register. *Journal of Neurology Neurosurgery and Psychiatry* **72**, 211–16.

Wong KS, Haung YN, Gao S, Lam WWM, Chan YL (2001) Cerebrovascular disease among Chinese populations—recent epidemiological and neuroimaging studies. *Hong Kong Medical Journal* **7**, 50–7.

Genetic predisposition

Dichgans M (2007) Genetics of ischaemic stroke. *Lancet Neurology* **6**, 149–61.

Jerrard-Dunne P, Cloud G, Hassan A, Markus HS (2003) Evaluating the genetic component of ischemic stroke subtypes: a family history study. *Stroke* **34**,1364–9.

Major modifiable stroke risk factors

Physical inactivity

Gillum RF, Mussolino ME, Ingram DD (1996) Physical activity and stroke incidence in women and men. The NHANES I Epidemiologic Follow-up Study. *American Journal of Epidemiology* **143**, 860–9.

Shinton R, Shipley M, Rose G (1991) Overweight and stroke in the Whitehall Study. *Journal of Epidemiology and Community Health* **45**,138–42.

Suk SH, Sacco RL, Boden-Albala B *et al.* (2003) Northern Manhattan Stroke Study. Abdominal obesity and risk of ischemic stroke: the Northern Manhattan Stroke Study. *Stroke* **34**, 1586–92.

Alcohol

Reynolds K, Lewis LB, Nolen JDL *et al.* (2003) Alcohol consumption and risk of stroke: A meta-analysis. *JAMA* **289**, 579–88.

Hypertension

Lewington S, Clarke R, Qizilbash N *et al.* (2002) Age-specific relevance of usual blood pressure to vascular mortality: a meta-analysis of individual data for one million adults in 61 prospective studies [published correction appears in] *Lancet* **360**, 1903–13.

PROGRESS Collaborative Group (2001) Randomised trial of a perindopril-based blood-pressure-lowering regimen among 6,105 individuals with previous stroke or transient ischaemic attack. *Lancet* **358**, 1033–41.

Metabolic syndrome

Burchfiel CM, Curb JD, Rodriguez BL, Abbott RD, Chiu D, Yano K. Glucose intolerance and 22-year stroke incidence: the Honolulu Heart Program. Stroke. 1994; **25**: 951–957

Lakka HM, Laaksonen DE, Lakka TA, Niskanen LK, Kumpusalo E, Tuomilehto J, Salonen JT. The metabolic syndrome and total and cardiovascular disease mortality in middle-aged men. JAMA. 2002; **288**: 2709–2716

Kernan WN, Inzucchi SE, Viscoli CM, Brass LM, Bravata DM, Horwitz RI. Insulin resistance and risk for stroke. Neurology. 2002; **59**: 809–815

Hypercholesterolaemia

Prospective Studies Collaboration (2007) Blood cholesterol and vascular mortality by age, sex and blood pressure: a meta-analysis of individual data from 61 prospective studies with 55 000 vascular deaths. *Lancet* **370**, 1829–39.

Sillesen H, Amarenco P, Hennerici MG *et al.* on Behalf of the SPARCL Investigators (2008) Atorvastatin reduces the risk of cardiovascular events in patients with carotid atherosclerosis: a secondary analysis of the stroke prevention by aggressive reduction in cholesterol levels (SPARCL) Trial. *Stroke* **39**, 3297–302.

The Stroke Prevention by Aggressive Reduction in Cholesterol Levels (SPARCL) Investigators (2006) High-dose atorvastatin after stroke or transient ischemic attack. *New England Journal of Medicine* **355**, 459–559.

Atherosclerosis

Executive Committee for the Asymptomatic Carotid Atherosclerosis Study (1995) Endarterectomy for asymptomatic carotid artery stenosis. *JAMA* **273**, 1421–8.

MRC Asymptomatic Carotid Surgery Trial (ACST) Collaborative Group (2004) Prevention of disabling and fatal strokes by successful carotid endarterectomy in patients without recent neurological symptoms: randomised controlled trial. *Lancet* **363**, 1491–502.

Röther J, Alberts MJ, Touzé E *et al.* (2008) REACH Registry Investigators. Risk factor profile and management of cerebrovascular patients in the REACH Registry. *Cerebrovasc Disease* **25**, 366–74.

Structural cardiac abnormalities

Harloff A, Olschewski M, Hetzel A, Geibel A (2007) Patent foramen ovale and cryptogenic stroke in older patients. *New England Journal of Medicine* **357**, 2262–8.

Overell JR, Bone I, Lees KR (2000) Interatrial septal abnormalities and stroke: a meta-analysis of case-control studies. *Neurology* **55**, 1172–9.

Messe SR, Silverman IE, Kizer JR *et al.* (2004) Quality Standards Subcommittee of the American Academy of Neurology. Practice parameter: recurrent stroke with patent foramen ovale and atrial septal aneurysm: report of the Quality Standards Subcommittee of the American Academy of Neurology. *Neurology* **62**, 1042–50.

Vaitkus PT, Barnathan ES (1993) Embolic potential, prevention and management of mural thrombus complicating anterior myocardial infarction: a meta-analysis. *Journal of the American College of Cardiology* **22**, 1004–9.

Minor modifiable stroke risk factors

Diet

Johnsen SP, Overvad K, Stripp C *et al.* (2003) Intake of fruit and vegetables and the risk of ischemic stroke in a cohort of Danish men and women. *American Journal of Clinical Nutrition* **78**, 57–64.

Steffen LM, Jacobs DR Jr, Stevens J *et al.* (2003) Associations of whole-grain, refined-grain, and fruit and vegetable consumption with risks of all-cause mortality and incident coronary artery disease and ischemic stroke: the Atherosclerosis Risk in Communities (ARIC) Study. *American Journla of Clinical Nutrition* **78**, 383–90.

Hyperhomocysteinaemia

Casas JP, Bautista LE, Smeeth L, Sharma P, Hingorani AD (2005) Homocysteine and stroke: evidence on a causal link from Mendelian randomisation. *Lancet* **365**, 224–32.

Wang X, Qin X, Demirtas H *et al.* (2007) Efficacy of folic acid supplementation in stroke prevention: a meta-analysis. *Lancet* **369**, 1876–82.

Inflammation and CRP

Di Napoli M, Schwaninger M, Cappelli R *et al.* (2005) Evaluation of C-reactive protein measurement for assessing the risk and prognosis in ischemic stroke: a statement for health care professionals from the CRP Pooling Project members. *Stroke* **36**, 1316–29.

Yaggi HK, Concato J, Kernan WN *et al.* (2005) Obstructive sleep apnea as a risk factor for stroke and death. *New England Journal of Medicine* **353**, 2034–41.

Infections

Espinola-Klein C, Rupprecht HJ, Blankenberg S *et al.* (2002) Impact of infectious burden on progression of carotid atherosclerosis. *Stroke* **33**, 2581–6.

Smeeth L, Thomas SL, Hall AJ *et al.* (2004) Risk of myocardial infarction and stroke after acute infection or vaccination. *New England Journal of Medicine* **351**, 2611–18.

Hormone replacement therapy

Chang CL, Donaghy M, Poulter N (1999) Migraine and stroke in young women: case-control study: the World Health Organization collaborative study of cardiovascular disease and steroid hormone contraception. *BMJ* **318**, 13–18.

Gillum LA, Mamidipudi SK, Johnston SC (2000) Ischemic stroke risk with oral contraceptives: a meta-analysis. *JAMA* **284**, 72–8.

MacClellan LR, Giles W, Cole J *et al.* (2007) Probable migraine with visual aura and risk of ischemic stroke: The Stroke Prevention in Young Women Study. *Stroke* **38**, 2438–45.

Simon JA, Hsia J, Cauley J *et al.* (2001) Postmenopausal hormone therapy and risk of stroke: The Heart and Estrogen-progestin Replacement Study (HERS). *Circulation* **103**, 638–42.

Viscoli CM, Brass LM, Kernan WN *et al.* (2001) A clinical trial of estrogen-replacement therapy after ischemic stroke. *New England Journal of Medicine* **345**, 1243–9.

Other drugs

Douglas IJ, Smeeth L (2008) Exposure to antipsychotics and risk of stroke: self controlled case series study. *BMJ* **337**, a1227. doi: 10.1136/bmj.a1227.

Kearney PM, Baigent C, Godwin J *et al.* (2006) Do selective cyclo-oxygenase-2 inhibitors and traditional non-steroidal anti-inflammatory drugs increase the risk of atherothrombosis? Meta-analysis of randomised trials. *BMJ* **332**, 1302–8.

Herrman N, Mamdani M, Lanctôt KL (2004) Atypical antipsychotics and risk of cerebrovascular accidents. *American Journal of Psychiatry* **161**, 1113–15.

Chapter 2

Neuroanatomy

Introduction

Stroke is a disease affecting the brain. Therefore, there is no escaping having to understand some neuroanatomy. However, stroke is a very practical subject and with a relatively simple understanding of the neuroanatomy and vascular anatomy, it is not difficult to localize the lesion and the arterial territory involved.

The most important aspects of neuroanatomy to understand are:

- The motor system
- The sensory system
- The visual system
- The brainstem
- Cortical function
- Neuroanatomy of stroke subtypes
- Neuroanatomy of vascular territories.

Basic neuroanatomy principles

These rules will sound overly simple but actually they are the cornerstone of your examination.

First, decide the side affected:

- The right side of the brain normally controls the left side of the body (and vice versa)
- The exception is the cerebellum which controls the same side of the body.

Second, decide the level of the lesion:

- The nervous system is arranged in a series of ascending levels
- You should learn enough neuroanatomy to be able to work out the level of the lesion.

These two principles allow you to think of the body as a grid and to pinpoint the lesion. After that, using a knowledge of the cerebral arterial territories, one can work out which vascular territory is involved.

Motor system

The motor system is an efferent system. It runs from the brain down and is organized as follows.

Motor cortex

- Located in the precentral gyrus in the frontal lobe
- As this is a relatively large area, small infarcts here may cause paralysis of an isolated region such as the hand or arm
- Complete paralysis of one side occurs if the infarct involves the whole motor cortex. This is the case for many middle cerebral artery infarcts.

Corticospinal tract

- The motor fibres from the cortex descend in this tract which passes through the centrum semiovale, on down through the internal capsule into the brainstem, and on to the spinal cord. Disruption at any of these sites can cause motor deficit (hemiparesis).

Centrum semiovale

- Here the fibres are gathered together from the cortex into a small bundle
- If infarcts involve the corticospinal tracts they cause hemiparesis which usually involves at least two areas of the body (e.g. face and arm or arm and leg). Lacunar infarcts are common at this site.

Internal capsule

- This is rather small and runs through the basal ganglia
- It is boomerang-shaped with an anterior and posterior limb
- Motor fibres run in the posterior limb
- The fibres are so tightly packed that small infarcts here usually cause paralysis of a whole side. Normally, at least two areas of the body are affected (e.g. arm and leg). Lacunar infarcts are common at this site.

Brainstem

- The motor fibres run through the brainstem
- This is the first time that fibres from *both* sides lie close together
- The cranial nerve nuclei are closely packed here
- Therefore, infarcts here may cause quadriparesis as well as affecting several cranial nerves.

Pyramids

- Here the fibres cross over to the other side.

Spinal cord

- The motor fibres run down in the cord until they reach their exit level
- They terminate at the anterior horn cell (the junction of the upper motor neuron and the lower motor neuron).

Peripheral nerve

- Here the motor fibre runs out to the muscle.

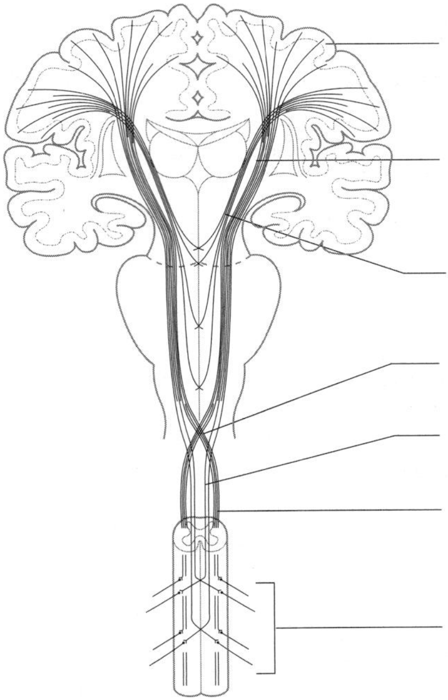

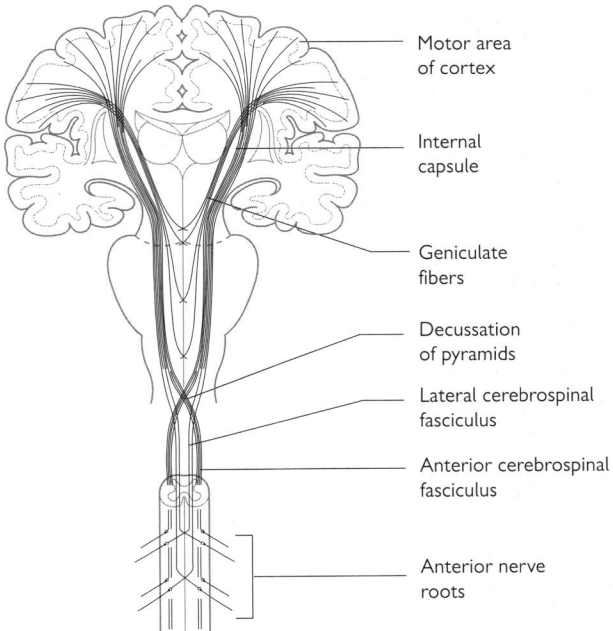

Fig. 2.1 Diagram of the motor system. The fibre tracts start from the cortex, run through the internal capsule and cross over in the pyramids (the pyramidal tracts). They then descend towards the anterior horn cells in the spinal cord. The nerve down to the ending on the anterior horn cell is the 'upper motor neuron'. From the anterior horn cell to the end muscle is the 'lower motor neuron'.

Sensory system

The sensory system is an afferent system. It runs from the periphery up to the brain and is organized as follows.

Peripheral nerves

- These arise from sensory receptors in the skin or end organs
- Some fibres are myelinated and fast conducting (e.g. joint position sense)
- Some fibres are unmyelinated and slow conducting (e.g. some pain fibres)
- The peripheral nerves enter the dorsal spinal cord.

Spinal cord

- Most fibres run up the same side of the spinal cord in the dorsal columns. These carry sensation for light touch, vibration, and joint position sense
- Some fibres cross over straight away. These are spinothalamic fibres and run in the spinothalamic tract. They carry sensation of pain and temperature.

Brainstem

- Here the fibres from the dorsal columns (light touch, vibration, joint position sense) cross over to the other side and run up in a tract called the medial lemniscus.

Thalamus

- This is the big group of nuclei where the sensory fibres end
- The fibres and nuclei in the thalamus are very tightly packed
- The thalamus relays the sensory information to the sensory cortex
- Because fibres are closely packed, a small infarct here usually results in complete hemisensory loss (i.e. affecting the face, arm, and leg).

Primary sensory cortex

- This lies in the postcentral gyrus of the frontal lobes
- Like the motor cortex, it is very extensive
- Therefore, infarcts may involve only part of the sensory cortex and result in sensory loss in only one limb or part of limb (e.g. arm or leg or face alone).

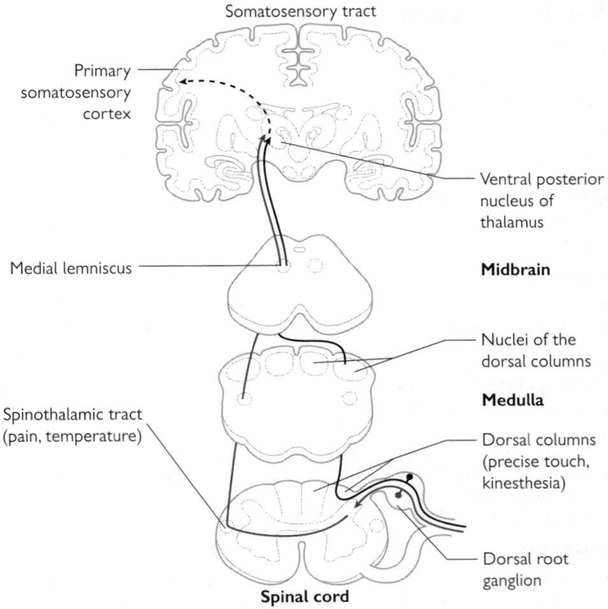

Fig. 2.2 Schematic diagram of the sensory pathway.

Visual system

The visual system is organized as follows.

The retina

- Detects light and converts this into transmissible electrical impulses
- The visual world is split into left and right. Half of each retina detects the left field and the other half of each retina detects the right visual field
- Retinal ischaemia may cause temporary monocular visual loss (amaurosis fugax) or permanent blindness (e.g. central retinal artery occlusion).

Optic nerve

- This runs from each eye to the optic chiasm
- A lesion here will cause blindness of one eye. The other eye will be unaffected.

Optic chiasm

- Here fibres from each optic nerve partially cross over (see Fig. 2.3)
- The important point is that the visual world is split into left and right
- A lesion affecting the whole chiasm will cause complete blindness
- A lesion pushing on the centre of the chiasm and therefore affecting the central crossing fibres (e.g. a pituitary tumour) will cause a bitemporal hemianopia.

Optic tract

- Each optic tract carries information from one visual field. Lesions here will cause visual disturbance affecting the same field in *both* eyes
- If the whole optic tract on one side is damaged, the entire hemifield may become blind, a homonymous hemianopia.

Optic radiation

- Each optic radiation stretches back to the visual cortex
- The radiation is actually quite wide. Therefore, small infarcts may affect only a small part of one radiation. This may damage the bottom (or top) half of the left or right visual field. This causes a quadrantanopia.

Visual cortex

- This occupies the occipital cortex
- Complete infarction of one side will produce a homonymous hemianopia.

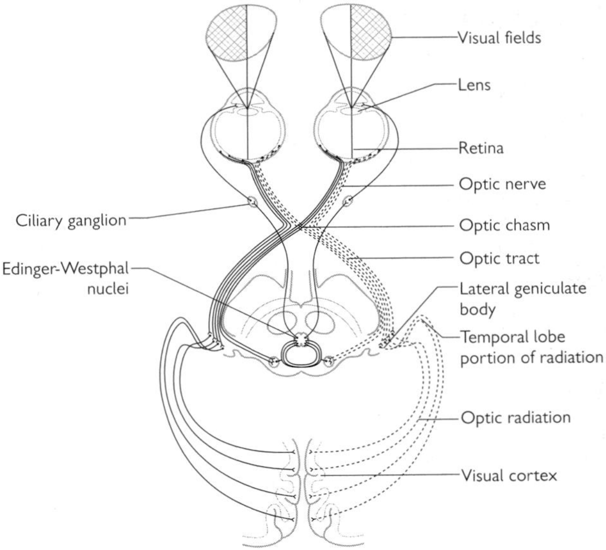

Fig. 2.3 The optic pathways.

Brainstem

The brainstem contains:

- A large number of cranial nerve nuclei and their interconnections
- The descending motor and ascending sensory pathways
- Cerebellar connections.

It can appear confusing. However, if one localizes the site and side of the lesion by knowing which cranial nerves it is affecting, and which ascending and descending pathways are involved, it becomes easier.

Think of the brainstem as a grid. Again you have left and right. The top to the bottom of the brainstem is divided by the cranial nerves, and as long as you know what the cranial nerves do it is quite easy to localize lesions to the brainstem.

Nerve	Function
Olfactory (1)	Olfaction (smell)
Optic (2)	Vision
Occulomotor (3)	Eye movements and pupillary responses
Trochlear (4)	Eye movements: superior oblique. "Look at your nose"
Trigeminal (5)	Facial sensation and muscles of mastication
Abducent (6)	Eye movements: lateral rectus. "Look to the side"
Facial (7)	Facial movement
Auditory (8)	Hearing and balance
Glossopharyngeal (9)	Pharyngeal sensation
Vagus (10)	Muscles of larynx and pharynx
Accessory (11)	Trapezius and sternocleidomastoid
Hypoglossal (12)	Tongue movement

The site of origin of the cranial nerves in the brainstem is shown in Figure 2.4. On subsequent pages, cross-sectional views of the brainstem at the different levels are shown.

When localizing a lesion, first work out which of the following are affected:

- Cranial nerves
- Motor pathway
- Sensory pathway
- Cerebellar function.

Then refer to these diagrams and it is usually possible to localize the lesions.

Examination of the individual cranial nerves is covered in 📖 Chapter 5, pp. 130–137.

Figures 2.4 and 2.5 show the positions of the cranial nerve nuclei in the brainstem.

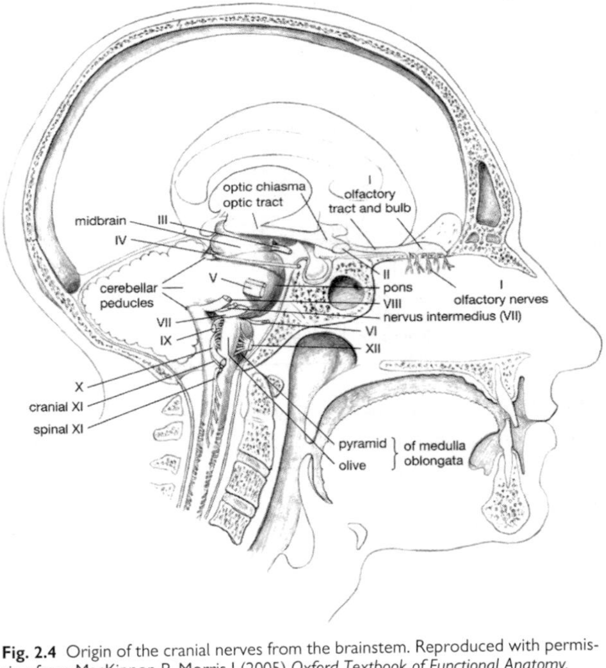

Fig. 2.4 Origin of the cranial nerves from the brainstem. Reproduced with permission from MacKinnon P, Morris J (2005) *Oxford Textbook of Functional Anatomy*, Vol. 3. Oxford, Oxford University Press.

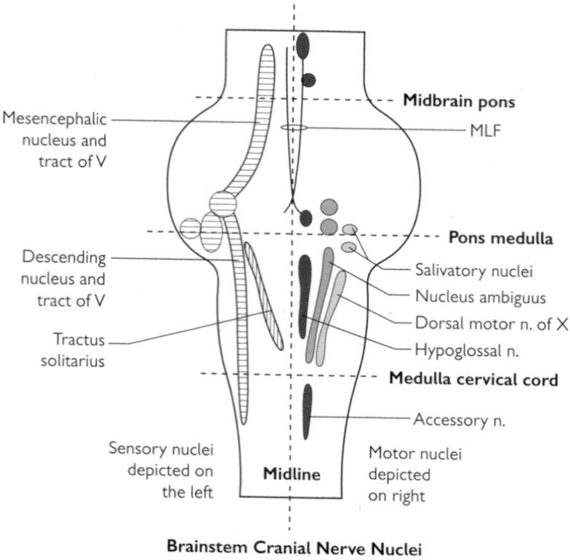

Fig. 2.5 Longitudinal diagram of the brainstem showing the cranial nerve nuclei and the position of the major tracts.

Cerebellum

- The cerebellum is located inferior to the tentorium
- It coordinates muscle activity and balance
- It is split into three lobes:
    - Flocculonodular lobe (archicerebellum) supports equilibrium
    - Anterior lobe (paleocerebellum) supports muscle tone
    - Posterior lateral lobes (neocerebellum) support coordination.

The motor tracts are doubly crossed so affect the ipsilateral side.
Major cerebellar tracts are:

- Spinocerebellar, connecting the spinal cord
- Vestibulospinal, connecting the vestibular system
- Corticopontocerebellar, connecting the cortex and pons
- Dentatorubrothalamic connecting to the red nucleus and thalamus.

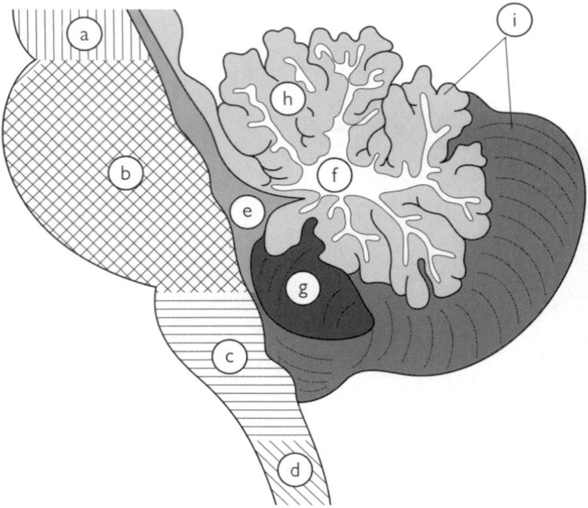

Fig. 2.6 Cerebellum and surrounding regions; sagittal view of one hemisphere. a, midbrain; b, pons; c, medulla; d, spinal cord; e, fourth ventricle; f, arbor vitae; g, tonsil; h, anterior lobe; i, posterior lobe.

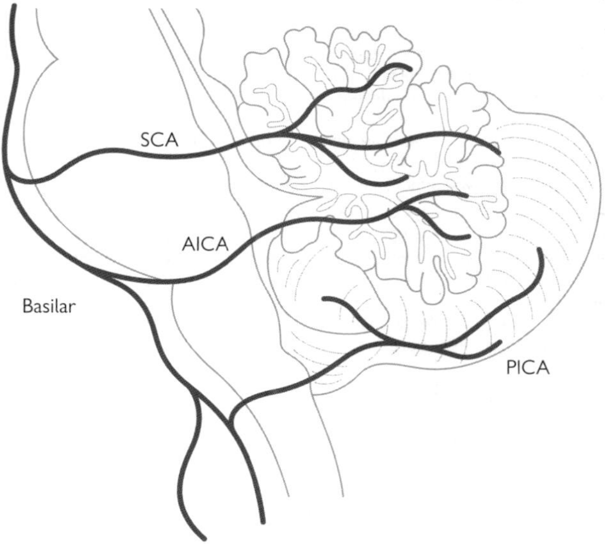

Fig. 2.7 Blood supply to the cerebellar regions. SCA, superior cerebellar artery; AICA, anterior inferior cerebellar artery; PICA, posterior inferior cerebellar artery.

Cortex

- Different functions are localized in specific cortical regions
- A knowledge of the different areas is essential to localize a brain infarct and subsequently determine which arterial territory is involved
- Figure 2.8 shows how different areas of the cortex control different functions
- Therefore you can see how infarcts in different regions could produce particular symptoms
- Large infarcts will affect multiple regions.

From Figure 2.8 it can be seen how a small infarct in the motor cortex may cause hand weakness alone. To paralyse the whole side would require a large infarct. From Figure 2.9, you can see it is impossible to paralyse the whole motor cortex alone; other areas such as the sensory cortex will also be involved. In contrast, where the motor fibres are closely packed in the internal capsule, a small lesion can damage them all and cause an isolated hemiparesis (pure motor stroke lacunar infarct).

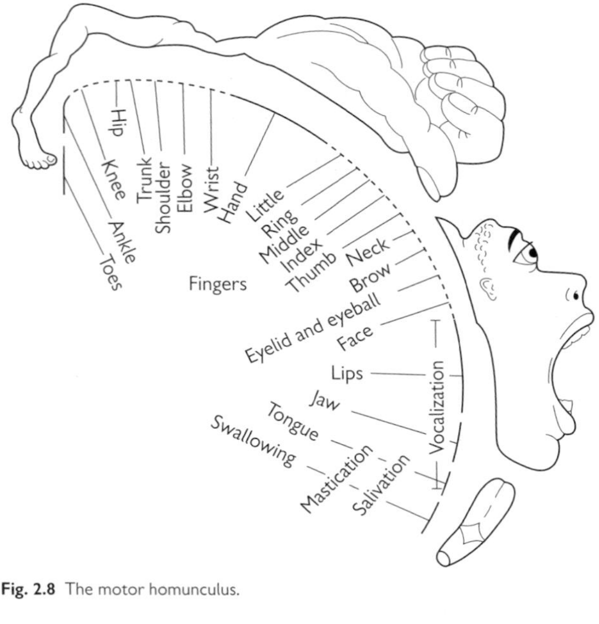

Fig. 2.8 The motor homunculus.

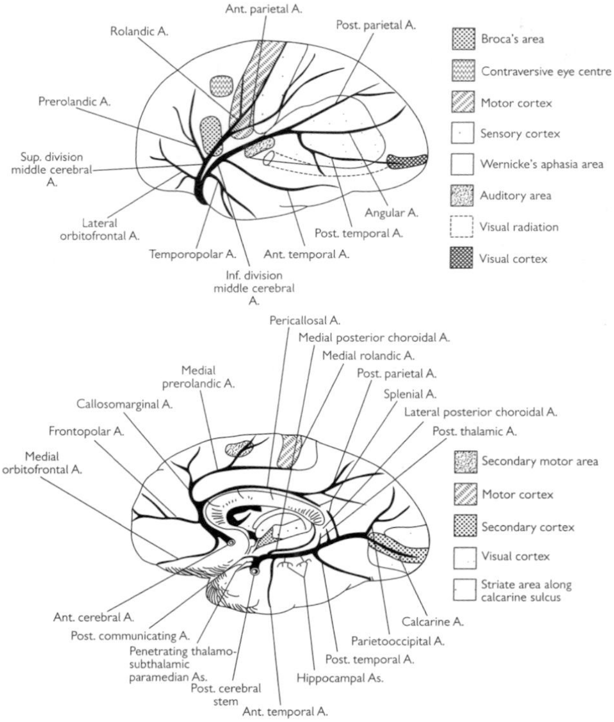

Fig. 2.9 Images showing lateral (above) and medial (below) views of the cerebral cortex. The different cortical regions are shown although it is not necessary to learn all their names. However, it is important to remember the location of the areas controlling the major functions which are shown in different shadings. The major arteries supplying the cortex are also shown. © Hugh Markus.

Fig. 2.9 [illegible]

Chapter 3

Vascular anatomy and stroke syndromes

Introduction

Stroke is a disease of blood flow. Therefore, it is very important to understand the blood supply of the brain. Most ischaemic stroke is embolic. Emboli may arise anywhere from the heart and the arterial tree connecting the heart to the brain.

The circulation is conventionally split into:

- Anterior circulation
  - Carotid artery distribution
- Posterior circulation
  - Vertebral and basilar artery distribution.

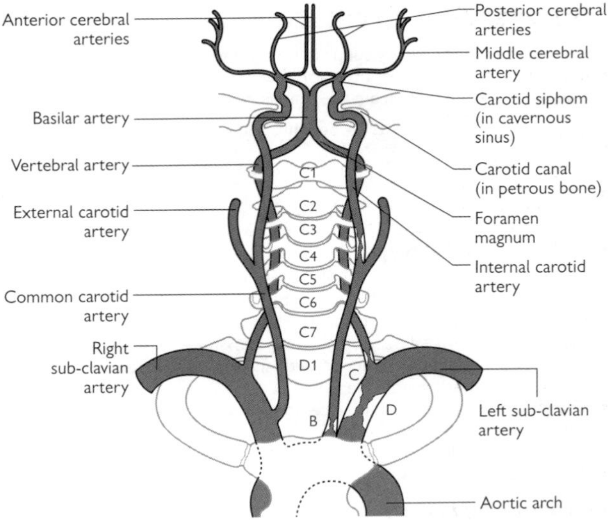

Fig. 3.1 The arterial supply of the brain with common sites of atheroma shown.

The anterior circulation

This comprises the territory supplied by the carotid arteries.

- The left carotid arises from the aorta
- The right carotid arises from the brachiocephalic artery.

The internal carotid artery is divided into four portions:

- Cervical
- Petrous
- Cavernous
- Cerebral.

Cervical carotid artery

- This runs from the bifurcation of the common carotid to the carotid canal within the petrous portion of the temporal bone
- Behind it is the superior cervical ganglion of the sympathetic trunk and the superior laryngeal nerve. The close proximity to the sympathetic fibres means a carotid dissection with an expanding artery often causes unilateral Horner's syndrome
- The glossopharyngeal, vagus, accessory, and hypoglossal nerves lie between the artery and the internal jugular vein. The hypoglossal artery is particularly vulnerable during carotid endarterectomy
- There are no branches.

Petrous carotid artery

- The carotid curves upward through the petrous bone to enter the skull cavity
- The artery is surrounded by the carotid plexus which contains sympathetic fibres from the superior cervical ganglion.

Cavernous carotid artery

- The artery runs through the cavernous sinus
- The artery is surrounded by the sympathetic fibres
- It lies close to crainal nerves 3, 4, 5a and 5b, and 6
- An important branch is the ophthalmic artery. Emboli passing into this artery are common in carotid stenosis and cause amaurosis fugax (fleeting uniocular loss of vision).

Cerebral carotid artery

- The artery penetrates the dura mater and passes between the second and sixth cranial nerves
- Terminal branches include:
  - Anterior cerebral artery
  - Middle cerebral artery—this supplies a very large part of the cerebral cortex
  - Posterior communicating artery
  - Choroidal artery.

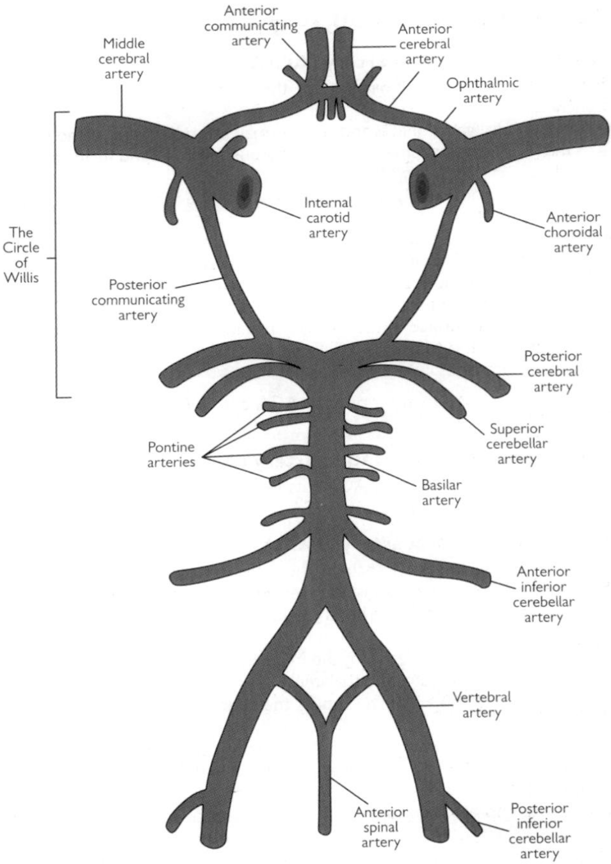

Fig. 3.2 The Circle of Willis and the major intracranial arteries.

Carotid arterial supply

The anterior cerebral artery (ACA)

The ACA is a major termination of the carotid artery. It has several branches.

- Anteromedial ganglionic branches are small arteries arising at the start of the ACA which supply part of the corpus callosum and head of caudate
- Inferior branches supply the orbital surface of the frontal lobe and the olfactory lobe
- Anterior branches supply a part of the superior frontal gyrus and send twigs over the edge of the hemisphere to the superior and middle frontal gyri and upper part of the anterior central gyrus
- Middle branches supply the corpus callosum, the cingulate gyrus, and the medial surface of the superior frontal and upper part of the anterior central gyrus
- Posterior branches.

The ACA lies close to the opposite ACA and is linked by the anterior communicating artery.

The anterior communicating artery (Acom)

The Acom connects the two ACAs. Its length averages about 4 mm. It is very variable and sometimes both ACAs arise from the same side.

The middle cerebral artery (MCA)

The MCA is the largest branch of the internal carotid. It runs laterally in the Sylvian fissure to the insula where it divides into several branches over the lateral surface of the hemisphere.

The branches include:

- Lenticulostriate branches from the MCA itself which supply the basal ganglia, internal capsule, and thalamus
- Inferior lateral frontal which supplies the inferior frontal gyrus (Broca's area)
- Ascending frontal which supplies the anterior central gyrus
- Ascending parietal which supplies posterior frontal and superior parietal lobule
- Parietotemporal which supplies the supramarginal and angular gyri, and the posterior parts of the superior and middle temporal gyri
- Temporal branches, two or three in number, which supply the temporal lobe.

The posterior communicating artery (Pcom)

The Pcom connects the internal carotid to the posterior cerebral artery. It is frequently larger on one side. It may be so large that the posterior cerebral artery appears to arise from the internal carotid rather than from the basilar. It gives off a few small branches.

The anterior choroidal artery

The anterior choroidal artery is a small branch which arises from the internal carotid near the Pcom. It supplies the choroid plexus and hippocampus.

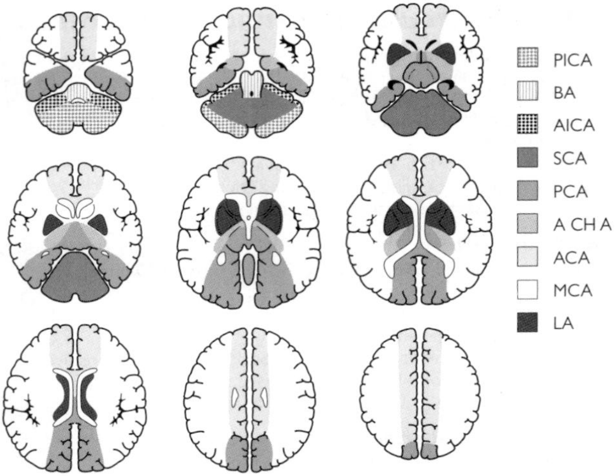

Fig. 3.3 Territories of the main cerebral arteries supplying the supratentorial structures. © Hugh Markus. PICA, posterior inferior cerebellar artery; BA, basilar artery; AICA, anterior inferior cerebellar artery; SCA, superior cerebellar artery; PCA, posterior cerebral artery; AChA, anterior choroidal artery; ACA, anterior cerebral artery; MCA middle cerebral artery; LA, lenticulostriate artery.

Anterior circulation clinical syndromes

By combining a knowledge of arterial anatomy, which brain regions are supplied by the different arteries (see Fig. 3.3), and which functions are located in which brain region (see Fig. 3.4), one can work out the consequences of occlusion of a particular artery.

Remember deficits can arise from:

- Involvement of cortical regions controlling specific functions
- Involvement of ascending or descending connections
- Involvement of subcortical and brainstem nuclei.

Ophthalmic artery

- Emboli from an internal carotid stenosis often pass down this artery
- Occlusion causes uniocular loss of vision
- Often transient amaurosis fugax
- Can result in permanent loss of vision
- Tight carotid stenosis can occasionally be associated with 'positive' retinal symptoms with flashing lights owing to haemodynamic compromise.

Anterior cerebral artery

- Leg and trunk weakness
- Relative sparing of the face
- Bilateral ACA infarction may cause weakness of both legs and gait apraxia (both ACAs can arise from a single ICA as a normal variant)
- Sensory disturbance (same distribution as motor weakness)
- Abulia (decrease in spontaneous speech and activity)
- Excessive or inappropriate crying or laughing
- Callosal disconnection
- Perseveration.

Middle cerebral artery

- Contralateral hemiplegia
- Eye deviation toward the side of the infarct (owing to disruption of frontal eye fields)
- Contralateral hemianopia
- Contralateral hemianaesthesia
- Global aphasia (dominant hemisphere)
- Expressive or motor aphasia (dominant hemisphere)
- Receptive or sensory aphasia (dominant hemisphere)
- Neglect
- Anosognosia (non-dominant hemisphere)
- Dyspraxia
- Movement disorders such as chorea and dystonia

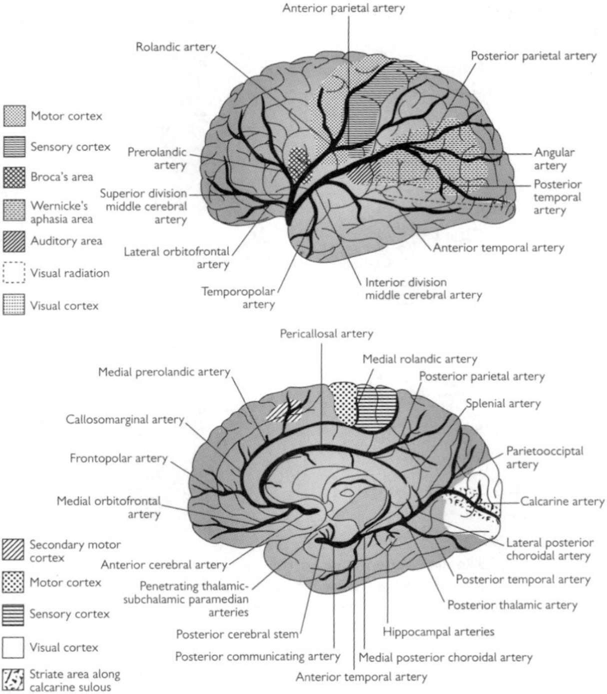

Fig. 3.4 Cortical brain regions supplied by the middle cerebral artery (above) and anterior and posterior cerebral arteries (below). © Hugh Markus.

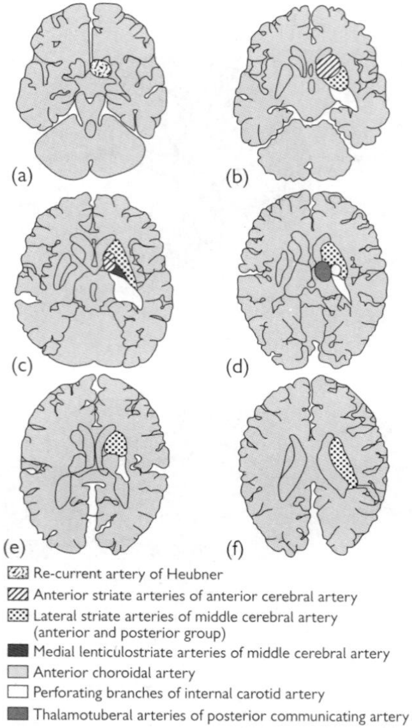

Fig. 3.5a Vascular supply of supratentorial subcortical regions. © Hugh Markus.

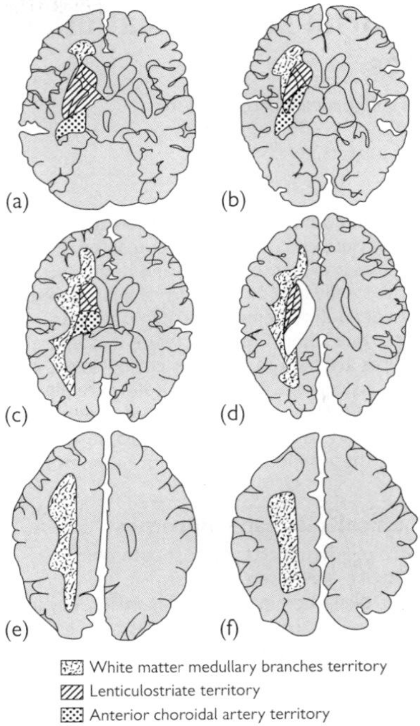

Fig. 3.5b Vascular supply of supratentorial subcortical regions. © Hugh Markus.

Supratentorial subcortical infarct syndromes

Specific types of subcortical infarcts include:
- Lacunar infarcts
- Striatocapsular infarcts.

Lacunar infarcts

- These are the most common type of subcortical infarcts occurring because of the occlusion of perforating end-arteries supplying the white matter, deep grey matter nuclei, and brainstem
- Named after the small lakes or 'lacunae' of infarction they cause
- Conventionally defined as being ≤1.5cm in diameter
- Symptoms occur due to disruption of white matter tracts
- Because the fibres are packed together closely in the descending and ascending tracts, usually the face, arm, and leg are affected together. Sometimes only two body parts are affected. However, it is unusual for a single body part (e.g. arm or hand alone) to be affected. MRI studies have shown that these syndromes are more commonly caused by small cortical infarcts.

Common 'classical' lacunar syndromes

- Pure motor stroke—hemiparesis (most common)
- Pure sensory stroke—hemisensory loss
- Sensorimotor stroke—hemiparesis and hemisensory loss
- Ataxic hemiparesis—ataxia and hemiparesis on the same side
- Clumsy hand and dysarthria syndrome.

A large number of atypical syndromes may occur.

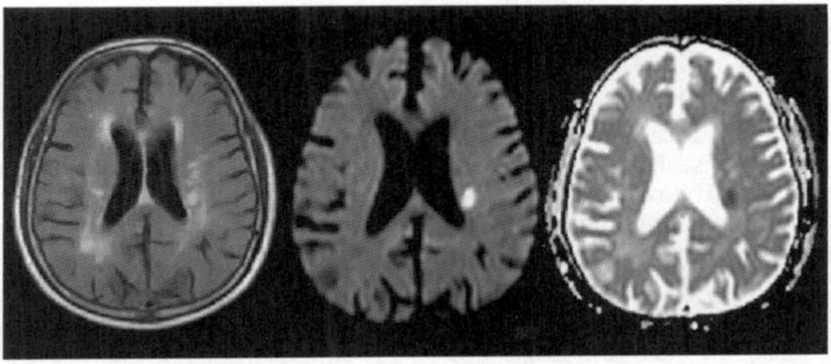

Fig. 3.6 MRI of an acute lacunar infarct. From left to right the scans show FLAIR and diffusion-weighted (DWI) images and an apparent diffusion coefficient (ADC) map. An acute lacunar infarct in the left corona radiate can been seen as high signal on DWI and corresponding low signal on the ADC map. It is in the corona radiata and resulted in right hemiparesis owing to disruption of the corticospinal tract. © Hugh Markus

Striatocapsular infarction

These are infarcts in the striatocapsular region which includes the corpus striatum and internal capsule. They are typically comma-shaped (see Fig. 3.7) and are larger than the upper limit for lacunar infarcts (>1.5 cm).

They arise from transient occlusion of the MCA, usually due to an embolus. This results in ischaemia in both:

- The territory of the perforating arteries coming off the MCA
- The regions of the cortex supplied by the MCA.

The perforating arteries arising from the trunk of the MCA (lentostriatal branches) are end-arteries with no collateral supply. Therefore, the area supplied by them (the striatocapsular region) rapidly dies. In contrast, the cortical regions receive some collateral supply and can survive for longer. If recanalization and reperfusion occurs before cortical infarction occurs, then the only region infarcted is the striatocapsular region.

Clinical features

Clinical features are caused by:

- Infarction in the striatocapsular region, causing hemiparesis and hemisensory loss. As these areas are infarcted, these deficits are usually permanent
- Ischaemia in cortical regions, e.g. dysphasia, neglect, hemianopia. As these areas are reperfused, the deficit is usually transient although it may take a few days to recover.

Causes

Striatocapsular infarction is usually due to either embolism from the heart or carotid artery or sometimes associated with MCA stenosis.

It often occurs in patients who are thrombolysed, when this results in reperfusion before cortical infarction has occurred.

This is an important diagnosis to be aware of because:

- Cardiac embolic sources with echocardiogram and ECG monitoring, and carotid stenosis should always be carefully sought
- It is not caused by small-vessel disease
- The symptoms and signs owing to transient cortical ischaemia usually improve rapidly.

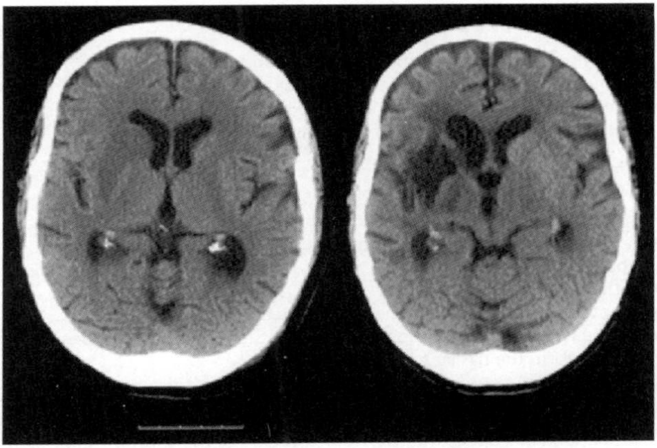

Fig. 3.7 Striatocapsular infarction. The scan on the left shows an early striatocapsular infarction with low density in the striatocapsular region. On the late scan on the right a much more well developed area of infarction can be seen. © Anthony Pereira.

The posterior circulation

This comprises the vertebrobasilar circulation.

- The vertebrals combine to form the basilar artery
- The basilar artery terminates in the two posterior cerebral arteries
- The anterior and posterior circulations are joined by the Circle of Willis.

The vertebral artery

- First branch of the subclavian artery
- It ascends through the foramina in the transverse processes of the upper six cervical vertebrae
- It then winds behind the atlas
- It enters the skull through the foramen magnum
- At the lower border of the pons it meets the vessel of the opposite side to form the basilar artery.

The vertebral artery may be divided into four parts:

- **V1**—The first part runs upward and backward behind the internal jugular and in front of the transverse process of the seventh cervical vertebra
- **V2**—The second part runs upward through the foramina in the transverse processes of the upper six cervical vertebrae, and pursues an almost vertical course as far as the transverse process of the atlas
- **V3**—The third part exits the foramen of the transverse process of the atlas and curves backward behind the atlas and enters the vertebral canal by passing beneath the posterior atlanto-occipital membrane
- **V4**—The fourth part pierces the dura mater and inclines to the front of the medulla oblongata. At the lower border of the pons it unites with the vessel of the opposite side to form the basilar artery.

V1–3 are extracranial. V4 is intracranial.

The most common site of atheromatous stenosis is at the origin, i.e. in the V1 section. Sometimes the origin itself is referred to separately as the V0 section.

Asymmetry is common between the vertebral arteries—unlike the carotids. Around 15% of the population have a hypoplastic or atretic single vertebral artery (less than 2 mm in diameter). This may be clinically significant if the dominant vessel becomes diseased.

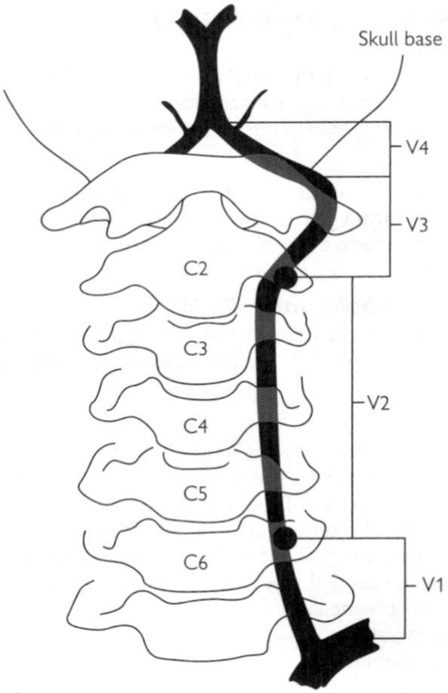

Fig. 3.8 The four segments of the vertebral artery.

The branches of the vertebral artery

Posterior spinal artery

This arises at the side of the medulla oblongata. Passing backward, it descends and is reinforced by a succession of small branches which enter the vertebral canal and it continues to the cauda equina.

Anterior spinal artery

This arises near the termination of the vertebral and, descending in front of the medulla oblongata, unites with its fellow of the opposite side at the foramen magnum to form a single descending trunk which stretches down to the cauda equina.

Posterior inferior cerebellar artery (PICA)

The PICA is the largest branch of the vertebral and winds back around the upper part of the medulla oblongata. It supplies part of the brainstem and cerebellum.

Basilar artery

This is a single trunk formed by the junction of the two vertebral arteries: it extends from the lower to the upper border of the pons, lying in its median groove under cover of the arachnoid. It ends by dividing into the two posterior cerebral arteries. Its branches include:

- Pontine vessels which come off at right angles from either side of the basilar artery and supply the pons
- Anterior inferior cerebellar artery
- Internal auditory artery
- Superior cerebellar artery.

Perforating arteries

End-arteries come off the intracranial vertebral and basilar arteries and supply the brainstem—occlusion of these results in brainstem lacunar infarcts.

Posterior cerebral arteries

These are the large terminal branches of the basilar artery. They are linked to the anterior circulation through the Pcom arteries. Their branches supply:

- Posterior choroidal branches to the choroid plexus
- A considerable portion of the thalamus
- Temporal cortex
- Occipital lobe.

An embryonic/normal variant seen in approximately 5% of the population is that the PCA arises directly from the ICA. This is clinically relevant as, in such circumstances, carotid stenosis can cause posterior circulation stroke symptoms.

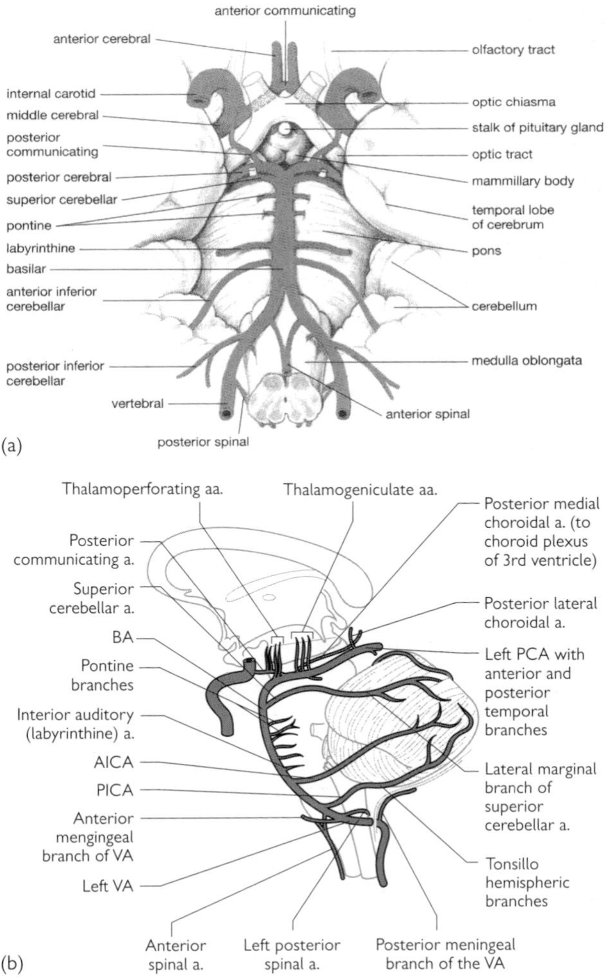

Fig. 3.9 The blood supply of the brainstem. **(a)** Anterior posterior view and **(b)** lateral view. Figure 3.9a is reproduced from MacKinnon P, Morris J (2005) *Oxford Textbook of Functional Anatomy*, Vol. 3. Oxford, Oxford University Press.

Posterior circulation clinical syndromes

Ischaemia in the posterior circulation can present with symptoms caused by damage to functions controlled by the:

- Cortex, most commonly the occipital cortex
- Thalamus
- Brainstem nuclei
- Descending motor and ascending sensory pathways
- Cerebellum.

Posterior cerebral artery infarction

The following areas may be involved as described below.

Parieto-occipital involvement

- Unilateral occipital infarction produces homonymous hemianopia
- Sparing of the macula may occur because of collateral vascular supply to the occipital pole from posterior branches of the MCA
- Bilateral infarctions of the occipital lobes produce cortical blindness
  - Anton syndrome, patients have very realistic visual hallucinations
- Balint syndrome
  - Bilateral parieto-occipital infarction
  - Simultanagnosia (patient identifies specific parts of a scene but cannot describe the entire picture), optic ataxia (a loss of hand—eye coordination) and apraxia of gaze
- Pure alexia may result from infarction of the dominant occipital cortex.

Thalamus

- Thalamic infarction may present with confusion or memory disturbance and, if isolated, the diagnois of stroke is sometimes missed. It often improves, particularly if the infarction is unilateral
- Pure hemisensory loss (infarction of the ventral posterolateral nucleus of the thalamus)
- Bilateral thalamic ('butterfly') infarction may cause an obtunded or comatose patient and/or severe memory dysfunction.

Other features

- Occlusion of the posterior choroidal artery may produce hemianopia, hemidysaesthesia, and memory disturbance
- In some cases the posterior limb of the internal capsule is supplied from the PCA and infarction then results in hemiparesis
- Infarction of the medial temporal lobe or medial thalamic nuclei may result in permanent anterograde amnesia (normally bilateral infarction needed).

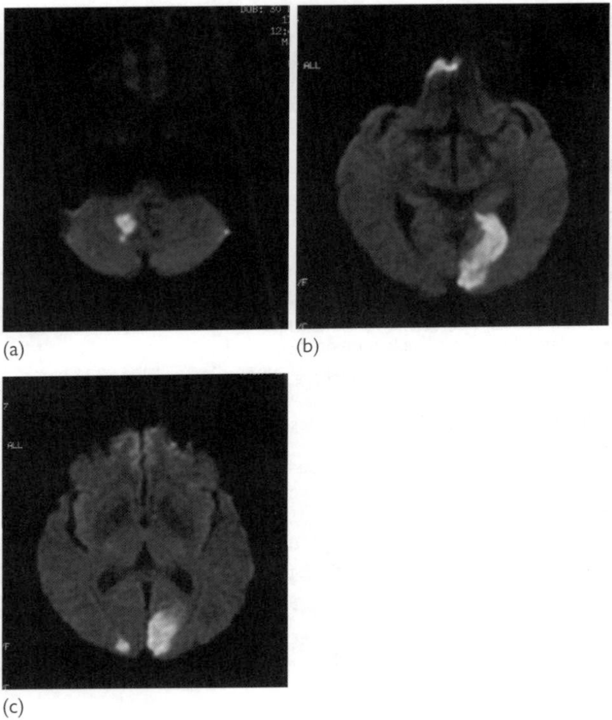

Fig. 3.10 Diffusion-weighted MRI showing multiple infarcts in the PCA territory involving the **(a)** right cerebellum; **(b)** the left cortical PCA territory; and **(c)** both occipital poles. © Hugh Markus.

Brainstem infarcts

These are special types of subcortical infarcts. From Figs 3.11 and 3.12, it can be seen that there are many nuclei and tracts densely packed in the brainstem. Therefore, infarction here tends to be accompanied by other features and damage to the cranial nerves.

- Vertigo
- Diplopia
- Sensorineural hearing loss
- Facial numbness or paraesthesias
- Dysphagia
- Dysarthria
- Syncope (loss of consciousness)
- Nystagmus
- Limb and trunk ataxia
- Contralateral pain and temperature loss
- Ipsilateral limb and trunk numbness.

Lateral medullary infarct (Wallenberg syndrome)

- Ipsilateral facial pain and numbness
- Ipsilateral ataxia (falling to side of lesion)
- Vertigo, nausea, and vomiting
- Contralateral pain and temperature loss
- Nystagmus
- Ipsilateral Horner's syndrome.

Basilar artery occlusion

- Decreased level of consciousness
- Locked-in state
- Tetraplegia
- Horizontal gaze palsy
- Bifacial and oropharyngeal palsy.

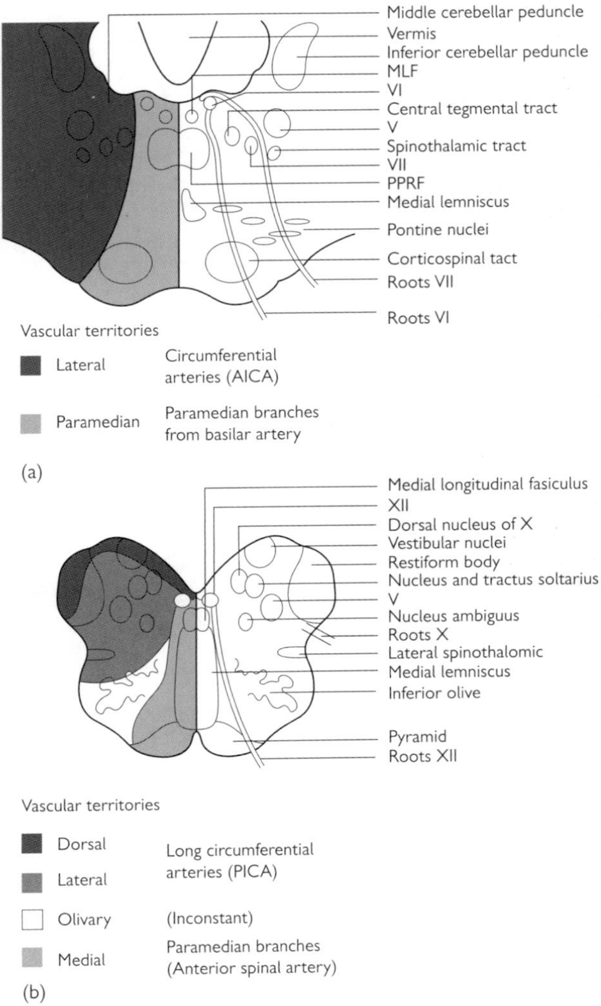

Fig. 3.11 Arterial supply of the pons (upper) and medulla (lower).

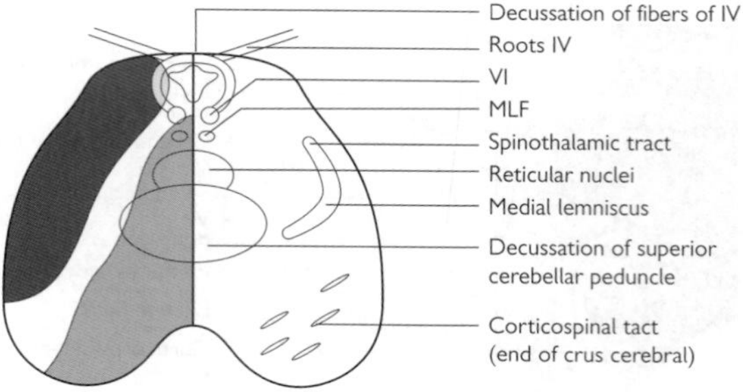

Vascular territories

■	Lateral	Circumferential arteries (SCA)
□	Intermediate	(Inconsistant)
▒	Paramedian	Paramedian branches from basilar artery

(c)

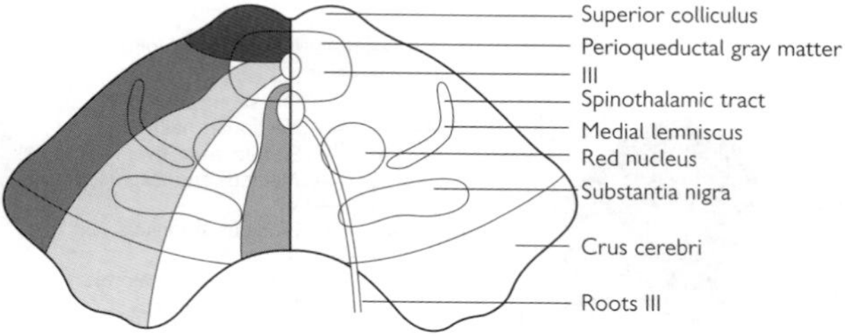

Vascular territories

■	Dorsal	Long circumferential arteries (SCA)
▓	Lateral	
░	Intermediolateral	Short circumferential from PCA (P_2 segment)
□	Intermediomedial	
▒	Medial	From the tip of basilar artery

(d)

Fig. 3.12 Arterial supply of the brainstem.

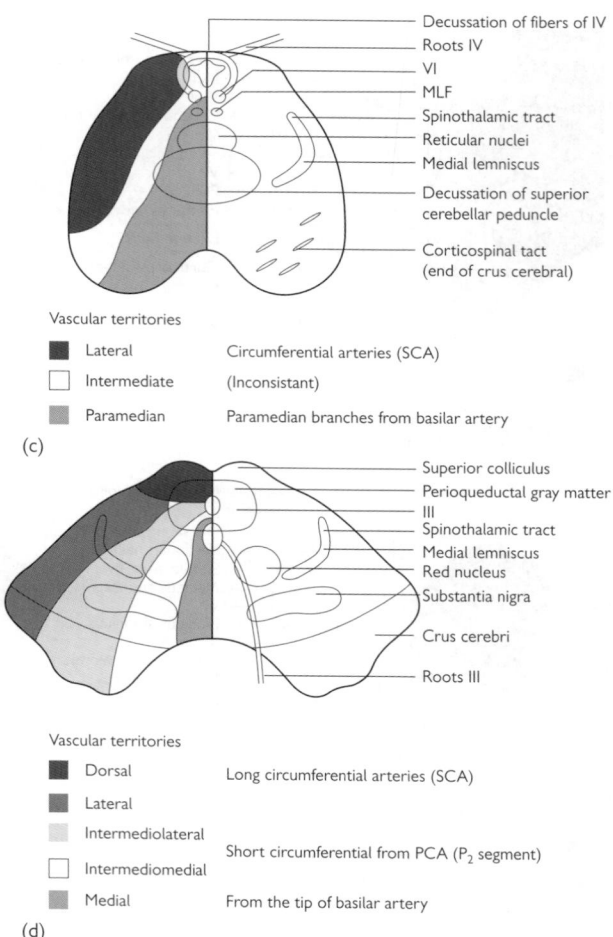

Cerebellar infarction

This presents with ataxia. In addition, frequently brainstem nuclei and their connections are also infarcted, resulting in cranial nerve deficits, and involvement of ascending sensory and descending motor pathways in the brainstem is common; this results in hemiparesis and/or hemisensory loss.

Syndromes associated with infarction in specific cerebellar artery territories include the following.

Superior cerebellar artery infarct

- Ipsilateral ataxia
- If upper brainstem/cortex is involved:
  - Hemianopia (or cortical blindness)
  - Memory loss
  - Confusion
  - Contralateral hemiparesis
- If brainstem is involved
  - Ipsilateral Horner's syndrome
  - Contralateral loss of pain sensation
  - Contralateral sixth palsy
  - Tremor.

Anterior inferior cerebellar artery

- Vertigo
- Dysarthria
- Ipsilateral facial palsy
- Ipsilateral Horner's syndrome
- Ipsilateral ataxia
- Contralateral pain loss
- Gaze palsy.

Posterior inferior cerebellar artery

- Wallenberg syndrome (see 📖 Brainstem infarcts, p. 88).

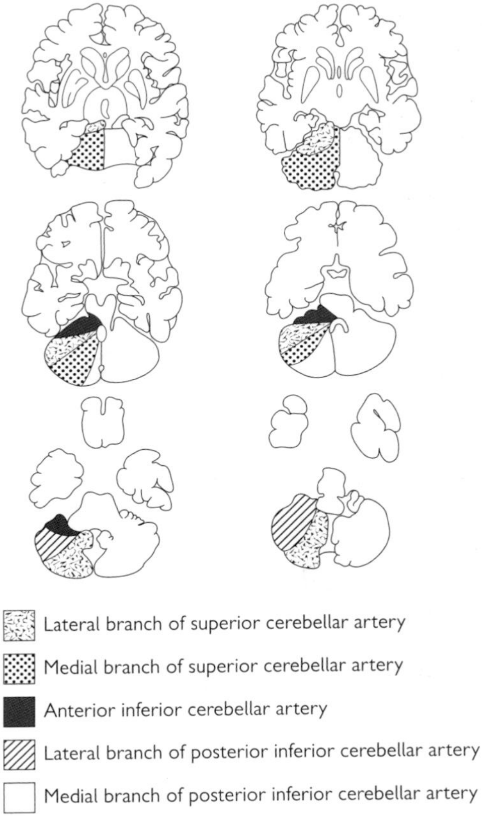

Fig. 3.13 Arterial supply of the cerebellum.

Border zone areas of the brain

These regions of the brain are at the extremities of the major vascular supply. Reduction in perfusion pressure either caused by systemic hypotension, and/or by tight stenoses, particularly if collateral supply is poor, may result in border zone (or watershed) infarction.

The classical border zone areas are:

- Cortical (dark grey in Figure 3.14)
  - Anterior border zone where the ACA meets the MCA
  - Posterior border zone where the MCA meets the PCA
- Subcortical (light grey in Figure 3.14)
  - Internal border zone which is found at the extremity of the arterial arcades supplying the white matter of the centrum semiovale.

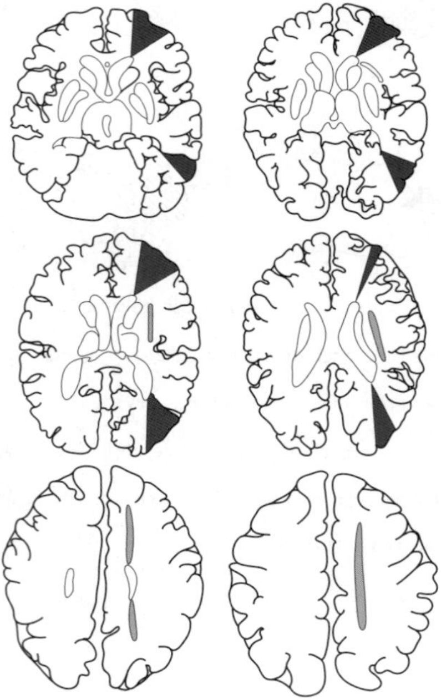

Fig. 3.14 The cerebral arterial border zone regions.

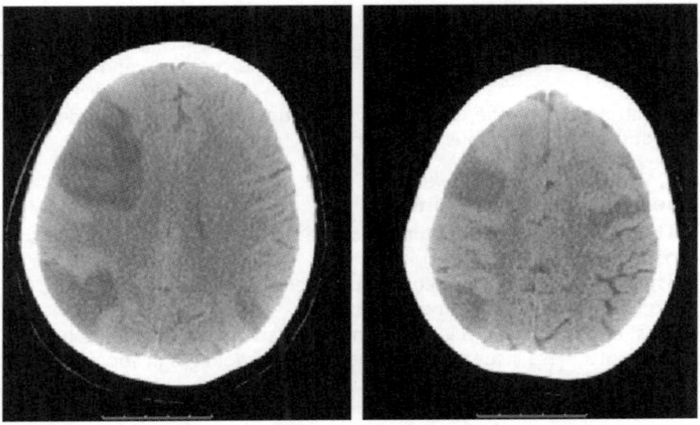

Fig. 3.15 Two slices of a CT brain scan in a patient who suffered cardiac arrest. The hypodense areas are regions of infarction. They are visible in the anterior and posterior border zones. © Hugh Markus.

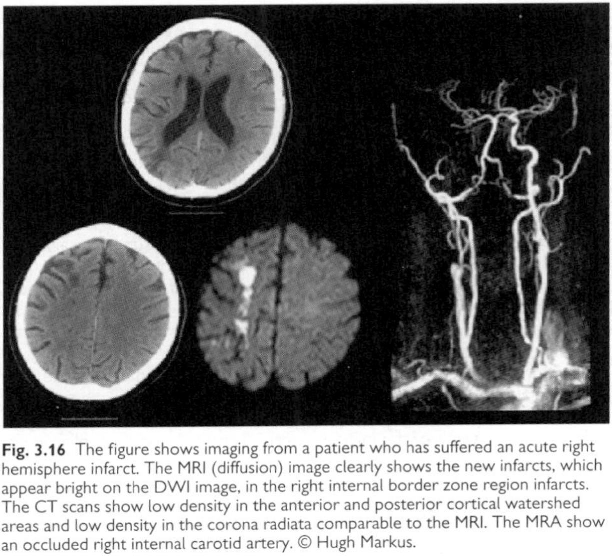

Fig. 3.16 The figure shows imaging from a patient who has suffered an acute right hemisphere infarct. The MRI (diffusion) image clearly shows the new infarcts, which appear bright on the DWI image, in the right internal border zone region infarcts. The CT scans show low density in the anterior and posterior cortical watershed areas and low density in the corona radiata comparable to the MRI. The MRA show an occluded right internal carotid artery. © Hugh Markus.

Venous drainage of the brain

The venous drainage of the brain is through the cerebral venous sinuses. They are:

- Situated between the two layers of the dura mater and are lined by endothelium continuous with that which lines the veins
- Devoid of valves.

The superior sagittal sinus

- This occupies the convex margin of the falx and runs from anterior to posterior
- There are usually three lacunae on either side of the sinus: a small frontal, a large parietal, and an occipital
- Most of the cerebral veins from the outer surface of the hemisphere open into these lacunae, and numerous arachnoid granulations (Pacchionian bodies) project into them from below
- It receives many dural draining veins and the superior cerebral veins.

The inferior sagittal sinus

- This runs in the posterior part of the free margin of the falx cerebri
- It ends in the straight sinus
- It receives several veins from the falx cerebri.

The straight sinus

- This is situated at the junction of the falx cerebri with the tentorium cerebelli
- It runs downward and backward from the end of the inferior sagittal sinus
- Its terminal part communicates with the confluence of the sinuses
- Besides the inferior sagittal sinus, it receives the great cerebral vein (great vein of Galen) and the superior cerebellar veins.

The transverse sinuses

- One, often the right, is the direct continuation of the superior sagittal sinus, while the other is a continuation of the straight sinus
- Each passes lateral and forward in the attached margin of the tentorium cerebelli
- It then leaves the tentorium and curves downward to reach the jugular foramen, where it ends in the internal jugular vein
- The portion which occupies the groove on the mastoid part of the temporal bone is sometimes termed the *sigmoid sinus*
- They receive the blood from the superior petrosal sinus
- They receive some of the inferior cerebral and inferior cerebellar veins.

The occipital sinus

- This is the smallest of the cranial sinuses
- It is situated in the attached margin of the falx cerebelli.

The confluence of the sinuses

- This is the dilated extremity of the superior sagittal sinus
- It receives blood from the occipital sinus
- It connects across the midline to the opposite transverse sinus.

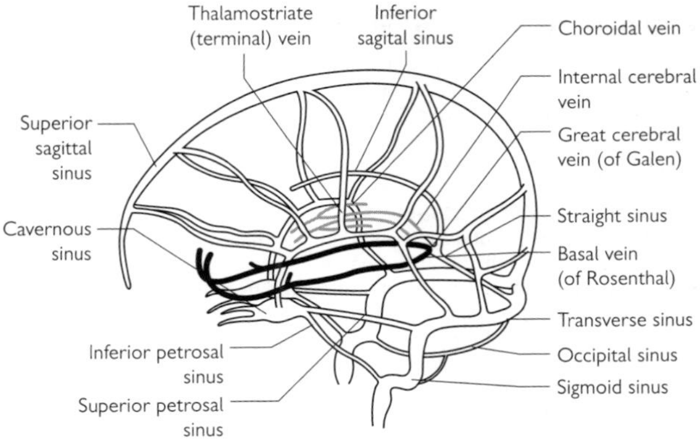

Fig. 3.17 The major cerebral venous sinuses.

The cavernous sinuses

These structures are anatomically important because thrombosis here results in a specific syndrome (see 📖 Chapter 12).

- They are so named because they present a reticulated structure
- They are traversed by numerous interlacing filaments
- They extend from the superior orbital fissure to the apex of the petrous portion of the temporal bone
- Each opens behind into the petrosal sinus
- On the medial wall of each sinus is the internal carotid artery
- Near the artery is the abducent nerve
- On the lateral wall are the oculomotor and trochlear nerves, and the ophthalmic and maxillary divisions of the trigeminal nerve are separated from the blood by the lining membrane of the sinus
- The cavernous sinus receives the superior ophthalmic vein through the superior orbital fissure
- It communicates with the transverse sinus by means of the superior petrosal sinus with the internal jugular vein through the inferior petrosal sinus
- The two sinuses also communicate with each other by means of the anterior and posterior intercavernous sinuses.

The superior petrosal sinus

- Small
- Connects the cavernous with the transverse sinus
- It joins the transverse sinus where the latter curves downward on the inner surface of the mastoid part of the temporal bone.

The inferior petrosal sinus

- It joins the cavernous sinus to the superior bulb of the internal jugular vein
- The inferior petrosal sinus receives the internal auditory veins and also veins from the medulla oblongata, pons, and undersurface of the cerebellum.

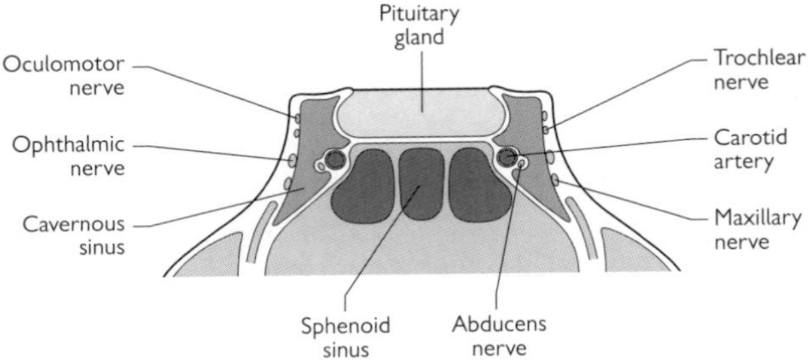

Fig. 3.18 Cross-sectional view through the cavernous sinus.

Chapter 4

History-taking in the stroke patient

General principles of history-taking in the stroke patient

Stroke is defined as a sudden-onset focal neurological deficit lasting for 24 hours or more, or leading to earlier death attributed to a vascular cause.

General points about history-taking

Make the patient central

Stroke affects a wide variety of patients but particularly older people. It can be very challenging to get a coherent history. By definition stroke is sudden onset—one moment a person is well and the next they are not, and so acute stroke patients are often frightened. Patients may be drowsy, disorientated, frightened, dysphasic or even demented as a result of the stroke or other comorbidity. Therefore, the history, the most vital part of clinical evaluation, may be very difficult.

Always start by allowing the patient to give their version of events. If allowed to speak, most patients will not talk for more than a couple of minutes and often that amount of time will provide all the information you need to make a diagnosis.

It cannot be overstated how important it is to get even a small amount of history from a patient. For example, it may provide a clue to the initial chest pain from the heart attack that led to the stroke—the heart attack which you are just about to miss because the stroke seems so obvious!

Always take a collateral history

This is particularly important in stroke patients, many of whom have communication or cognitive problems that limit their ability to give a complete history.

Therefore, consider talking to:

- Witnesses who saw the event
- Ambulance personnel who brought the patient to the emergency department
- Family members who may provide important information on the patient's premorbid state and whether there were pre-existing cognitive problems
- The family doctor, who may provide important information on past medical history, particularly if an informant is unavailable.

Scheme of history-taking in stroke

Skilful history-taking should not take more than a few minutes but it is important to have in mind a scheme of what you are looking for to help you find it.

- First, make the diagnosis
- Second, look for a cause
- Third, look for the risk factors.

Making the diagnosis

Key points to determine are:
- Is it a stroke?
- Could it be a mimic?
- What vascular territory is affected?

Some useful principles in stroke diagnosis

- The attack on the brain happens suddenly
- The brain stops working, i.e. a loss of function (e.g. weakness or visual field defect) rather than a gain of function (e.g. involuntary movement or positive visual phenomena) usually occurs
- The symptoms the patient experiences will parallel the underlying pathological process: the symptoms are 'telling' you the pathology
- An important feature of the history is the time course of symptoms, which indicates the time course of the pathological process.

Transient ischaemic attack (TIA)

TIA is defined as a sudden-onset focal neurological deficit which is fully recovered within 24 hours, i.e. it has a similar presentation to stroke and a similar pathophysiology.
- Although patients with TIA recover within 24 hours, the average length of TIA is about 15 minutes and most last less than 1 hour
- With MRI it has been shown that many TIAs which last longer than an hour are associated with new infarction
- During the acute phase, particularly within the first 3 hours when decisions on thrombolysis are being made, TIA and stroke cannot be differentiated with certainty
- Patients with TIA may not present for several days or weeks after the event, as transient symptoms are often ignored by patients. Then, obtaining a history of only 15 minutes of illness can be very difficult.

Time of onset

- With the advent of thrombolysis, it is imperative that you establish the time of onset of stroke
- If the stroke is noticed on awakening, for the purposes of deciding whether to give thrombolysis, the time of onset is considered to be the time the patient was last seen well

Consider the time courses of disease

There are several time courses seen in neurology and keeping them in the back of your mind when tackling the history will help distinguish stroke from its mimics.

Sudden onset

Few pathological processes are sudden in onset, the main ones being:
- Stroke
- Epilepsy
- Trauma.

Subacute
Here symptoms build up either over hours or days or perhaps weeks. The underlying pathology here may be:
- Infectious
- Inflammatory
- Metabolic
- Malignant.

Chronic and progressive
Symptoms which progress relentlessly over months or years are usually due to:
- Malignancy
- Degenerative disease, e.g. Alzheimer's disease or motor neuron disease.

Relapsing and remitting
A good example of this is multiple sclerosis.

The 'normal' stroke history

Stroke is almost always sudden in onset. If the symptoms are not sudden-onset then you should be very wary of diagnosing stroke.

The normal history for stroke is a sudden-onset loss of function of something. Most commonly, this will be loss of power down one side.

Sometimes there are a multiplicity of symptoms which appear confusing. The way to tackle this is to deal with each symptom individually and try to work out the time course of the start of each symptom. It may then be possible to ascertain that all the symptoms started at approximately the same time but had differing time courses thereafter.

Differentiating stroke/TIA from mimic conditions

The main differential diagnoses of TIA in the emergency department are:
- Blackouts/syncope
- Epilepsy
- Migraine with aura
- Metabolic, particularly hypoglycaemia.

Isolated loss of consciousness
This is seldom due to stroke or TIA. Loss of consciousness in stroke occurs with:
- Massive supratentorial stroke
- Brainstem stroke. Other posterior circulation neurological signs are almost always present (e.g. eye signs, ataxia, vertigo, vomiting)
- Seizures (possibly complicating the stroke).

Epileptic seizures
These may occur secondary to the acute stroke, but seizures in the absence of stroke can also present as a stroke mimic.
- Normally occur with sudden onset
- Sometimes there may be an aura and if patients have had previous attacks they may recognize the aura

- The aura is normally quite short
- The patient will lose consciousness
- The most common seizure type is the generalized tonic/clonic fit. This is aptly named as the patient will exhibit a tonic stage where the body goes stiff, usually in extension, followed by a clonic phase when all four limbs shake rhythmically
- Most seizures last only a couple of minutes
- The patient may bite the tongue or be incontinent during the seizure
- They will usually be confused and disorientated afterwards
- Post-ictal neurological symptoms and signs may occur—most commonly Todd's paresis, a hemiparesis which can last hours to days. This is more common in patients with previous stroke
- A careful eyewitness history is very helpful in diagnosis.

Migraine with aura

A typical migraine attack with aura accompanied by severe unilateral headache, nausea, and vomiting is easy to differentiate from stroke. However, migraine can present with aura alone and this can present diagnostic difficulty.

- The time course for migraine aura is usually about 30 minutes
- There may be several symptoms, and typically the patient may notice flashing lights, zigzag lines or castellations moving across the visual field, followed by difficulty finding words, followed by tingling in the arm
- There is what is termed a characteristic 'march' of symptoms: the visual phenomenon occurs first followed by the other phenomena, one subsiding while the next one starts. Similarly, motor symptoms may march along the limbs.

What vascular territory is affected?

Occlusion of a cerebral artery will result in ischaemia in the territory of that artery, therefore all symptoms and signs will be caused by failure of brain regions supplied by the affected artery. The pattern of symptoms (and signs) will help identify which arterial territory is affected. This may be of clinical importance, e.g. in determining whether a carotid stenosis is symptomatic and therefore requires urgent endarterectomy.

It is helpful to think in terms of the vascular territories so that you can relate the symptoms to a vascular region. Initially try to determine whether the stroke has affected the anterior or posterior circulation. More details on vascular anatomy and associated stroke syndromes are given in 📖 Chapter 3. Some symptoms and signs (e.g. hemiparesis) can be caused by both anterior and posterior circulation ischaemia, while others are specific to one arterial circulation. This is detailed below and illustrated in Table 4.1.

Anterior circulation stroke

- Eighty per cent of cerebral blood flow and therefore 80% of ischaemic stroke
- Anterior cerebral artery
    - Can be asymptomatic
    - If hemiparesis, the leg is affected more
    - Dysphasia can occur, predominantly expressive

- Middle cerebral artery
  - Face and arm more affected, visual disturbance, speech disturbance (language)
  - Dysphasia, expressive and/or receptive
  - Dyspraxia, present with infarction in either hemisphere
- It is important to check handedness of patients. Most patients are right-hand dominant and left hemisphere language-dominant. In those who are left-hand dominant, 50% will still be left hemisphere language-dominant.

Posterior circulation stroke

- Sometimes termed vertebrobasilar territory infarction or vertebrobasilar insufficiency; the latter term is better not used
- Most ischaemic stroke is embolic or due to small-vessel disease
- Haemodynamic insufficiency is a rare cause
- The vertebral arteries unite to form the basilar artery which terminates in the posterior cerebral arteries. These vessels supply the brainstem, pons, cerebellum, occipital lobes, and, to a varying degree, the posterior thalamus

Common symptoms and signs of posterior circulation ischaemia follow.

- Brainstem and cerebellar involvement
  - Vertigo
  - Diplopia and nystagmus
  - Nausea and vomiting
  - Unsteadiness and ataxia
  - Dysarthria
  - Hemiparesis—but will spare face if below pons
  - Hemisensory loss
  - Loss of consciousness
  - Bilateral or crossed weakness/sensory disturbance
- Posterior cerebral artery involvement
  - Hemianopia
  - Cortical blindness (owing to basilar occlusion and disruption of both posterior cerebral arteries)
  - Confusion/amnesia (owing to branches supplying posterior thalamus).

A good rule of thumb is that *two* symptoms and signs should be present to make one suspect posterior circulation infarction.

A crucial point is that hemiparesis may be caused by a lesion anywhere along the motor pathway from the motor cortex to the cervical cord. However, only if it is in the brainstem would it become accompanied by vertigo, diplopia, nausea, vomiting, and possibly loss of consciousness.

Isolated vertigo is rarely due to stroke or TIA and is far more commonly caused by peripheral labyrinthine disturbance.

Table 4.1 Symptoms and signs associated with anterior and posterior circulation stroke

Symptom/sign	Anterior circulation	Posterior circulation
Hemiparesis	Yes	Yes
Hemisensory loss	Yes	Yes
Hemianopia	Yes	Yes
Slurred speech	Yes	Yes
Neglect	Yes	No
Dysphasia	Yes	No
Apraxia	Yes	No
Drowsy	Yes	Yes
Loss of consciousness	No	Sometimes
Diplopia	No	Yes
Nystagmus	No	Yes
Ataxia	No	Yes
Nausea/vomiting	No	Yes
Vertigo	No	Yes
Crossed signs	No	Yes
Quadriparesis	No	Yes

What caused the stroke—clues from the history

A key question, which is of major importance later when planning management, is 'What has caused this stroke in this person'; i.e. is it embolism from a carotid artery, cardioembolism, small-vessel disease, dissection, etc.

This is *not* the same as asking for risk factors, although the two do overlap. Go through the normal history.

Past medical history

- Previous stroke or TIA
- Heart disease:
  - Past myocardial infarct (MI)
  - Recent chest pain suggesting recent MI (or thoracic root aortic dissection)
  - Atrial fibrillation
  - Rheumatic fever as a child
  - Valvular heart disease or valve replacement
  - Symptoms of heart failure
  - Palpitations
  - Pacemaker
- Peripheral vascular disease
- Diabetes
- Recent injury (e.g. to the neck). Ask if the patient has had any trauma of the head or neck in the last few weeks and investigate whether they have noticed any neck pain or pain behind the eye that may identify dissection
- Evidence of thrombophilia (e.g. DVT, PE, recurrent miscarriages).

Drug history

- Oral contraceptive pill
- Hormone replacement therapy
- Illicit drug use, e.g. cocaine

Family history

This must be taken in full. A full family history is important for two reasons.

- It may detect rare monogenic causes of stroke (📖 p. 325)
- Family history is a risk factor for 'sporadic' stroke

This should be taken in a systematic fashion.

- For first degree relatives (parent and sibs) ask:
  - Are they are alive—if so, what age?
  - If dead, age and cause of death
  - Have they had stroke—if so, at what age?
  - Have they had MI—if so, at what age?
  - Have they had other neurological disease (e.g. stroke in the young can be misdiagnosed as multiple sclerosis; vascular dementia is often misdiagnosed as Alzheimer's disease
- For more distant relatives, ask if any had stroke, MI, dementia or other neurological diseases and, if so, record age of onset and death
- It helps to record family history on a family tree visually using standard symbols (Fig. 4.1).

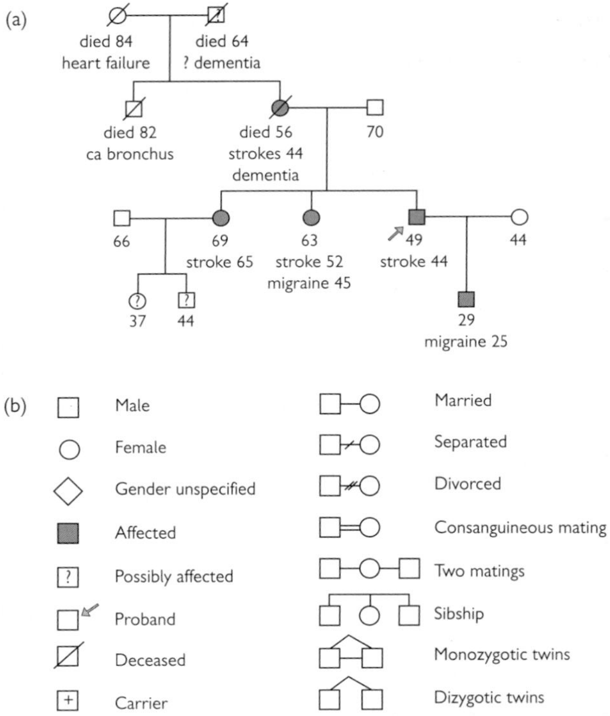

Fig. 4.1 (a) An example of a family tree from a family with CADASIL, an autosomal dominant form of stroke (📖 p. 326). (b) Standard symbols illustrated are used to indicate the status of individuals. Reproduced from Markus H (ed.) (2003) *Stroke Genetics*. Oxford, Oxford University Press.

Risk factors

History of risk factors

Next, move on to the risk factors. This will be identified by both history and examination and investigation. Ask about:

- Hypertension
- Diabetes
- Angina
- Peripheral vascular disease
- Cholesterol
- Smoking
- Alcohol
- Family history of stroke.

Social history

It is very important to have some idea of the person who now has the disease.

- Do they live alone?
- Do they work; if so, what is their job?
- Do they drive?
- Are they married?
- What is their social support network?
- Are they in receipt of social services or reliant on others for domestic or personal care?
- What sort of a house do they live in?

Functional enquiry

Lastly, go through the functional enquiry. This is a good chance to catch anything missed.

- Cardiovascular system
- Respiratory system
- Abdominal system
- Urinary system and continence
- Problems with skin or joints. Previous level of mobility/falls.

Summary

- Stroke is almost always sudden in onset
- Determine the time of onset
- The time course of symptoms is essential.

First, make the diagnosis:
- Is it a stroke?
- Could it be a mimic?
- What vascular territory is affected?

Second, look for a cause, e.g:
- Heart disease
- Drug use

Third, look for the risk factors:
- Hypertension
- Diabetes
- Smoking
- Heart disease
- Cholesterol
- Age
- Family history

Make sure you take as much history from the patient as possible.

Find out about the patient's premorbid state and home situation, and determine what are the immediate problems for the patient.

Take an eyewitness report if available.

Always take a collateral history.

Remember to talk to the family doctor.

Summary

Chapter 5

Examination

Introduction

The examination must seek specific information to:

- Understand the anatomy of the disease
- Form a diagnosis
- Plan management
- Anticipate possible complications.

The neurological examination provides information to aid diagnosis:

- Is there evidence of single or multiple lesions?
- Is the stroke in an arterial territory supplied by the carotid or vertebral artery?
- Has the stroke damaged or spared the cerebral cortex?
- Is this a lacunar syndrome?

Examination may also identify aetiological factors:

- Atrial fibrillation
- Hypertensive end-organ damage
- Diabetes mellitus
- Carotid bruits
- Absent peripheral pulses
- Cigarette tar-stained fingers.

The answer to these questions will help in making a diagnosis and may be very useful when interpreting the further investigations.

The examination is important in planning management and rehabilitation:

- Is swallowing impaired?
- To what extent is communication affected?
- Is the patient continent?
- Is there function left in the hands/arms?
- Can the patient sit/stand/walk?

The systemic examination is an equally important part of the evaluation of the stroke patient. Like the neurological examination, it must be directed to look for signs that may identify the cause of the stroke or other comorbidity, which will have a direct effect on the management of the patient and their potential complications. For example:

- Is the patient in atrial fibrillation?
- Is there evidence of pneumonia?
- Is there a palpable bladder?
- Does the patient have arthritis?

> The examination of the stroke patient should not be considered as a voyage of discovery but should be used to identify features that will complement the history to secure a diagnosis and guide patient management. The purpose of the neurological examination is to differentiate normal and abnormal anatomy within the nervous system.

Neurological examination

Follow a conventional neurological examination. Start at the top and work down.

Neurological examination

- Inspection
- Conscious level
- Speech and language
- Higher mental function
- Cranial nerves
- Peripheral nervous system
- General examination

Inspection

This is an important part of any examination. Stand back and look at the patient for a few moments. It can pay dividends. For example, you may see focal twitching of a limb and make a diagnosis of epilepsy.

It is best to have a system for inspection. We do the following:

- Is the patient alert or drowsy?
- Is the patient having absences?
- Is the speech abnormal?
- Is the head normal size and shape? Is there evidence of head injury?
- Is there pallor or cyanosis?
- It there abnormal facial asymmetry?
- Is there eye deviation to one side or a squint?
- Are the limbs normal length? A fractured limb may be apparent from observation
- Are all limbs moving or is there a particular pattern of lack of movement (e.g. hemiplegia/paraplegia/tetraplegia)?
- Is there resting tremor or jerking of any limbs?

Higher mental function and conscious level

Higher mental function

Many trainees find this difficult to assess. It is best to examine using a systematic approach, as described below. If some parts cannot be examined due to dysphasia, other cognitive deficits or reduced conscious level, record this and move on.

Examination of higher mental function should be considered as examination of different parts of the brain itself. For example, Broca's aphasia would indicate damage to the dominant frontal lobe.

Domains which should be assessed include:

- Conscious level
- Speech: dysarthria or dysphonia or dysphasia
- Orientation (time, place, and person)
- Memory
- Neglect
- Ability to think and calculate
- Ability to mime simple tasks
- Ability to read, write, and copy drawn shapes.

Conscious level

This should be assessed using the Glasgow Coma Score (GCS). This gives some indication of the size of stroke and has some predictive value regarding the long-term outcome. Unconscious patients have a much worse prognosis.

Glasgow Coma Score (see Table 5.1)

- This scale is widely used to assess, and monitor, conscious level
- It is scored between 3 and 15, 3 being the worst, and 15 being the best
- It contains three domains: best eye response, best verbal response and best motor response
- It is better to think about the composition of the GCS rather than just a number
- Remember all dysphasic patients will have a reduced GCS but may not be drowsy.

Orientation

Test this by asking the current time, current place, and if the patient can identify an appropriate person (e.g. doctor or nurse). Stroke patients are seldom confused without also being dysphasic. Ensure they are not merely dysphasic and not confused (see 📖 Speech and language, p. 120).

Table 5.1 Glasgow Coma Score

Best eye response (maximum 4 points)	
No eye opening	1
Eye opening to pain	2
Eye opening to verbal command	3
Eyes open spontaneously	4
Best verbal response (maximum 5 points)	
No verbal response	1
Incomprehensible sounds	2
Inappropriate words	3
Confused	4
Orientated	5
Best motor response (maximum 6 points)	
No motor response	1
Extension to pain	2
Flexion to pain	3
Withdrawal from pain	4
Localizing pain	5
Obeys commands	6

From Teasdale G, Jennett B (1974) *Lancet*, **ii**, 81–3.

Speech and language

Listening carefully to spontaneous speech during history-taking may already have identified a speech problem. Specific questions during the examination will then allow the nature of the speech problem to be fully determined.

Speech problems can be divided into:
- Dysarthria
- Dysphonia
- Dysphasia.

Dysarthria

- This describes slurred speech
- The commonest cause of this is weakness of the face, and a facial palsy may be apparent
- Patients can be very difficult to understand but usually one can discern that their words are appropriate but slurred
- They will be able to use 'yes' and 'no' correctly and consistently—either verbally or by head nods/shakes or gesture
- With experience, one can distinguish:
  - Lower motor neuron (bulbar) dysarthria with air escape through nose
  - Upper motor neuron, pseudobulbar, spastic dysarthria; the patient sounds as though they are speaking with a boiled sweet in their mouth
  - Cerebellar dysarthria has a characteristic 'Mon-o-syl-lab-ic' quality
  - Parkinsonian, extrapyramidal dysarthria: quiet, monotonous, and slow.

Dysphonia

- A problem with sound production
- Speech articulation is normal, as is the content but the sound is abnormal (e.g. bovine cough)
- May be caused by vocal cord paralysis.

Dysphasia

- This is a problem with language
- Examination for dysphasia includes testing spontaneous speech, naming, and repetition. Also remember to test comprehension, reading, and writing
- Dysphasia is normally split into expressive or receptive problems
- Usually in stroke, both coexist. Where there is no verbal output and no understanding of language, the condition is termed global aphasia.

Receptive dysphasia

- Caused by a lesion in the dominant temporal lobe affecting Wernicke's area, superior temporal gyrus posterior to the Sylvian fissure
- To test a receptive dysphasia, start by testing comprehension
- Ask the patient to perform a single stage command such as touch their nose or put a hand on their head, and then to do more complex tasks such as ordering objects on the bedside table

- Patients with a severe receptive dysphasia tend to be fluent in their speech but use wrong words. Sometimes this can manifest as real words used in the wrong context, or made up words (neologisms) or just plain gibberish
- If the patient is truly receptively dysphasic, they will be distant and unable to communicate either verbally or by writing or by using behavioural cues (e.g. pointing to the mouth to indicate hunger).

Expressive dysphasia

- Caused by lesion in the dominant dorsal frontal lobe affecting Broca's area
- An impairment of the speech production or the ability to 'think of words'
- Comprehension is better and in pure forms or as patients understand that what they are saying is wrong, they frequently become frustrated
- Communication with these patients can be improved by tailoring the consultation to simple 'yes' and 'no' questions and by using cues and gestures
- If receptive abilities are preserved, there is greater capacity for recovery
- Nominal dysphasia is a subtype of expressive dysphasia. It is the inability to identify names of objects. This is most easily tested by asking the subject to name different parts of a watch or pen or object by the bedside.

Conduction dysphasia

- Caused by subcortical lesion of the arcuate fasciculus which joins Broca's and Wernicke's areas. Speech is fluent and comprehension is intact but there is a severe inability to repeat words or phrases.

Transcortical aphasias

- Here patients have the ability to repeat words although they may not be able to speak otherwise
- The transcortical motor aphasia is characterized by reasonable understanding of speech but difficulty producing words
- The transcortical sensory aphasia is characterized by an ability to make words but a lack of understanding of their meaning
- Transcortical dysphasia indicates a subcortical lesion.

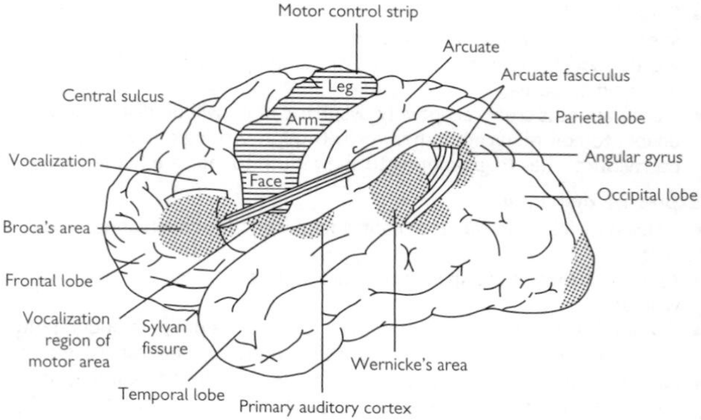

Fig. 5.1 Diagram of the speech areas.

Apraxia and agnosia

Apraxia

Here there is loss of ability to perform a previously learned or well practised motor task. For example, the loss of the ability to walk in spite of normal power, sensation, and coordination may be described as gait apraxia.

Types of apraxia to consider are:

- Gait apraxia where walking is very abnormal although the legs may move well enough in the bed
- Dressing apraxia where the patient's dressing routine becomes disordered
- Ideomotor apraxia where a patient cannot mime a response to your command but may do the movement spontaneously (e.g. 'scratch your nose')
- Ideational apraxia where the patient cannot plan a series of movements and cannot perform a three-part command
- Constructional apraxia where the patient cannot copy.

Apraxia normally indicates a dominant hemisphere parietal lesion. However, the inability to copy interlocking shapes indicates a deficit in the right parietal lobe.

In stroke it is unusual to have a pure apraxia. More commonly in a middle cerebral artery infarct, apraxia coexists with dysphasia and hemiparesis.

It is helpful to have a list of examination routines to use if you think the patient is apraxic. We ask the patient to:

- Make a fist
- Scratch their nose
- Imitate combing their hair
- Imitate using scissors to cut something
- Imitate how they would pay for their shopping
- Mimic the examiner interlocking the fingers of both hands
- Copy two interlocking shapes drawn by the examiner.

Agnosia

This is the failure to recognize objects in spite of normal working afferent input (e.g. normal sensation or vision).

Forms of agnosia to consider are:

- Visual agnosia—here patients can see an object and describe it but may not be able to say what it is
- Prosopagnosia—here one cannot recognize a famous face
- Anosagnosia—here a stroke patient may not realize they have had a stroke or that the affected limbs are weak. (This usually indicates a right parietal lesion causing left-sided anosagnosia)
- Astereognosis—here a patient will not be able to distinguish coins of differing value placed in their hand. Sensation in the hand must be preserved and the hand must retain some dexterity.

Location of lesion in agnosias

- Usually indicates a parietal lesion
- Visual agnosia may be attributed to a parieto-occipital lesion
- Anosagnosia is caused by a frontoparietal lesion. The patient may deny they have the resulting (obvious) hemiplegia
- A form of visual anosagnosia (Anton syndrome) is seen in patients with bilateral occipital infarction; these patients have bilateral cortical blindness but may deny that they are blind.

Neglect and inattention

Here patients fail to recognize or attend to stimuli on one side of the body.

- Neglect may indicate a lesion of either parietal lobe but is classically described with right-sided lesions
- It is important to detect as it has implications for rehabilitation, e.g. the patient may only attend to people and stimuli on one side. It is associated with worse outcome from rehabilitation.

Neglect may be:

- Sensory
- Visual
- Auditory.

It may be assessed by:

- Careful observation during history-taking and examination
  - You may notice the patient is not attending to one side
- Systematic examination
  - Stimuli are presented to both sides simultaneously and the patient fails to identify the stimulus on the neglecting side
  - First it is essential to determine that the patient can detect the stimulus when presented to the neglecting side alone, i.e. if they have a hemianopia, it is not possible to test for visual neglect
  - Therefore, to detect visual inattention move finger in one hemifield, then the other hemifield. If they can detect both, then move fingers in both simultaneously. If they have neglect they will not notice it in the neglecting field on bilateral simultaneous presentation
  - For sensory inattention, touch both hands in turn and then both simultaneously.

Memory and frontal tests

Memory

During normal examination a screen, including memory tests, is performed, such as the mini mental state examination (MMSE) or the abbreviated mental test score (aMTS). This is useful to identify gross deficits and dementia. If deficits are uncovered, more detailed testing is required, and this is often performed with the assistance of a neuropsychologist.

The simple schema suggested here for bedside testing relies on memory being subdivided into the following subtypes.

Episodic memory

This is the ability to learn new memories and recall them after minutes or days. It is split into:

- Anterograde memory, the ability to remember new things. Ask the patient to repeat the names of three objects (e.g. apple, pen, tie) and then recall them after 5 minutes
- Retrograde memory, the recall of past events
- It usually indicates damage to the temporal lobe and hippocampus, and may be profound if bilateral.

Working memory

Working memory is the temporary storage of information while manipulations are performed on the memorized information.

- This can be assessed by determining digit span backwards
- It is often caused by disruption of cortical–subcortical circuits due to subcortical stroke or leukoaraiosis.

Semantic memory

This is the recall of meanings and general knowledge. Test historical data (e.g. years of World War 2, name of the last prime minister).

Implicit memory

This is the recall of learned patterns (e.g. riding a bicycle).

Calculation

Ask the patient to subtract 7 serially from 100 (or 3 from 20 for an easier task). This tests concentration and memory as well as calculation.

Frontal tests

The frontal lobes are involved in planning and execution of tasks. Lesions of the frontal lobes may, therefore, produce problems with executive tasks. Cortical lesions often only result in these deficits if they are bilateral. Executive deficits are common in subcortical vascular disease, particularly bilateral lacunar stroke and/or leukoaraiosis caused by small-vessel disease. This is due to disruption of white matter pathways and disruption of frontocortical projections.

Frontal lobe lesions may be identified by the following.

Perseveration

- Patients may continue to repeat a past movement when asked to do something else. They have difficulty changing sequence. This can be demonstrated using Luria's hand sequence task. The patient is asked to tap with their fist, palm, and the side of their hand in sequence. Patients with frontal dysfunction have difficulty with this or when asked to change the sequence.

Utilisation behaviour

- Here, handing the patient an object may stimulate them to use it no matter how inappropriate. For example, patients may put on a second or even third (!) set of spectacles.

Emotional lability

- Inappropriate laughing and crying often in response to the most minor stimuli or even no stimulus at all.

Inaccurate cognitive estimates

- The patient loses the ability to reason and may guess wildly inaccurately. For example, one can ask:
  - How high is Nelson's column (185 feet, 56 metres)?
  - How fast does a race horse run (not 100 mph)?
  - How many elephants are there in England?

Clues from the history to executive dysfunction

- Loss of motivation; 'sits in front of the TV all day'
- Loss of ability to multitask
- Loss of planning ability.

In addition to these tests, there are frontal release signs indicating bilateral frontal damage or disconnection:

- Grasp reflex—stroke the patient's palm with the handle of the tendon hammer. The patient may grasp it and not be able to let go
- Rooting reflex—here stroking the side of the mouth will make the subject turn their head towards the stimulus. The subject may also start sucking
- Palmar mental reflex—here a contraction of the mentalis muscle of the chin is elicited following a brief scratch of the thenar side of the palm.

Examination of the cranial nerves

There are twelve cranial nerves.

Table 5.2 Cranial nerves

	Name	Function	Clinical
I	Olfactory	Sense of smell	Anosmia
II	Optic	Vision and direct pupillary light reflex	Blindness, loss of direct pupillary light reflex
III	Oculomotor	Medial rectus, superior rectus, inferior re ctus, inferior oblique levator palpebrae	Dilated, fixed pupil, ptosis, ipsilateral gaze fixed 'down and out'
IV	Trochlear	Superior oblique intorts eye and rotates down and out	Weakness of down gaze
V	Trigeminal	Ophthalmic, maxillary, mandibular branches	Loss of sensation in the face, eyes, nose, and mouth. Loss of corneal reflex. Deviation of the jaw to the ipsilateral side
VI	Abducent	Lateral rectus muscle	Exotropia
VII	Facial	Facial movement, taste, salivation, and lacrimation	Facial palsy, loss of blink, loss of taste from the anterior two-thirds of the tongue
VIII	Acoustic (Vestibulocochlear)	Balance and hearing	Vertigo, tinnitus, and deafness
IX	Glossopharyngeal	Taste, salivation, and swallowing	Loss of pharyngeal and gag reflex, loss of taste from posterior third of tongue
X	Vagus	Larynx and swallowing	Dysarthria
XI	Spinal accessory	Larynx and muscles in the neck	Difficulty in turning the neck; drooping shoulder
XII	Hypoglossal	Tongue movement	Ipsilateral tongue paralysis

Examination of the cranial nerves should encompass

- Visual acuity and visual fields
- Eye movements
- Pupillary responses, corneal reflex, and fundoscopy
- Facial movement (expression and biting)
- Facial sensation
- Hearing
- Palatal and tongue movement and gag reflex
- Shoulder shrug, head turning, and neck flexion

Cranial nerve 1 (olfactory)

- Unmyelinated fibres going from the olfactory epithelium in the nose, through the cribriform plate of the ethmoid bone to the olfactory bulb
- Seldom affected in stroke
- Damage causes loss of smell (sometimes manifesting in the patient's perception as loss of taste)
- Test by getting the patient to identify the smell of fruit.

Cranial nerve 2 (optic)

- Connects the retina to the superior colliculi and lateral geniculate nuclei
- There is a decussation at the optic chiasm
- The lateral fibres continue on the ipsilateral side
- The nasal fibres decussate to the opposite side
- Proximal to the decussation, damage results in blindness in one eye
- Distal to the decussation and in the ensuing optic radiation which terminates in the occipital cortex, damage results in loss of information for the right or left visual field and hence hemianopia
- The pupillary light reflex fibres bypass the geniculate body and go to the pretectal area and the parasympathetic part of the third nerve nucleus: the arc for the consensual pupillary reflex.

The examination of the optic nerve includes:

1. Acuity, using the Snellen chart
2. Visual fields to confrontation (do each eye separately)
3. Colour, with an Ishihara chart (sensitive to optic neuropathy or demyelination)
4. Fundoscopy (vessel changes, retinopathy, emboli)
5. Pupil examination—shine a bright torchlight into each eye separately. Look for the response to direct light and then the consensual response to light directed into the contralateral eye. Next ask the patient to follow your finger as it is moved back and forth. Observe the pupil constrict as the finger nears the patient's nose and the pupil dilate as it is moved away again.

- Sympathetic dysfunction produces Horner's syndrome where the pupil is small but reacts to light. This is accompanied by partial ptosis and is common in carotid dissection
- Parasympathetic dysfunction produces a large and poorly reacting pupil

- Damage to the ciliary ganglion or short ciliary nerves produces a tonic pupil where the pupil reacts very slowly to light and then may remain contracted. The response to accommodation is rapid
- Marcus–Gunn pupil: this is demonstrated by the swinging flashlight test. The abnormal pupil appears to dilate (paradoxically) when the light is switched back to the abnormal eye. It is seen in a relative afferent pupillary defect.

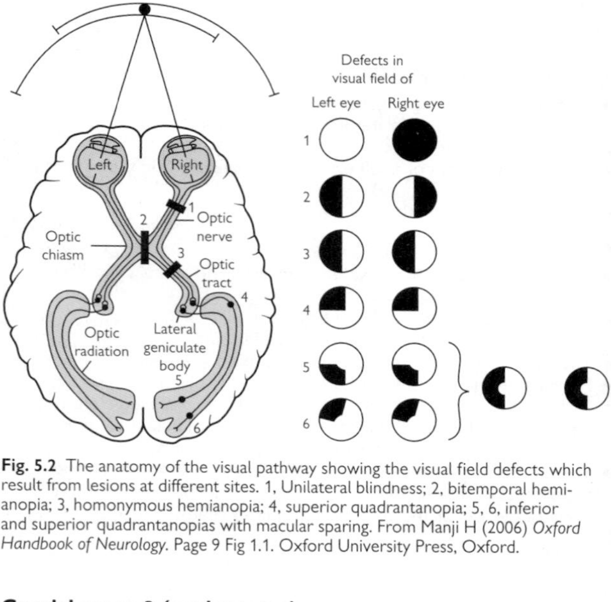

Fig. 5.2 The anatomy of the visual pathway showing the visual field defects which result from lesions at different sites. 1, Unilateral blindness; 2, bitemporal hemianopia; 3, homonymous hemianopia; 4, superior quadrantanopia; 5, 6, inferior and superior quadrantanopias with macular sparing. From Manji H (2006) *Oxford Handbook of Neurology*. Page 9 Fig 1.1. Oxford University Press, Oxford.

Cranial nerve 3 (oculomotor)

This comes from its nucleus in the midbrain. It supplies:

- The pupil constrictors (damage causes a dilated pupil)
- Levator palpebrae superioris (damage causes ptosis)
- Superior, inferior, and medial rectus and inferior oblique (damage causes ophthalmoplegia).

In a complete palsy, the eye will often be in a down and out position. Damage to the nerve or its nucleus causes diplopia in more than one direction of gaze. Also, as the medial rectus is involved, adduction of the eye is difficult.

Cranial nerve 4 (trochlear)

This comes from the midbrain and runs over the trochlea pulley. It controls superior oblique and tips the eye down and in. It enables you to look at the end of your nose.

- Lesions result in the eye drifting out
- If the right superior oblique is affected, the diplopia is worse when the eye tries to look to the left or the head is tilted to the right
- Often, if asked to look down, the patient notes diplopia with two images, one above the other. If the two images are horizontal, they appear angulated, like an arrow head and it points towards the bad side
- If the patient's head is tilted toward the side of a superior oblique palsy, the separation of the images increases (Bielschowsky sign).

Cranial nerve 5 (trigeminal)

This nerve has a long nucleus. The nucleus lies in the midbrain and pons with part of it reaching down to the cervical region (the spinal tract of the trigeminal nerve). It provides sensation from the face and the muscles of mastication. There are three divisions of the trigeminal nerve:

- Ophthalmic (V1)—damage results in sensory loss over the forehead
- Maxillary (V2)—damage results in loss of sensation over the cheek
- Mandibular (V3)—damage results in loss of sensation in the jaw back towards the ear.

In stroke, if complete paralysis of the trigeminal nerve occurs, this results in sensory loss over the ipsilateral face and weakness of the muscles of mastication. Attempted opening of the mouth results in deviation of the jaw to the paralysed side.

Cranial nerve 6 (abducens)

The nucleus of the nerve is located in the paramedian pontine region in the floor of the fourth ventricle. It innervates the lateral rectus which abducts the eye.

- Damage results in failure of abduction of the eye and diplopia on lateral gaze
- Abducens nerve palsy may result from raised intracranial pressure and pressure on the nerve.

Cranial nerve 7 (facial)

The nucleus of the nerve lies in the floor of the fourth ventricle (facial colliculus).

- The fibres wind around the nucleus of the sixth nerve
- The facial nerve exits the cranial cavity through the stylomastoid foramen
- It sends branches to the muscles that control facial expression
- It also innervates a small strip of skin at the back of the pinna and around the external auditory canal
- The nervus intermedius conducts taste sensation from the anterior two-thirds of the tongue
- It also supplies autonomic innervation to the salivary and lacrimal glands

- Lower motor neuron lesions occur in Bell's palsy
- Upper motor neuron lesions occur in stroke.

These are sometimes confused, resulting in Bell's palsy being diagnosed as stroke. They can usually easily be differentiated:

- A lower motor neuron facial palsy paralyses the whole side of the face
- In an upper motor neuron lesion the forehead is spared.

Isolated facial palsies are not uncommon in stroke. Exceptionally, a brainstem stroke affecting the facial nerve can cause a lower motor neuron facial palsy but this is very rare.

Other tricks to help the differentiation are:

- If the lesion is proximal to the nerve to the stapedius, hyperacusis, loss of taste in the anterior two-thirds of the tongue, loss of lacrimation, and facial weakness occur
- If the lesion is distal to the nerve to the stapedius but before the chorda tympani, loss of taste in the anterior two-thirds of the tongue and facial weakness occur
- If the lesion is distal to the nerve to the chorda tympani, facial weakness occurs.

Cranial nerve 8 (vestibulocochlear)

This arrives in the brainstem at the pontomedullary junction. It serves hearing and vestibular function.

Hearing

- Tested by whispering numbers into one of the patient's ears while covering the other ear and asking the patient to repeat those numbers heard
- Alternatively, hold a tuning fork close to each ear and ask the patient to say when they cannot hear it any longer. If you can still hear it but they cannot, then there is a problem
- If hearing loss is identified, then one has to distinguish conductive loss from sensorineural loss. There are two common tests used:
  - **Rinne's test**—a vibrating tuning fork is placed at the opening of the ear canal and then on the mastoid bone. It is normally louder when heard at the mouth of the ear canal. If there is a conductive problem (such as damage to the ossicles), sound is better heard when the tuning fork is placed on the mastoid bone
  - **Weber's test**—the tuning fork is placed on the forehead in the midline. Normally sound is heard equally in the centre. In conductive hearing loss, sound is better heard in the 'bad' ear. If the patient is deaf in one ear, it will be heard in the good ear.

Therefore, to test hearing quickly:

1. Can you hear this tuning fork?
2. Which side is louder? (Weber's test)
3. Is it louder in front or behind the ear? (Rinne's test).

Vestibular function

The vestibular nerve links the utricle and saccule (linear acceleration) and the cristae in the ampullae of the semicircular canals (angular acceleration) with the vestibular nucleus. This is a complex nucleus. The superior, lateral, medial, and inferior nuclei project to the:

- Pontine gaze centre through the medial longitudinal fasciculus
- Cervical and upper thoracic levels of the spinal cord through the medial vestibulospinal tract
- Lumbosacral regions of the ipsilateral spinal cord through the lateral vestibulospinal tract
- Ipsilateral flocculonodular lobe, uvula, and fastigial nucleus of the cerebellum through the vestibulocerebellar tract.

(Hallpike) Bárány test

Here the patient reclines from the sitting position with the head turned to one side and hanging over the end of the bed. If positive, the patient experiences nystagmus after a latent period. The nystagmus increases to a crescendo and then dissipates. The test is repeated on the other side. A positive test shows an abnormality in the peripheral vestibular function. It is particularly useful in detecting benign positional vertigo, which is commonly mistaken for TIA.

Cranial nerve 9 (glossopharyngeal)

The nucleus lies in the medulla closely apposed to the nuclei of cranial nerves 10 and 11 (nucleus ambiguous).

- It provides sensory innervation of the posterior third of the tongue and the pharynx
- The motor side supplies the pharyngeal muscles
- Glossopharyngeal nerve lesions cause loss of taste and sensation in the posterior third of the tongue.

Cranial nerve 10 (vagus)

This nerve has a long course.

- It supplies the pharyngeal muscles and the larynx
- It innervates smooth muscle in the trachea, bronchi, oesophagus, and gastrointestinal tract
- Stretch afferents from the aortic arch and carotid sinus travel in the nerve of Herring to join the glossopharyngeal nerve, terminating in the nucleus ambiguous, and thence the dorsal nucleus of the vagus, resulting in neural control of blood pressure.

It is tested by testing pharyngeal and palatal sensation with an orange stick:

- The gag reflex occurs when the posterior wall of the pharynx is touched. The response of retraction of the tongue and elevation of the palate is lost if nerves 9 and 10 are damaged
- You should touch either the right or left side of the palate. If only one side is affected, the good side contracts and pulls the uvula over
- In the palatal reflex, touching the soft palate will result in elevation of the soft palate on that side.

Cranial nerve 11 (spinal accessory)

- The cranial part of the nerve stems from the nucleus ambiguous and joins the vagus nerve to form the recurrent laryngeal nerve which innervates the larynx
- The spinal portion of the nerve arises from motor nuclei in the upper five cervical segments, enters the skull through the foramen magnum, and exits through the jugular foramen:
  - It supplies sternocleidomastoid and trapezius. Remember, the sternocleidomastoid pushes the face towards the other side
  - Therefore, weakness of head turning to the left is due to paralysis of the right sternocleidomastoid.

Cranial nerve 12 (hypoglossal)

- This nucleus lies in the lower medulla
- The nerve exits the skull through the hypoglossal canal
- It supplies the muscles of the tongue
- Ask the patient to protrude their tongue. Deviation to one side indicates paralysis on the same side.

Eponymous cranial nerve syndrome details

The important thing is to localize the lesion and determine the arterial territory affected rather than identify rare eponymous syndromes. A number of syndromes were described before the advent of the ability to localize brainstem infarcts accurately with MRI. We list them in Table 5.3 for those interested.

Table 5.3 Eponymous cranial nerve syndromes

Weber	Oculomotor palsy and contralateral hemiplegia from corticospinal tract damage
Claude	Oculomotor palsy with contralateral cerebellar ataxia and tremor
Benedikt	Oculomotor palsy with contralateral cerebellar ataxia, tremor, and hemiplegia from corticospinal tract damage
Nothnagel	Ocular palsies, paralysis of gaze, and cerebellar ataxia. This is at the level of the superior cerebellar peduncles
Parinaud	Supranuclear paralysis of upward gaze and accommodation with fixed pupils
Millard–Gubler and Raymond–Foville	This is at the level of the facial nerve (and abducens). There is a facial palsy and contralateral hemiplegia with a gaze palsy to the side of the lesion sometimes
Avellis	Paralysis of soft palate and vocal cord and contralateral hemianaesthesia with a Horner's syndrome. It is at the level of the spinothalamic tracts
Jackson	Tongue paralysis with contralateral hemiplegia
Wallenberg	This affects the lateral medulla at the level of nerves 9, 10, and 11, and spinal 5. Ipsilateral 5, 9, 10, and 11 palsies, Horner's syndrome, cerebellar ataxia. Contralateral loss of pain and temperature

Peripheral nervous system examination

The scheme for testing the peripheral nerves is as follows:
- Inspection
- Tone
- Power
- Sensation
- Reflexes and plantar responses.
- Coordination
- Gait.

Think as you go along how the signs will help localize the lesion.

Peripheral nervous system examination—inspection

Involuntary movements

These include:
- Seizures—always stop and look for evidence of seizures. They may manifest as subtle chewing movements or blinking or jerking of the arms
- Fasciculations are random muscle twitches seen under the skin. They may indicate serious neuromuscular disease such as motor neuron disease
- Myoclonus is a very brief muscle jerk. It may be focal or generalized
- Dystonia is abnormal, prolonged muscle contraction where part of the body adopts an abnormal posture
- Hemiballismus is a violent flinging movement of one side of the body. It is associated with lesions of the subthalamic nucleus
- Chorea comprises short movements that flit from different parts of the body. Often the patient looks fidgety
- Asterixis is where there are brief, jerky downward movements of the outstretched, pronated, dorsiflexed hands when the eyes are closed. It usually signifies a metabolic encephalopathy.

Muscle bulk

In a stroke patient, muscle bulk will usually be normal. Therefore, careful examination for wasting or fasciculation will pay dividends. Wasting suggests a lower motor neuron problem or a chronic upper motor neuron problem with disuse atrophy. There should be a system of inspection, e.g. start at the top and work down. Look at the temples; look at the tongue; look for the pattern of wasting. Wasting can be:
- Unilateral
- Symmetrical
- Proximal
- Distal wasting affecting the small muscles of the hands.

Pronator drift

Pronator drift is a very good way of bringing out subtle pyramidal abnormalities. Ask the patient to hold their arms outstretched in front of them with the palms facing upwards. Look for any overshoot on one side that may indicate a cerebellar lesion. The patient should hold the position for at least 30 seconds and a drift of one side down and into pronation may be observed. If present, follow up with examination of the limb for evidence of weakness which may be slight and otherwise overlooked.

Peripheral nervous system examination—tone

Muscle tone is the steady state of partial muscle contraction. It is assessed by passive movement.

- Hypotonia is defined as decreased tone (lower motor neuron lesions, early acute stroke and spinal shock)
- Hypertonia may manifest as spasticity or rigidity
  - Spasticity with the clasp-knife phenomenon
  - Rigidity with increased tone associated with extrapyramidal lesions; it may result in a cogwheel (stepwise) or lead-pipe (uniform) resistance to passive movement
  - Gegenhalten where resistance increases in flexion and extension (commonly seen in advanced dementia).

Peripheral nervous system examination—power

The MRC grading scale is simple and useful to describe weakness severity. Category 4 is a large category, from mild weakness to disabling weakness. It is sometimes subdivided into 4– and 4+.

0. No movement
1. Flickers of movement
2. Weak but can move with gravity eliminated
3. Weak but can move against gravity
4. Weak but can move against resistance
5. Full strength.

The pattern of weakness following stroke is often in a pyramidal distribution: power in the arm muscle flexors is greater than in the extensors; the reverse is true in the legs. In mild stroke, weakness may only be manifest in finger abduction and hip flexion.

Peripheral nervous system examination—sensation

This comprises light touch, pin-prick, joint position sense, and vibration and astereognosis.

- Look for a hemisensory loss. This is the commonest and is caused by a hemispheric lesion
- Look for crossed signs. This is seen in a brainstem stroke
- If the patient is diabetic, there will usually be a stocking neuropathy
- Always think about cord compression.

If the signs seem to stop at the neck you *must* look for a sensory level and you *must* go all the way up to the head. The common mistake is only to look for a sensory level on the chest and abdomen and forget to go up the neck.

Peripheral nervous system examination—reflexes

Primitive reflexes

These include the glabellar tap, rooting, snout, sucking, and palmomental reflexes. They are termed frontal release signs and are seen in cases of dementia.

Jaw jerk

This is elicited by placing the examiner's index finger on the patient's lower jaw and then striking it with the reflex hammer. An exaggerated reflex indicates the presence of a supra-pontine lesion. When the rest of the examination findings are normal, it may indicate physiological hyperreflexia.

Superficial reflexes

The most important superficial reflex is the plantar reflex. This may be elicited by stroking the lateral aspect of the sole with a sharp object. The normal response is plantar flexion of the big toe. Dorsiflexion of the big toe and fanning of the other toes suggests an upper motor neuron lesion.

Deep tendon reflexes

These are monosynaptic spinal segmental reflexes. When present, the cutaneous input, motor output, and descending cortical control must be intact. You are looking for asymmetry of the sides.

- Biceps—musculocutaneous nerve C5, 6
- Brachioradialis—radial nerve C6
- Triceps—radial nerve C7
- Knee jerk—femoral nerve L2–4
- Ankle jerk—tibial nerve S4.

Important points to remember

- After stroke (resulting in an upper motor neuron lesion), reflexes are increased. However, in the acute phase they may not be increased
- Determining physiologically increased reflexes from pathologically increased reflexes can be difficult. They are pathological if:
  - There is asymmetry
  - There is also sustained clonus
  - Plantar responses are extensor.

Anatomical basis of the different reflexes

Reflex	Afferent	Centre	Efferent
Corneal	Trigeminal (CN5)	Pons	Facial (CN7)
Pharyngeal	Glossopharyngeal (CN9)	Medulla	Vagus
Abdominal (upper)	T7, 8, 9, 10	T7, 8, 9, 10	T7, 8, 9, 10
Abdominal (lower)	T10, 11, 12	T10, 11, 12	T10, 11, 12
Cremasteric	Femoral	L1	Genitofemoral
Plantar	Tibial	S1, 2	Tibial
Anal	Pudendal	S4, 5	Pudendal
Deep reflexes			
Jaw	Trigeminal	Pons	Trigeminal
Biceps	Musculocutaneous	C5, 6	Musculocutaneous
Triceps	Radial	C6, 7	Radial
Supinator	Radial	C6, 7, 8	Median
Patellar	Femoral	L2, 3, 4	Femoral
Achilles	Tibial	S1, 2	Tibial
Visceral			
Light	Optic	Midbrain	Oculomotor
Carotid sinus	Glossopharyngeal	Medulla	Vagus

Coordination and gait

Coordination

Look for both lateralizing cerebellar signs (indicating damage to one side of the cerebellum or its brainstem connections) and truncal ataxia.

Lateralizing cerebellar signs:

- Tapping the outstretched arms while the eyes are closed may lead to rebound of the affected arm
- Patients may not be able to match the position of one arm in space using the other, a sign termed dysmetria
- Finger–nose test—ask the patient to point to the nose and then to your finger. Make sure they have to stretch out their arm to reach your finger. Intention tremor and past pointing indicates a cerebellar lesion
- Heel–shin test—ask the patient to place their heel on their knee and slide it down the shin
- Remember if a limb is weak that it is very difficult to test coordination
- Ataxia and mild hemiparesis in the same side suggest the ataxic hemiparesis lacunar syndrome. This is caused by a small infarct in the internal capsule, the pons, or in between.

Truncal ataxia

This may be evident on walking but more subtle deficits can be detected by testing heel-to-toe tandem gait. Ask the patient to walk with one foot directly in front of the other.

If the patient cannot walk, sit them up in bed and see if they can maintain balance when pushed gently to one side.

Gait

It is important to look at gait if at all possible. There are several gaits to identify.

Hemiparetic gait

- The shoulder is adducted, the elbow flexed, and the forearm pronated with the wrist and fingers flexed. In the leg, the knee is extended and then plantar-flexed. To walk, the patient circumducts the affected leg.

Ataxic gait

- The patient spreads their legs to widen the base of support and compensate for the lack of balance. This is a wide-based gait. If you are not sure, ask the patient to walk heel-to-toe (tandem gait) and this should magnify the ataxia. Subtle ataxia may be missed unless the patient is assessed (if possible) while seated, standing, and walking.

Shuffling gait

- The patient shuffles, taking small steps. This is seen in Parkinson's disease where the patient's step may become faster and faster (festinant) and in subcortical cerebrovascular small-vessel disease where it is thought to be a type of gait apraxia ('marche a petit pas'). It is commonly associated with other aspects of dysexecutive function such as poor sequencing and planning, and is a cause of falls. To test if it is apraxia, ask the patient to mime walking or cycling while lying on the bed. They should be able to do this without problem.

High stepping

- This is caused by bilateral foot drop usually owing to severe peripheral neuropathy. This sort of gait can normally be heard.

Spastic gait

- Here the legs are very stiff and there is little bending of the knees when walking. If very bad, there is adductor spasm and the legs are pulled together as the patient walks. The knees may knock together or even cross (a scissoring gait).

Antalgic gait

- This is basically a limp caused by a unilateral painful leg. The patient puts most weight on the good leg.

Examination of the unconscious patient

Trainees often find this difficult, but if a systematic approach is taken, a useful assessment can be made.

- Remember to look for neck stiffness, essential in the unconscious patient
- Observe the patient's response to pain, produced by pressing just under the roof of the orbital cavity or on a patient's fingernail. The responses may be:
  - Decorticate posturing—adduction of the arms, flexion of the fore-arms, wrists, and fingers
  - Decerebrate posturing—adduction of the arms, extension and pro-nation of the forearms, and extension of the legs
- Pupil responses are tested as usual
- Visual fields may be tested by moving your fingers into the visual field suddenly. There may be a sudden closure of the eyelid to threat
- Look at the resting position of the eyes
  - This is particularly important in the drowsy or comatose patient
  - Deviation to one side often indicates a frontal lesion, ipsilateral to the side of eye deviation. (The eyes 'look towards' the sound limb)
  - A skew deviation indicates a pontine lesion
  - Absence of the 'doll's eye reflex' is an ominous sign of severe brainstem damage but Guillain–Barre syndrome or myasthenia gravis may mimic it
  - If a patient cannot follow the examiner's hand or other target, ask them to follow their own hand as you guide it back and forth to assess eye movement
  - Failure of gaze to one side indicates a lesion of the pontine gaze centre
- Extraocular muscles may be evaluated by inducing eye movements via reflexes
  - The doll's eye reflex, or oculocephalic reflex, is produced by moving the patient's head side to side or up and down
    - The eyes will normally remain stationary in spite of the head moving
    - The afferent arc consists of the vestibular apparatus and neck proprioception
    - The efferent part consists of cranial nerves 3, 4 and 6, and eye muscles
    - The two parts join in the pons and medulla
    - If this reflex is damaged, turning the head from side to side moves the eyes in the same manner
  - In caloric testing, cold water is infused into the patient's ear
    - The patient's eyes turn towards the ear of injection (the same effect as turning the patient's head away from the injection). An absent reflex indicates severe damage in the medulla or pons or nerves that control eye movements
- The corneal reflex tests the afferent trigeminal nerve pathway and the efferent facial nerve pathway
- The gag reflex tests nerves 9 and 10.

The motor system is assessed by testing for:

- Spasticity—it takes some practice to be able to elicit spasticity
  - The speed of the movement is important. For example, examine the forearm and arm around the elbow joint. Extending the flexed forearm at moderate speed will normally result in a 'catch' as the tone suddenly seems to increase
  - Continued traction on the forearm will result in an equally sudden 'give' in the resistance: the clasp knife phenomenon
  - If the manoeuvre is too slow, the 'catch' will be missed. Too fast and the limb will appear rigid. This clasp knife phenomenon is best seen in arm flexors and leg extensors
  - Withdrawal responses to pain may be asymmetric, indicating a hemiparesis
- Reflexes may be increased (but early on may be reduced)
- Plantar responses may be extensor.

Criteria for 'brainstem death' are discussed in 📖 Chapter 17.

Examination of swallowing

This must be performed in all patients. It is best to test the overall action of swallowing. Relying on the presence or absence of the gag reflex is very misleading. Many units have local swallowing protocols which should be applied. However, a simple test is to observe whether aspiration occurs when a patient sips water from a cup. The patient must be alert and able to sit up or be so positioned.

Swallowing is divided into four stages:

1. Oral preparatory stage—here food and liquid entering the mouth are retained in the mouth while moving from side to side and being chewed
2. Oral stage—here food and liquid move from the front to the back of the mouth
3. Pharyngeal stage—here food and liquid move through the throat into the oesophagus. This is the stage where the airway has to be protected from aspiration
4. Oesophageal stage—here food and liquid move through the oesophagus to the stomach.

To assess swallowing, the patient must be conscious and alert long enough to swallow. Then:

- Sit the patient upright in a comfortable position
- Give 5 ml water
- After each swallow, ask the patient to talk.
- Look out for signs of poor or unsafe swallowing.
- Coughing or choking
- Water pooling in mouth
- Absent swallow
- Reduced laryngeal elevation
- Evidence of respiratory distress
- Change in voice.

If the swallow looks unsafe, then ensure the patient is kept 'nil by mouth'.

An algorithm for ongoing management of an unsafe swallow is found on 🕮 p. 268.

General examination

A thorough general examination is essential and may identify possible aetiological factors for stroke as well as possible complications. Relevant abnomalities include the following.

Cardiovascular

- Blood pressure
- Arrhythmias, particularly atrial fibrillation
- Evidence of cardiac failure
- Valvular heart disease
- Peripheral sign of endocarditis
- Peripheral pulses/evidence of peripheral vascular disease
- Complications of diabetes in the feet.

Respiratory

- Pneumonia, especially following aspiration
- Pleural effusion or pleural rub.

Abdominal

- Organomegaly, especially liver (metastases)
- Enlarged bladder (urinary retention).

Skin

- Rashes, e.g. facial photosensitive rash of SLE
- Livedo reticularis
- Evidence of pressure sores over bony prominences.

Musculoskeletal

- Hypermobility or other evidence of collagen vascular disease, e.g. Ehlers–Danlos type IV associated with cervical dissection
- Inflammatory arthritis associated with a vasculitis
- Arthritis that may have functional consequences and hamper rehabilitation.

Further reading

Examination

Harrison MJH (1996). *Clinical Skills in Neurology*. Butterworth-Heinemann, Oxford.

Oommen KJ (2008). *Neurological History and Physical Examination*. eMedicine, available online at http://emedicine.medscope.com/article/1147993-overview.

Wasman SG (2009). *Clinical Neuroanatomy*, 26th edition. McGraw-Hill Medical, New York.

Chapter 6

Investigation of the stroke patient

Investigation of the stroke patient

Investigation of acute stroke patients can be categorized into five sections.

1. Emergency investigation of the patient
2. Investigation to confirm or refute the diagnosis of stroke
3. Investigation of the aetiology of stroke
4. Investigation of risk factors (see 📖 Chapters 1 and 10)
5. Anticipation of complications of stroke.

This chapter provides an overview of stroke investigation. 📖 Chapter 7 provides detail, particularly on imaging in stroke.

Emergency investigation of the patient

It is *impossible* to distinguish between infarction and haemorrhage on clinical grounds alone. Therefore, urgent brain imaging is essential.

Imaging

- A brain scan should be performed as soon as possible after admission
- Aspirin or other specific treatment is not normally given until the result of the admission scan is known.

Blood tests

- Full blood count
- Electrolytes (renal disease)
- Blood glucose
- Clotting screen (if haemorrhage is suspected).

Cardiac test

- ECG (myocardial infarction or atrial fibrillation).

Radiology tests

- Chest X-ray (heart failure or suspected pneumonia).

Other tests

- Sometimes a blood gas analysis is necessary.

Investigation to confirm or refute the diagnosis of stroke

Brain imaging with either CT or MRI is the key investigation here.

Computed tomography (CT)

CT scanning is usually most easily available.

- It is cheap
- Widely accessible
- Non-invasive
- It can reliably identify intracerebral haemorrhage early
- However, it may be difficult to identify early cerebral infarction
- Posterior fossa and brainstem lesions may not be visible
- It may not detect small infarcts, particularly lacunar infarcts
- It cannot differentiate between old infarcts and old intracerebral haemorrhage (once blood has been resolved and an area of infarction remains).

Magnetic resonance imaging (MRI)

MRI offers better resolution as well as a number of other advantages. A typical examination uses several sequences, each of which contribute different information.

- It is much better at visualizing the posterior fossa
- It is more sensitive to small infarcts, particularly lacunar infarcts
- The most useful sequence in acute stroke is diffusion-weighted imaging (DWI). This becomes positive within minutes or a couple of hours of stroke onset and the new stroke appears bright ('light bulb' sign on the DWI image). It therefore allows:
  - Early detection of ischaemia
  - Differentiation of old infarction from recent infarction; the latter appears as a bright region on DWI imaging for 2–3 weeks after stroke onset. This is particularly useful in a patient with an old stroke in whom you want to know if they have had a new stroke or merely an exacerbation of existing deficit, as for example can happen following a seizure
- Sometimes very small lesions in the brainstem may be missed, but over 95% of acute ischaemic infarcts can be competently and quickly diagnosed with this modality
- MRI with gradient echo is also sensitive to both new and old haemorrhage; the latter feature allows one to determine whether an old lesion was initially caused by infarction or haemorrhage. This can sometimes be impossible to differentiate using CT.

In many ways it makes more sense to use MRI first rather than CT as diffusion-weighted changes are so apparent that they make diagnosis relatively easy for the non-specialist. However, availability often means CT is the first line approach.

Brain imaging is covered in more detail in 📖 Chapter 7.

Investigation into the aetiology of stroke

The aetiology of stroke is:
- Ischaemic (80%), of which 60–80% is embolic
- Haemorrhagic (up to 20%).

In ischaemic stroke, it is important to look for a source of embolism or site of thrombosis. Emboli can arise anywhere in the arterial tree from the heart to the brain. Common sites are:
- The carotid artery at the bifurcation of internal and external carotid
- The vertebral artery, particularly at its origin
- The intracranial vessels, particularly in certain ethnic groups (e.g. Chinese, African-American)
- The heart
- The aortic arch.

Therefore potential embolic sources can be detected by:
- Imaging of the extracerebral vessels with duplex ultrasound, CTA or MRA
- Imaging of the intracerebral vessels with CTA or MRA
- Cardiac investigation
  - ECG
  - Echocardiography (transoesophageal echocardiography (TOE) also allows detection of aortic atheroma).

Imaging of the extracerebral and intracerebral arteries is covered in 📖 Chapter 7.

The aortic arch outside of cases of suspected aortic root dissection (see 📖 Chapter 11) is not normally routinely imaged, although there is research currently looking specifically at management of aortic arch atherosclerotic embolism.

A variety of blood tests and other tests may be required in stroke patients—these are listed in Table 6.1.

Table 6.1 A list of investigations in the stroke patient

	In all patients	Selected patients
All strokes	**Blood tests**	
	Full blood count (esp. platelet)	
	ESR	
	Urea and electrolytes	
	Glucose, HbA1c	
	Liver function tests	
	Thyroid function	
	Other tests	
	ECG	
	Brain CT or MRI	
	Chest X-ray	
	Urinalysis	
Cerebral infarction	**Blood tests**	
	Lipids	Sickle cell screen
		Thrombophilia, including anticardiolipin antibody
		Homocysteine and vitamin B12
		Drug screen (urine + blood)
		Syphilis serology
		HIV
		Autoantibody screen
		Blood cultures
		Genetic tests (e.g. CADASIL, Fabry)
	Other tests	**Other tests**
	Imaging of extracranial arteries	Echocardiography
		24-hour ECG
		Imaging of intracerebral arteries MRA/CTA
		Cerebral angiography
		Temporal artery biopsy
		CSF examination
Cerebral haemorrhage	**Blood tests**	**Blood tests**
	Clotting screen	Sickle cell screen
		Drug screen
		Other tests
		Imaging of intracerebral arteries MRA/CTA
		Cerebral angiography

Cardiac investigation

ECG

- 12-lead ECG should always be performed
- Left ventricular hypertrophy measured by voltage criteria can be a marker of hypertensive end-organ damage or a racial variant. An abnormal ECG may also indicate a source of cardiac embolism, e.g. persistent ST segment elevation may represent left ventricular aneurysm
- A 'baseline' ECG is helpful should complications arise after stroke; these include myocardial infarction or pulmonary embolus
- Occasionally, subarachnoid bleeding can induce ECG changes which mimic acute myocardial ischaemia
- It is helpful to be able to monitor the cardiac rhythm continuously for a few days after stroke, seeking atrial fibrillation or paroxysmal tachycardia or bradycardia.
- 24-hour ECG may identify paroxysmal atrial fibrillation
- An abnormal 12-lead ECG should generally be further investigated with echocardiography.

Echocardiography

This may identify a potential embolic source. Some units perform it in most patients while others argue that, while it may detect abnormalities relatively frequently, it does not often alter management (as supported by some case series). Therefore, they do not perform it routinely. If access is limited, we would recommend performing transthoracic echocardiography (TTE) in cases with:

- Cardiac abnormality on examination or ECG
- Ischaemic stroke aged under 65 years
- Strokes or cerebral infarcts on imaging in multiple territories. This suggests a cardiac or aortic arch embolic source
- A cerebral infarct that looks as if it may be embolic (e.g. a wedge-shaped cortical infarct or subcortical striatocapsular infarct) and no other obvious embolic source.

Transoesophageal echocardiography

- This has a greater sensitivity than TTE. In particular, it is better at looking for left atrial abnormalities, a PFO, vegetations in infective endocarditis, and aortic arch atheroma
- A specialized probe containing an ultrasound transducer at its tip is passed into the patient's oesophagus
- It does have disadvantages
  - The patient must fast
  - The technique requires a team of medical personnel and takes longer to perform
  - It is uncomfortable for the patient and usually requires sedation
  - There are some risks associated with the procedure: oesophageal perforation occurs in 1 in 10 000.

Investigations to anticipate complications

Complications after stroke include:

- Infections (pneumonia, urinary tract infection, cellulitis)
- Myocardial infarction or arrhythmia
- Electrolyte imbalance
- Re-feeding syndrome
- Deep vein thrombosis and pulmonary embolus
- Progressive swallowing disturbance over the week following a large cortical stroke.

Patients should be monitored with regular:

- Temperature
- Blood pressure
- Dipstick urine
- Full blood count
- Urea and electrolytes
- CRP
- Liver function tests (always check before starting statin therapy and remember to check again 6–12 weeks after to exclude significant transaminitis).

It may be helpful to perform a:

- Chest X-ray as a baseline investigation in a stroke patient who is likely to be hospitalized for a long time
- Videofluoroscopy or fibreoptic endoscopic examination of swallowing in anticipation of the patient needing a percutaneous endoscopic gastrostomy (PEG).

Chapter 7

Imaging in stroke

Introduction

Imaging plays a central role in diagnosis of stroke, planning treatment, and identification of the underlying pathophysiology.

Functions of imaging

Imaging in stroke has a number of major functions.

Diagnosis

- Identification of infarction
- Identification of haemorrhage
- Identification of structural stroke mimics.

Examination of the vasculature and vascular lesion leading to the stroke syndrome

- Detection of stenosis
- Identification of collateral supply
- Detection of aneurysms and other vascular malformations.

Planning treatment

- Selecting patients for thrombolysis

Imaging can also provide information on:

- Brain perfusion and haemodynamics
- Plaque and arterial wall morphology
- Circulating cerebral embolism.

Methods

Methods of imaging the brain include:

- Computed tomography (CT) techniques
- Magnetic resonance (MR) techniques
- Single photon emission computed tomography (SPECT)
- Positron emission tomography (PET).

The former two are the most widely used, the latter two have little applicability in normal clinical practice.

Methods of imaging the cerebral vessels include:

- Ultrasound
- CT angiography
- MR angiography
- Intra-arterial angiography.

Computed tomography (CT)

Brain CT scanning was first introduced in 1971 (first scan) at Atkinson Morley's Hospital in Wimbledon, UK by the radiologist Jamie Ambrose and the scientist Geoffrey Hounsfield who later went on to win the Nobel Prize for the development.

- It is the most widely available method of brain imaging
- The patient lies on a table
- A beam of X-rays revolves around the patient delimiting a slice through the subject (usually axial)
- The X-ray beam is attenuated by passing through the patient's tissues
- The exit beam is detected
- Computerized algorithms then reconstruct the image of the slice
- The slice thickness can be varied
- Changing the window level changes the contrast appearance, making structural identification easier (e.g. differentiating grey and white matter or bone).

Advantages of CT

- Easy to use
- Cheap
- Dysphasic or comatose patients can be imaged safely
- Safe in patients with metallic implants and not claustrophobic
- The quality of the pictures is usually good when looking at the cerebral hemispheres or the skull vault. Most things that are eventually identified on MR will have been visible on the initial CT scan
- Blood is well visualized very soon after haemorrhage onset.

Disadvantages of CT

- It may miss subtle features of brain pathology
- Artefacts produced in the posterior fossa make it poor for examination of the brainstem and cerebellum
- May miss small infarcts, particularly lacunar ones
- It can be difficult to tell whether an old stroke is due to previous haemorrhage or infarct
- Not as sensitive as MRI for hyperacute ischaemia
- Involves ionizing radiation—a routine CT scan exposes the patient to the equivalent of 10 months of background radiation (2 days for chest X-ray).

Modern CT scanners

- These acquire data much quicker and with higher resolution than earlier generations
- Spiral scanners—these draw the subject into the scanner as the beam rotates around the subject. This allows continuous spiral acquisition
- Modern scanners can investigate a large block of tissue (rather than a single slice at a time). These scanners can do blocks of 32 slices or 64 slices during a single set of acquisitions.

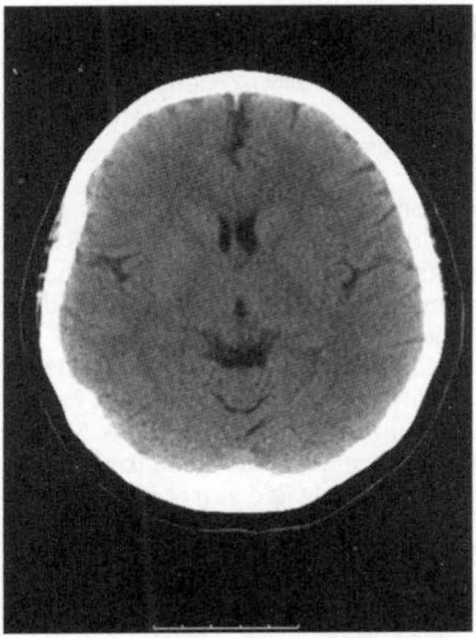

Fig. 7.1 CT scan of the brain. This is a normal section through the brain. The internal capsule and basal ganglia are clearly visible. © Anthony Pereira.

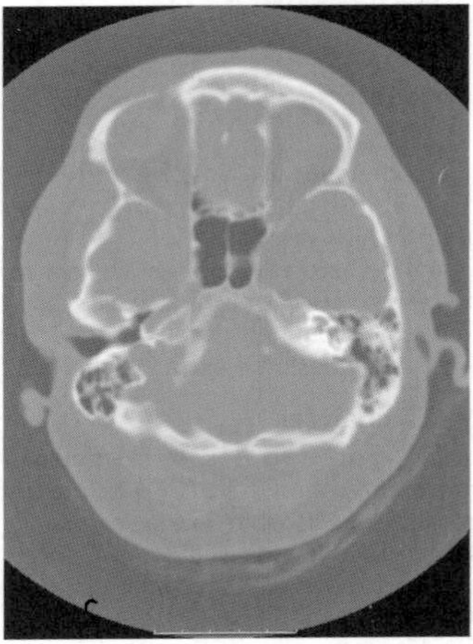

Fig. 7.2 This is a different slice through the brain with the CT windowing set to show the bones. This is used to seek fractures (e.g. after a fall and head injury). © Anthony Pereira.

CT in acute stroke

- CT is not very sensitive for early ischaemia (<6 hours)
- However, ischaemic changes are visible relatively early after stroke
  - Loss of the gray–white matter interface
  - Loss of sulci
  - Loss of the insular ribbon
- Early mass effect and areas of hypodensity suggest irreversible injury and identify patients at higher risk of post-thrombolysis haemorrhage
- Significant hypodensity on the baseline scan should prompt the physician to question the time of onset
- Hypodensity in an area greater than one-third of the MCA distribution is considered by many to be a contraindication for thrombolytics
- A dense MCA sign suggests a clot in the MCA. Similar appearances can be seen in other intracerebral vessels due to clot, although sometimes differentiating this from a calcified vessel can be difficult.

CT is very sensitive to acute blood which is visible soon after haemorrhage onset as high signal (white). One can see both:
- Intracerebral haemorrhage
- Subarachnoid haemorrhage.

CT may demonstrate other causes of the patient's symptoms:
- Neoplasm
- Epidural and subdural haemorrhage
- Aneurysm
- Abscess
- Arteriovenous malformation
- Hydrocephalus.

Extra information is sometimes available by the addition of intravenous contrast:
- This identifies areas of high vascularity
- Also identifies regions where the blood–brain barrier is leaky
- Contrast-enhanced scans also highlight all major intracranial vessels
- However, contrast is not routinely used in cross-sectional imaging in acute stroke as it usually adds little extra information (see Fig 7.3).

Images of early CT changes

When examining a CT, you should look for five findings:
- Look for evidence of thrombus in the MCA or other major intracerebral arteries (seen as white in the vessels)
- Look at the basal ganglia and internal capsule. Compare one side to the other. They have clearly been disrupted on the right in Fig. 7.3.
- Look at the insular ribbon and see if it is still intact
- Look at the grey white matter on the higher slices and see if it is lost.
- Look at the sulci and gyri and see if the sulci have been compressed on one side (by cerebral oedema).

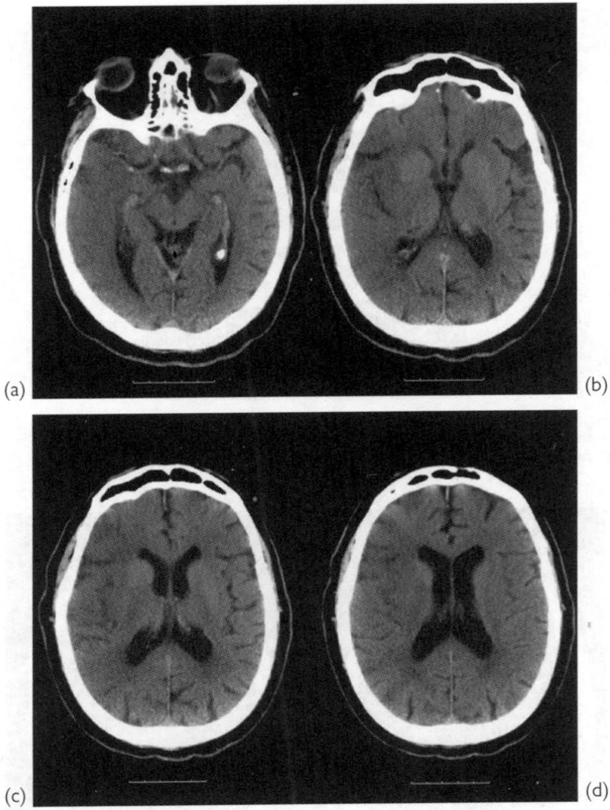

Fig. 7.3 Early CT appearances of a right middle cerebral artery infarct. Low density and loss of tissue definition is seen on all slices. There is loss of sulci and grey-white matter is not so easily distinguished.

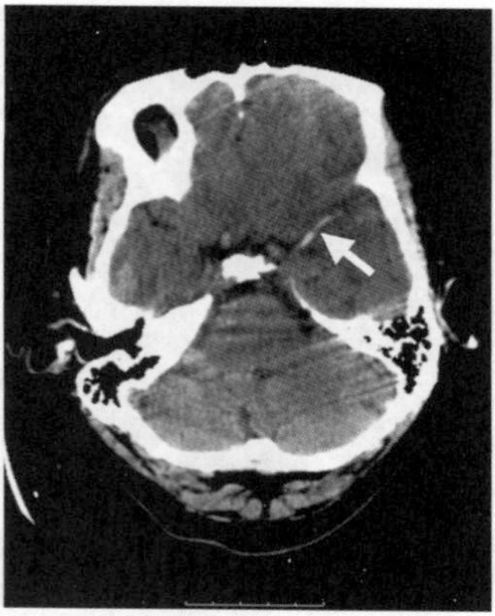

Fig. 7.4 The dense middle cerebral artery sign is seen on the left here. High signal representing thrombus can be seen in the left middle cerebral artery (arrowed). © Anthony Pereira.

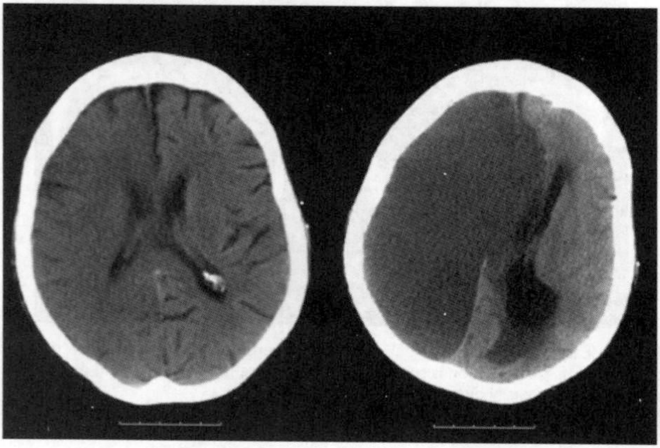

Fig. 7.5 Pair of CT images. The slice on the left shows subtle signs of an early large right carotid territory infarct. After 3 days, the infarct has swollen massively and is compressing the left hemisphere with midline shift and hydrocephalus. © Anthony Pereira.

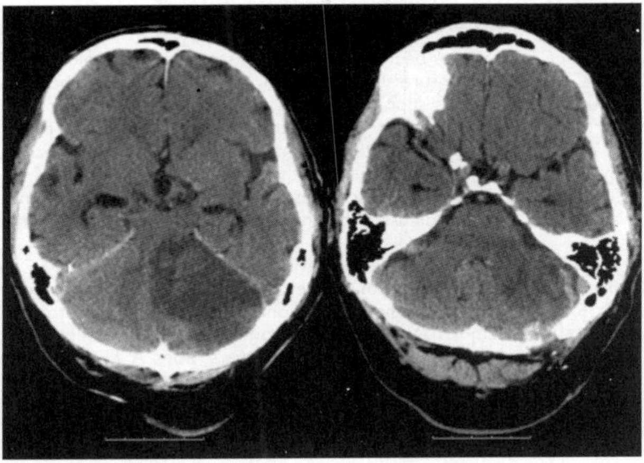

Fig. 7.6 Pair of images showing a left cerebellar hemisphere infarct. This swelled and caused mass effect and required neurosurgery. The break in the skull is visible on the left. © Anthony Pereira.

ASPECTS scale

The ASPECTS scale has been devised to help structure the evaluation of acute CT scans and ensure the clinician looks at all aspects of the scan, although it only covers supratentorial regions and is primarily designed for MCA infarction. The territory of the MCA is allotted 10 points (Fig. 7.7). One point is subtracted for an area of early ischaemic change, such as focal swelling, or parenchymal hypoattenuation, for each of the defined regions. A normal CT scan has an ASPECTS value of 10 points. A score of 0 indicates diffuse ischaemia throughout the territory of the MCA.

In the initial evaluation, baseline (on pre-thombolysis scans) ASPECTS score correlated inversely with stroke score on the NIH Stroke Scale ($r=0{\cdot}56$, $p<0{\cdot}001$) and predicted functional outcome and symptomatic intracerebral haemorrhage following thrombolysis ($p<0{\cdot}001$, $p=0{\cdot}012$, respectively). Agreement between observers for ASPECTS, with knowledge of the affected hemisphere, was good (kappa 0·71–0·89). It was suggested an ASPECTS score of 7 might separate a group with a much higher risk of post-thrombolysis haemorrhage.

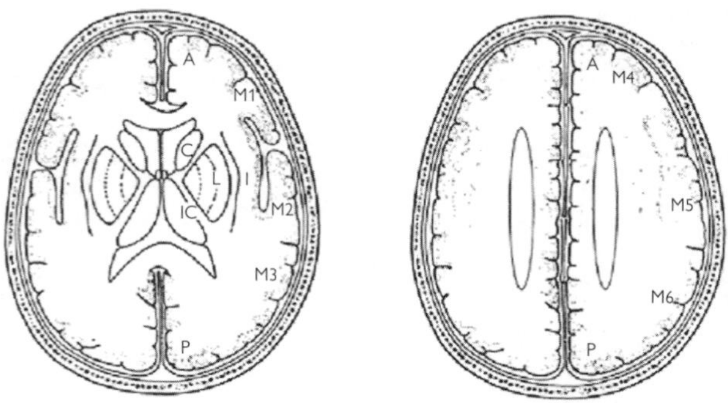

Fig. 7.7 The ASPECTS scale. A, anterior circulation; P, posterior circulation; C, caudate; L, lentiform; IC, internal capsule; I, insular ribbon; MCA, middle cerebral artery; M1, anterior MCA cortex; M2, MCA cortex lateral to insular ribbon; M3, posterior MCA cortex; M4, M5, and M6 are anterior, lateral, and posterior MCA territories immediately superior to M1, M2, and M3, rostral to basal ganglia. Subcortical structures are allotted 3 points (C, L, and IC), MCA cortex is allotted 7 points (insular cortex, M1, M2, M3, M4, M5, and M6). Reproduced from Barber PA, Demchuk AM, Zhang J, Buchan AM (2000) Validity and reliability of a quantitative computed tomography score in predicting outcome of hyperacute stroke before thrombolytic therapy. ASPECTS Study Group. Alberta Stroke Programme Early CT Score. *Lancet* **355**, 1670–4, with permission from Elsevier.

Practising reading acute stroke CT scans

There are a number of interactive websites where you can review CT images of acute stroke patients online. This is a useful way to gain experience in this area. Two can be found at www.dcn.ed.ac.uk/ist3/

Once on the website click either on the BASP CT Training Series or the ACCESS study.

Magnetic resonance (MRI)

- Nuclear magnetic resonance signals have been used to study physics and chemistry since the 1940s
- In the 1970s it became possible to localize the signal and generate images
- For clinical applications, the 'nuclear' has been dropped
- The terms 'magnetic resonance (MR)' and 'magnetic resonance imaging (MRI)' are preferred
- The technique produces very high quality images of brain parenchyma and individual structures. Small infarcts are well visualized
- In addition, different sequences can be tuned to identify very subtle brain pathology such as early brain ischaemia, and to look at brain function (e.g. fMRI).

Advantages of MRI

- Images are more detailed than CT
- Small infarcts are better detected
- Posterior fossa is better visualized
- Best technique for imaging the spinal cord
- Sensitive to acute ischaemia within minutes/hours of ischaemia onset (diffusion-weighted imaging)
- Can detect evidence of old haemorrhage (haemosiderin seen as black holes on gradient echo sequences—also called T2* imaging
- It can also provide information on brain biochemistry (spectroscopy), brain function (functional MRI, fMRI) and white matter pathways (diffusion tensor imaging, DTI).

Limitations of MRI

- Relatively expensive
- Not as widely available as CT
- Longer scanning times than CT, although echo planar MRI allows very rapid acquisition although with lower resolotution
- Contraindications (e.g. pacemakers, metal in the eyes)
- Some patients are too claustrophobic in the 'tunnel'. Open magnets can overcome this but are not widely available. They also often have a lower magnetic field strength and may produce less clear images.

Recent advances in MRI

- Higher strength of magnetic field (3.0 Tesla field strength); provides higher resolution and better signal to noise
- More sequences to examine different underlying pathologies
- Open MRI for patients who are claustrophobic or overweight
- Intraoperative MRI scanner

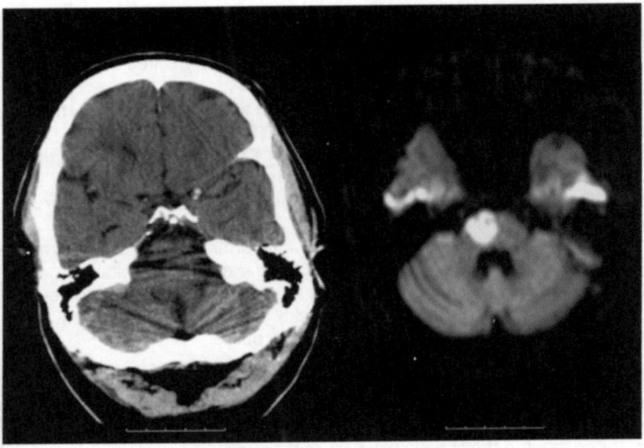

Fig. 7.8 A brainstem infarct on CT and MRI showing the much better sensitivity of MRI to lesions in the posterior fossa. The CT image on the left is very difficult to interpret. On the right is the DWI MR image which clearly shows the abnormal area of infarction. The symmetrical areas of high signal in the temporal lobes on MRI are due to artefact caused by nearby air cells in the bone. © Anthony Pereira.

Physics of MRI

- Atomic nuclei ^{1}H, ^{13}C, ^{19}F, and ^{31}P have a property called 'spin'
- The nucleus spins about its own axis
- Spinning creates a small magnetic field like a tiny bar magnet with its axis along the axis of rotation
- When an external magnetic field is applied (i.e. the MR scanner), the nuclei line up and spin at a given frequency
- When they are excited by a pulse of energy deliberately emitted from the MR scanner, two things happen:
  - They spin in a higher energy state and continue to do so until they give off that energy and return to their resting energy state
  - The energy pulse makes them all spin together in phase. However, they cannot maintain this and quickly spread out. They will still be in the high energy state but no longer in phase.

T1

- The time it takes for the nuclei spins to return from the high energy state to the resting energy state is the *T1 relaxation time*
- It depends on the actual structure of the brain
- Images based on this are called *T1-weighted images*
- T1 pictures tend to produce good anatomical definition of the structure of the brain and are often used to estimate brain volume.

T2

- The time it takes for the spins to dephase is the *T2 relaxation time*
- It is very short
- Spins in solids dephase fast but spins in liquids are much slower
- Images based on this are *T2-weighted images*
- Therefore, altered water content in tissues (e.g. brain oedema) is seen well
- T2-weighted images are good for looking at the pathological brain
- The scanner can be tuned to the spin frequency of different nuclei
- The main nucleus is ^{1}H (i.e. a proton)
- The commonest chemical containing this in the body is water
- Therefore, MR images often show the distribution of water molecules in different tissues in the body.

Commonly used MRI sequences

T1-weighted imaging

- Good for anatomical structure of normal tissue
- Used to measure whole brain volume or changes due to atrophy
- Sensitive to haemorrhage.

T2-weighted imaging

- Sensitive to oedema and increased water content
- Good for showing most pathology
- Small lesions around the ventricles may be missed.

Fluid-attenuated inversion recovery (FLAIR)

- Essentially a T2 image with an added inversion recovery sequence. This supresses signal from free water, i.e. in the ventricles and CSF. This improves contrast and visualization, particularly of white matter
- Lesions along the edges of brain and ventricles are more clearly seen.

Gradient echo imaging (T2*, pronounced 'T2 star')

- Sensitive to the presence of blood and blood products (i.e. haemorrhage) which are paramagnetic and degrades the image quality
- Haemorrhage appears as a large black 'hole' in the image
- Useful for looking at acute haemorrhage
- The most sensitive technique which can detect old haemorrhage—blood is degraded to haemosiderin which is deposited and results in areas of signal loss (black). This also enables microhaemorrhages to be detected—they are particularly seen in small-vessel disease and cerebral amyloid. Only larger lesions are seen on other sequences.

Diffusion-weighted imaging

- Very good for acute ischaemic stroke
- The infarct on DWI is bright
- The infarct on apparent diffusion coefficient (ADC) is dark
- ADC in ischaemic areas may be 50% lower than normal
- Changes in the ADC occur as early as 10 minutes after onset of ischaemia
- In old stroke the lesion will appear low signal on DWI—tissue breakdown results in increased diffusion.

Contrast can be added to MR sequences

- The contrast (gadolinium, a heavy metal) is paramagnetic
- It shortens the T1 signal and therefore appears bright
- It can be used to identify breakdown in the blood–brain barrier
- It is used to increase signal to noise for angiographic imaging (contrast-enhanced MRA).

Perfusion imaging

- This can be performed either using a contrast injection (exogenous contrast) or using 'endogenous contrast'
- Exogenous contrast perfusion uses a very rapid gadolinium injection and echo-planar imaging to acquire very frequent images over the next 2–3 minutes. This allows passage of the 'bolus' of contrast through the brain to be tracked and from this a perfusion map can be constructed. It is a good technique to detect perfusion deficits in acute stroke, and the signal changes seen are large. However, it is only semi-quantitative
- The following measures are commonly obtained—cerebral blood flow (CBF), cerebral blood volume (CBV), and mean transit time (MTT)
- Endogenous perfusion imaging creates 'contrast' in the tissue using a radiopulse. It is potentially quantitative but takes much longer to acquire and signal changes are much smaller. It is largely used as a research technique.

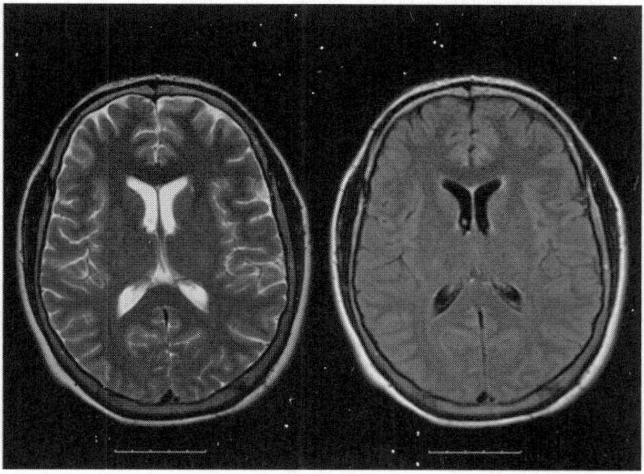

Fig. 7.9 T2 (left) and FLAIR (right) imaging. Both are good at detecting altered water content in brain tissue. In the FLAIR image the free water in the CSF and ventricles is suppressed. © Anthony Pereira.

Diffusion-weighted imaging (DWI)

This sequence is very useful in early diagnosis of ischaemic stroke, and in differentiating recent stroke from old stroke and other pathologies.

It is an essential sequence to include in MRI in any acute stroke patient.

Physics

- Water molecules in the tissue are in a continuous state of Brownian motion
- Therefore, the ^1H (protons) in water are also in continuous motion
- When the protons in a selected slice are excited by the scanner RF (radio frequency) pulse, some of them will diffuse out of the slice
- Restriction of diffusion results in molecules rephasing in a more coherent fashion and giving off a stronger signal, whereas free diffusion results in them becoming out of phase and a weaker signal
- This phenomenon is used in DWI
- If diffusion of water molecules is impaired (after acute ischaemia), more stay in the slice and the signal acquired is altered
- This is called restricted diffusion. The mathematical value calculated is the apparent diffusion coefficient (ADC) and it will be low because there is less diffusion. By convention, restricted diffusion is shown as dark as the ADC is low, whereas increased or free diffusion is shown bright as the ADC is high
- In clinical practice, a DWI image is often used for interpretation. For this the contrast is inverted so the dark areas of reduced ADC look bright—the light bulb sign of acute ischaemia.

DWI in acute stroke

- Restricted diffusion occurs rapidly (within an hour or two and can be in minutes) after stroke owing to cell swelling. This means DWI abnormalities are seen soon after stroke and it is the most sensitive technique to detect acute infarction
- The reduced diffusion remains for 1–3 weeks on average. As tissue breakdown occurs, diffusion increases. Therefore, an old infarct is characterized by increased diffusion (dark on a DWI image). This makes DWI very useful in:
  - Differentiating acute ischaemia from old infarcts—e.g. to determine if a new deficit is caused by a new stroke or a Todd's paresis (post-epileptic) in a patient with an old stroke
  - Differentiating acute ischaemia from non-stroke pathology, e.g. migraine, hysteria
- As well as the extent of diffusion, the directionality of diffusion can be determined using diffusion tensor imaging (DTI). This is enabled by acquiring the diffusion data in multiple planes. Because diffusion is greater along white matter tracts, rather than across them, this allows visualization of white matter tract anatomy. It is very sensitive to white matter tract damage, although is largely used as a research tool.

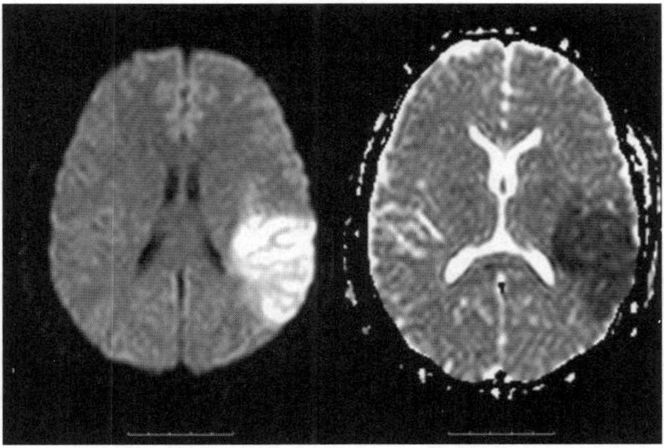

Fig. 7.10 DWI MRI in acute stroke. The left picture shows the DWI image of a slice through a left frontoparietal ischaemic infarct. It can be seen as high signal (white) on the DWI image. On the ADC map (right), the acute infarct is seen as a corresponding area of low signal. © Anthony Pereira.

Temporal profile of DWI in acute stroke

The mean diffusion of water molecules in the infarct changes over time. Fig. 7.11 shows how the ADC changes. Note that it is low for about 7–10 days and then increases.

There are a number of phases:

1. Initially restricted diffusion is seen—high signal on DWI
2. This DWI high signal persists for about 2 weeks
3. After this, diffusion increases as tissue breakdown occurs, allowing increased diffusion of water molecules—eventually the stroke appears dark on DWI. During the few days when the the ADC is around normal, the image of the infarct may appear normal. But this will not be the case on structural sequences, so it is important not to use DWI alone except in special circumstances.

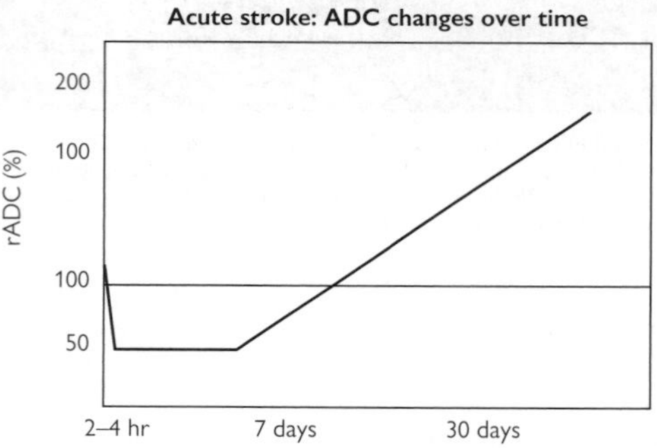

Fig. 7.11 ADC changes over time after acute ischaemic stroke. Remember that a reduction in ADC corresponds to an increase in signal on the DWI image.
© Hugh Markus.

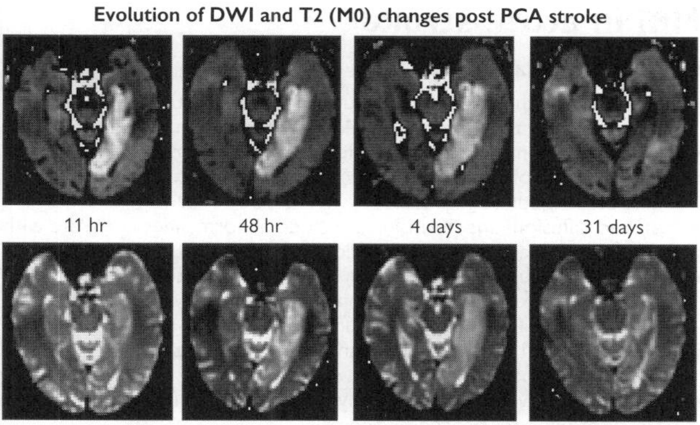

Fig. 7.12 DWI imaging of a posterior cerebral artery infarct at different time points after stroke. At 11 hours the infarct is clearly seen on DWI (top row) but is much less well seen on the T2 image (bottom row). By 48 hours it is visible on both DWI and T2. By 31 days the DWI image shows low signal (consistent with tissue breakdown and increased water diffusion). © Hugh Markus.

MRI in acute stroke

Very early (0–24 hours)

- DWI detects ischaemia within minutes of onset. Reduced water diffusion is detected as decreased ADC/increased signal on DWI
- Early perfusion imaging detects reductions of CBF and CBV and increased MTT of blood. CBV may rise in non-infarcted ischaemic areas whilst tissue is still salvageable
- Matched diffusion- and perfusion-weighted abnormalities correlate with the region of infarction and are indicative of permanent neuronal death
- Mismatched diffusion and perfusion abnormalities with the perfusion abnormality larger than the diffusion abnormality may be indicative of a region of reversible ischaemic penumbra
- At 2–4 hours, T1-weighted image shows subtle effacement of the sulci owing to cytotoxic oedema
- At 8 hours, T2-weighted image shows hyperintense signal caused by both cytotoxic and vasogenic oedema
- At 16–24 hours, T1-weighted image shows hypointense signal caused by both cytotoxic and vasogenic oedema
- Contrast-enhanced images show arterial enhancement followed by parenchymal enhancement. The arterial enhancement can be very early and is caused by slow blood flow; it typically disappears after 1 week
- Although conventional MRI sequences most often do not show evidence of stroke in the hyperacute phase, conventional MRI may show signs of intravascular thrombus such as absence of flow void on T2-weighted, and vascular hyperintensity on FLAIR, which can be an indication of patent vessels but altered flow.

MRI findings 1–7 days

- Oedema increases at 48–72 hours and MRI abnormality becomes more prominent and well demarcated on the T2 images
- The ischaemic area appears hypointense on T1-weighted and hyperintense on T2-weighted images
- The mass effect can be appreciated in this phase
- Reperfusion occurs. Sometimes haemorrhage (petechial or larger accumulations of frank haemorrhage) can be observed, typically 24–48 hours after the onset of the stroke.

MRI 7–21 days

- Mass effect becomes less marked
- The ischaemic area appears hypointense on T1-weighted and as a hyperintense area on T2-weighted images
- In contrast-enhanced images, the arterial enhancement usually improves but the parenchymal enhancement may persist
- DWI signal reduces in intensity, the infarct transiently becomes isointense and then increased diffusion is seen (low signal on DWI)
- T2 high signal lesions may normalize and not be visible before becoming identifiable again.

MRI findings >21 days

- Oedema completely resolves
- The ischaemic area appears hypointense on T1-weighted and hyperintense on T2-weighted images
- There is usually some T1 hyperintensity as well by this stage (if not earlier) owing to haemorrhagic transformation. This can be gyriform or localized depending on the type of infarct and extent of transformation. The equivalent on T2 or T2* is hypointensity, which is usually visible to some degree even on the spin echo sequences
- Infarct becomes low intensity on DWI
- In contrast-enhanced images, parenchymal enhancement typically persists throughout this phase; it usually disappears by 3–4 months.

Table 7.1 MRI findings in acute ischaemic stroke

Time	MRI	Finding	Cause
2–3 minutes	PWI	Reduced CBF, CBV, MTT	Decreased CBF
2–3 minutes	DWI	Reduced ADC	Decreased motion of protons
0–2 hours	T2 FLAIR	Absent flow void signal most sensitively seen on FLAIR	Slow flow or occlusion
0–2 hours	T1	Arterial enhancement	Slow flow
2–4 hours	T1	Subtle sulcal effacement	Cytotoxic oedema
2–4 hours	T1	Parenchymal enhancement	Incomplete infarction
8 hours	T2 FLAIR	Hyperintense signal—more sensitive on FLAIR	Vasogenic and cytotoxic oedema
16–24 hours	T1	Hypointense signal	Vasogenic and cytotoxic oedema
5–7 days		Parenchymal enhancement	Complete infarction

MRI and CT in cerebral haemorrhage

- MRI is as sensitive as CT for detecting acute haemorrhage. However, haemorrhage on MRI is more difficult to interpret than on CT for the inexperienced clinician
- Gradient echo MRI is very useful in the diagnosis of haemorrhage and it is recommended to include it in any acute stroke MRI—blood appears as a 'black hole'
- Haemorrhage can appear bright on DWI (admittedly with a black ring round it but can be subtle), and therefore acute stroke imaging cannot be DWI alone or you can thrombolyse bleeds in error. To avoid this, other MRI sequences, particularly T2*, must be performed with DWI
- Gradient echo MRI (GRE) is the most sensitive sequence for detecting intraparenchymal haemorrhage (primary intracerebral haemorrhage and haemorrhagic transformation) in the hyperacute stages
- Conventional T1-weighted and T2-weighted sequences may show subacute and chronic bleeding
- FLAIR is the most sensitive MRI sequence for detecting acute subarachnoid haemorrhage.

Table 7.2 Temporal sequence of appearances of cerebral haemorrhage on CT and MRI subject to variability depending on size and location of clot, haematocrit, sequences, etc

	Immediate	Hours	Days	Weeks	Months
CT	Dense	Dense	Dense	Isodense >1 week	Hypodense
T1 MRI	Isodense		Bright	Bright	Dark eventually
T2 MRI	Bright	Bright	Dark around 2 days	Bright after about 2 weeks	Dark
GRE	Dark hole	Dark hole	Dark hole	Dark hole	Dark hole

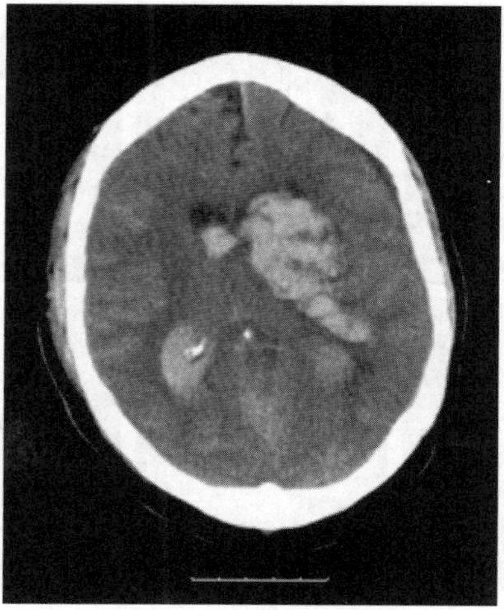

Fig. 7.13 CT in cerebral haemorrhage. A left subcortical haemorrhage can be seen with extension of blood into the ventricles and subarachnoid space. © Anthony Pereira.

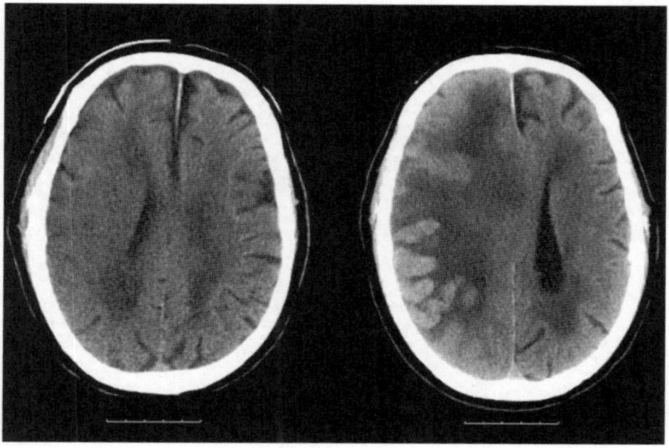

Fig. 7.14 Haemorrhagic transformation on CT. A pair of images show haemorrhagic transformation into a large infarct. The left-hand scan is in the first 24 hours. At this time no haemorrhage is present. The scan on the right is after a few days. © Anthony Pereira.

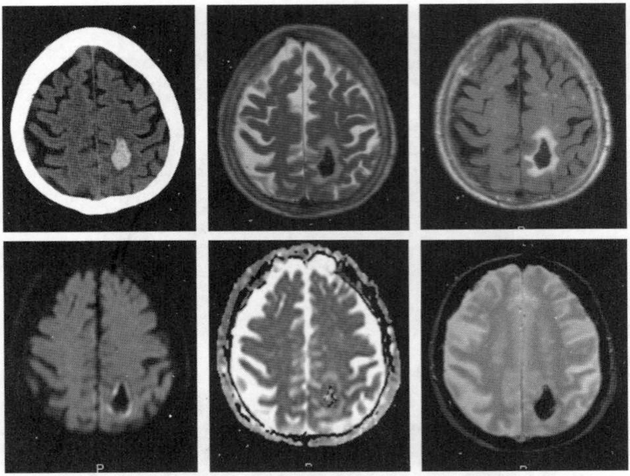

Fig. 7.15 CT and MRI images of an acute left parietal acute intracerebral haemorrhage. The top left hand image is CT. The remaining images are all MRI sequences and are from left to right. Top row: T2-weighted, FLAIR; bottom row: DWI, ADC map, gradient echo. © Anthony Pereira.

CT and MRI cerebral perfusion

Cerebral perfusion imaging has a number of applications.
- Assessing the perfusion deficit in acute stroke and calculating perfusion-diffusion mismatch
- Assessing cerebral perfusion prior to revascularization for cerebral occlusive disease
- Research.

A number of techniques can be used. These differ in that some are quantitative and some are semi-quantitative. Some techniques measure tissue perfusion with a high spatial resolution while others estimate volume flow in major vessels (e.g. transcranial Doppler (TCD) and MRA methods).

Quantitative
- PET
- Xenon CT
- Endogenous contrast MRI (potentially).

Semi-quantitative
- Exogenous contrast perfusion MRI
- CT perfusion
- SPECT
- TCD—flow in major cerebral vessels.

The two most applicable to acute stroke are:
- CT perfusion
- Contrast MR perfusion

TCD ultrasound can also be used to assess relative changes in perfusion—it measures flow velocity rather than flow but if MCA diameter stays the same, changes in velocity are directly proportional to changes in flow.

CT perfusion

- CT perfusion uses newer generation CT scanners to measure brain parenchymal perfusion in a brain slice/block. Whole brain coverage is currently not possible on routine clinical scanners, but coverage is increasing with newer scanners
- It requires an IV contrast infusion
- Contrast is followed as it passes through the brain
- The first pass of the contrast bolus is monitored
- A feeding artery and draining vein are selected to provide input functions
- The following parameters can be calculated:
  - Cerebral blood flow (CBF)
  - Cerebral blood volume (CBV)
  - Mean transit time (MTT)
- They can be displayed as a colour-coded image to identify areas of reduced cerebral perfusion
- Potentially, absolute quantification of CBF should be possible but, in practice, this is difficult and the technique is primarily semi-quantitative.

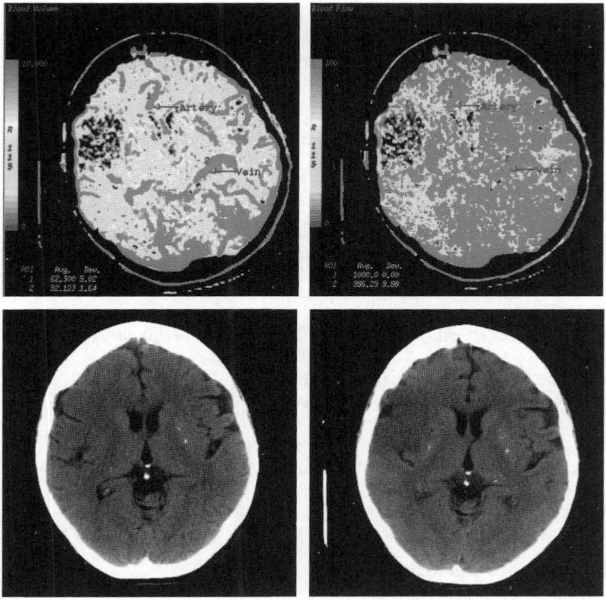

Fig. 7.16 CT perfusion in a patient presenting with a right frontal infarct. On the initial structural CT (bottom left) there are very early ischaemic changes. At this time a CT perfusion scan was performed. The cerebral blood volume and blood flow maps are shown on the upper left and right, respectively. There is a perfusion defect in the right frontal cortex. On the follow-up CT scan (bottom right), there is an established infarct in this area. © Anthony Pereira.

Perfusion-weighted MRI (PWI)

This allows assessment of brain parenchymal perfusion. Two methods are used.

Endogenous contrast PWI (bolus tracking)

- Requires an intravenous infusion of an MRI contrast agent. Gadolinium is used
- Gadolinium is rapidly injected and images are acquired as it passes through the cerebral circulation. A bolus tracking technique is used to obtain maps of:
  - CBF
  - CBV
  - MTT
  - Time to peak (TTP)
- CBF measurements require an input function to be obtained from a feeding artery
- Whole brain coverage can be obtained
- A robust technique with good signal to noise
- The technique is claimed to provide quantitative CBF maps but in practice it is best thought of as semi-quantitative. Similar to CT perfusion, this may be very helpful in showing reduced perfusion in areas of acute stroke
- It is most often used clinically in acute stroke to determine the size of the perfusion deficit, and calculate diffusion–perfusion mismatch.

Endogenous perfusion MRI

- This uses flowing blood as the contrast agent—it is labelled using a spin labelling technique
- The technique can potentially provide quantitative CBF values
- Signal to noise is low
- Whole brain coverage is often not possible
- Acquisition times can be long
- Signal to noise is higher with 3T scanners
- This is largely used as a research technique
- Can label individual arteries and potentially produce arterial territory maps.

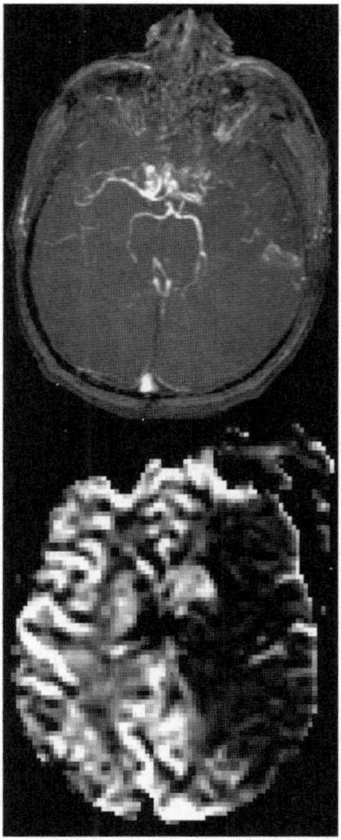

Fig. 7.17 An endogenous contrast MR perfusion study. On the upper image an MRA shows occlusion of the left MCA (arrowed). On the perfusion image below a large perfusion defect (low density) can be seen in the MCA territory. © Hugh Markus.

Positron emission tomography (PET) and single photon emission computed tomography (SPECT)

PET

- This uses radionuclear isotopes that emit positrons
- As they decay they emit a positron
- As soon as the positron collides with an electron it will disintegrate
- The resulting disintegration produces two photons
- They travel in diametrically opposite directions
- These photons can be detected by gamma camera detectors
- These positron-emitting isotopes have a very short half life; isotopes have to be made in a cyclotron and many have such a short half life that the cyclotron has to be on site
- Multitracer 15O PET can be used to measure CBF, CBV, MTT, oxygen consumption, and then to derive oxygen extraction. The combination of CBF and oxygen consumption measurements allowed it to be used to perform seminal work investigating the ischaemic penumbra in man
- Pharmacological compounds can be labelled to investigate neuropharmacology. For example, fluoroDOPA is used to look at presynaptic integrity of the dopaminergic system in Parkinson's disease
- ^{11}C-flumazenil is a central benzodiazepine receptor labelled with ^{11}C. It detects neuronal damage in the cortex in the first few hours after acute stroke and is used increasingly in acute stroke research as a marker of tissue integrity.

PET scanning is a very expensive and complicated process. It is also a useful technique for detecting neoplastic malignant cells and may identify small tumours in the body.

SPECT

- This uses a gamma camera
- Drugs labelled with gamma-emitting ligands are injected. A variety of ligands can be used depending on the requirement. For example, ligands taken up across the blood–brain barrier where they are fixed in the tissues give pictures of CBF (e.g. HMPAO). Other ligands are taken up by dopaminergic recpetors and are used in movement disorders to look at the basal ganglia
- Gamma radiation is emitted from the patient's brain
- The camera rotates around the patient and detects the gamma rays and their position in space from which it recreates a spatial map of the brain
- The resolution is much less than that of CT or MRI and therefore images often need to be viewed with either CT or MRI scans to identify where the areas of high signal occur
- Measurements of CBF with HMPAO SPECT are relative (to a selected reference region) and do not give absolute quantitative values.

Cerebrovascular ultrasound

Ultrasound (US) is widely used in non-invasive imaging of the cerebral circulation. It has a number of applications.

- Identifying stenoses in both the extracranial and intracranial circulation
- Imaging the arterial wall, primarily the carotid artery, to look both at intima–media thickness (IMT), a marker of cardiovascular risk, and at the morphology of established atherosclerotic plaque
- Studying haemodynamics; for example, looking at reactivity or perfusion reserve in the MCA distal to a carotid stenosis or occlusion
- Monitoring circulating emboli.

Extracranial US (carotid and vertebral)

This is widely used to screen for carotid and vertebral stenosis.

It uses higher frequency transducers (5–10 MHz) which allow higher spatial resolution. This is in contrast to transcranial Doppler ultrasound (TCD) where lower frequencies are required to allow penetration through the skull with a corresponding reduction in resolution.

It provides information on both structure (B-mode) and on flow (Doppler). The combination of the two is referred to as Duplex ultrasound.

B-mode

A transducer (probe) is placed on the patient's neck over the artery being studied. It emits ultrasound waves. Every time the waves cross a boundary where the tissues have different densities, some of the waves are reflected back or back-scattered. The transducer also detects the reflected waves and their position and a computer image is generated. This image is continually updated, giving the real-time B-mode image. This is used to obtain anatomical data (e.g. identify the carotid or vertebral artery or measure the IMT).

Doppler

The next stage is to use the Doppler principle to identify flowing blood.

This relies on a shift in the frequency of the ultrasound waves as they are back-scattered and reflected back from the moving blood (red cells).

From this frequency shift, combined with a knowledge of the angle between the ultrasound beam and the vessel, one can calculate the blood flow velocity.

The Doppler information is conventionally colour-coded (red for arterial blood, blue for venous blood).

Stenoses initially result in turbulence of blood flow and, as they become tighter, an increase in flow velocity.

Detection of stenoses on Duplex ultrasound

- A stenosis can be identified from visualization of plaque and also its effect on flow velocity. Measuring flow velocity is the most reliable way to determine the degree of stenosis
- Stenoses result in turbulent flow and loss of the spectral window. This reflects the fact that most blood flow is at a similar velocity with little flow at low velocities. With turbulence caused by stenosis, flow occurs at all velocities, including low velocities, and therefore flow is seen at

lower velocities where the acoustic window was. This change is seen before velocity starts to rise

- As stenosis increases above 50–60%, velocity increases (through the narrowed lumen). From the Doppler frequencies, the blood flow velocity and the degree of stenosis in the arterial lumen can be determined
- The usual parameter recorded is the peak systolic velocity (PSV). Sometimes the ratio of the PSV over the end-diastolic velocity (EDV) is used. A conversion chart is used to convert this to stenosis: this may vary between laboratories
- If there is contralateral carotid occlusion, normal flow in the ipsilateral carotid will increase. In such cases, PSV measurements alone will overestimate stenosis and one should use the PSV:EDV ratio
- With very tight stenosis, velocities can fall. Sometimes differentiating tight stenosis from occlusion can be difficult. MRA or CTA is then useful
- Ultrasound contrast (which relies on injection of minute air bubbles which are echogenic) can also help to differentiate
- The degree of stenosis can also be determined from the B image. This gives a useful idea for lesser degrees of stenosis when velocities are not increased but is not as accurate as velocities for tighter stenoses.

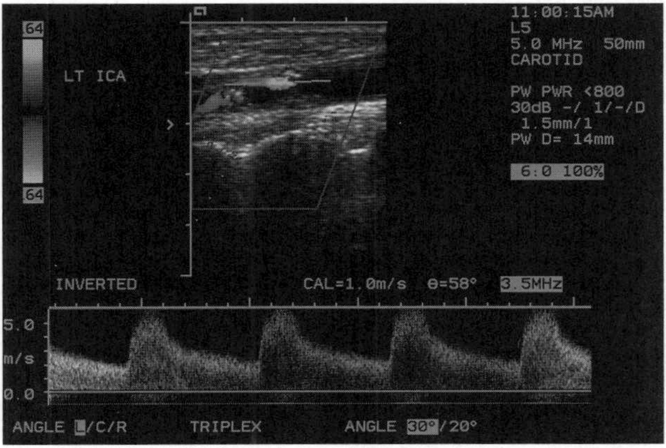

Fig. 7.18 Duplex ultrasound from a tight internal carotid stenosis. On the upper image the colour Doppler outlines the plaque and shows turbulent flow. On the lower image the peak systolic velocity is increased to above 5 m/s (normal up to 1.4 m/s). © Hugh Markus.

Ultrasound plaque morphology

B-mode ultrasound also gives information on plaque morphology. There are three main types of plaque:

- Echolucent plaques (appear black) contain lipid and have highest stroke risk
- Echogenic plaques (appear white) are fibrous and have the lowest stroke risk
- Mixed.

Plaques may also be calcified, in which case the calcium casts an acoustic shadow and the artery cannot be fully visualized.

Although plaque morphology relates to risk it is observer-dependent and has not been widely adopted in risk prediction.

Advantages and disadvantages of carotid and vertebral duplex

Advantages

- Quick
- Non-invasive
- Relatively inexpensive
- Widely available
- No radiation.

Disadvantages

- Experienced and skilled operator is required
- Inaccurate for stenoses below 50%
- Calcification of the artery may make it less accurate
- Distal carotid stenoses cannot be visualized (although abnormal flow patterns may give a clue to their presence)
- It is also not very reliable at looking at the vertebral arteries—it can only visualize the vertebral origin well and sometimes even this is poorly seen.

Carotid intima–media thickness (IMT)

- The thickness of the intima–media complex is measured on the far wall of the common carotid artery using high resolution B-mode ultrasound
- The IMT measured ultrasonically correlates well with the intima–media complex determined histologically
- Increased IMT is seen in patients with carotid stenosis, stroke, and ischaemic heart disease
- Increased IMT is an independent predictor of stroke and MI risk
- It is used as a screening test to assess vascular risk by some clinicians.

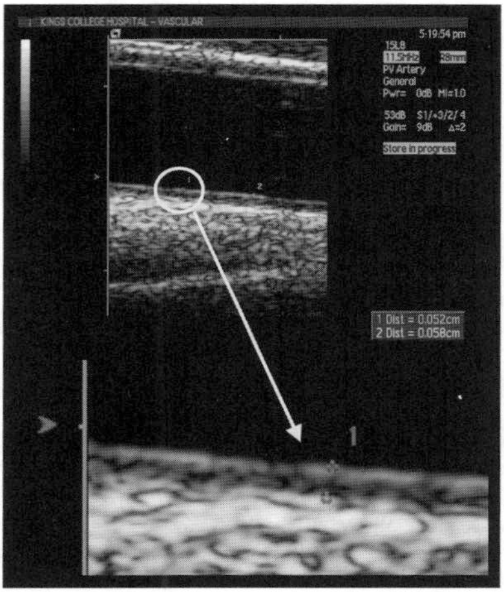

Fig. 7.19 Carotid artery intima–media thickness (IMT). On the posterior wall (lower wall) the intima–media complex can be seen. IMT is measured between the two interfaces as indicated on the lower magnified image by crosses. © Hugh Markus.

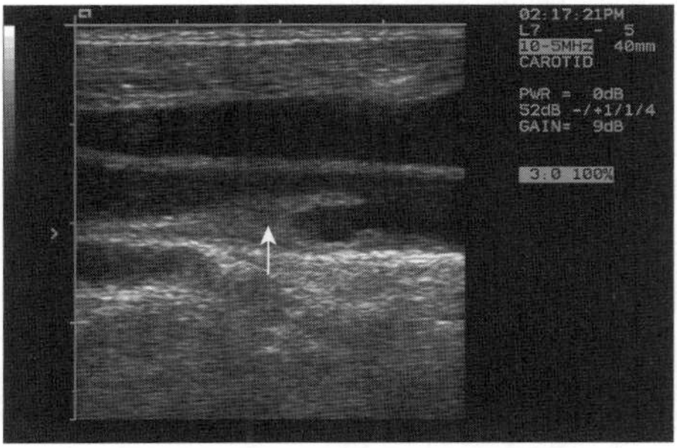

Fig. 7.20 Picture of an irregular plaque on B-mode ultrasound (arrowed). © Hugh Markus.

Further reading

Lorenz MW, Markus HS, Bots ML, Rosvall M, Sitzer M (2007) Prediction of clinical cardiovascular events with carotid intima–media thickness: a systematic review and meta-analysis. *Circulation* **115**, 459–67.

Transcranial Doppler ultrasound (TCD)

Transcranial Doppler (TCD) allows detection of stenoses in the intracranial circulation.

Transmission of ultrasound through the skull is much less good than that through the skin. This means:

- A lower frequency ultrasound (2 MHz) which is transmitted through the skull better has to be used
- This provides lower spatial resolution.Therefore while limited information on structure can be obtained from the B-mode images, TCD primarily gives information on flow velocity
- Insonation has to be made through bone windows which are thinner and therefore allow better transmission of ultrasound
- The most commonly used is the transtemporal window which allows insonation of the MCA, distal ICA, and PCA
- In 10–20% of individuals, no signals can be detected through this window (described as absent acoustic window). This absence of a TCD window is increased in the elderly, and in women
- A posterior window allows insonation of the basilar artery
- An orbital window allows insonation of the ophthalmic artery but insonating through the lens is associated with increased risk of cataracts.

Advantages

- Non-invasive
- Suitable for repeated measurement of flow velocity and for continuous monitoring, e.g. during carotid endarterectomy
- High temporal resolution.

Disadvantages

- Operator-dependent
- Poor spatial resolution
- Provides information on flow velocity, not absolute flow. Velocity correlates with flow if vessel diameter stays unaltered
- Does not allow visualization of all major intracerebral vessels
- Takes longer than CTA or MRA.

Clinical uses

- Screening for intracranial stenoses
- Monitoring for vasospasm in patients after subarachnoid haemorrhage (SAH)
- During carotid endarterectomy monitoring flow in the ipsilateral MCA to determine whether shunting is necessary, and monitoring for emboli in the immediate postoperative phase.

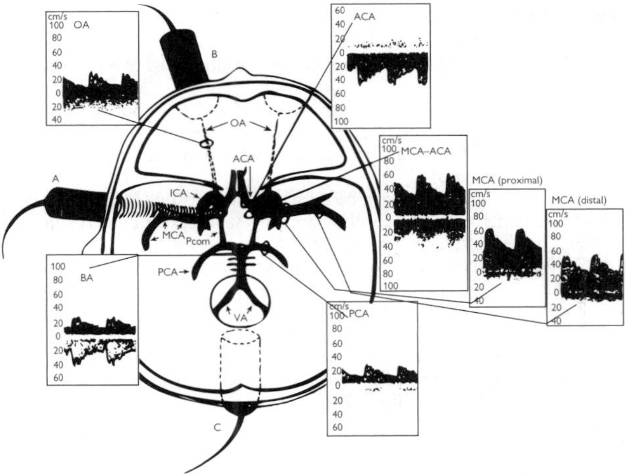

Fig. 7.21 A schematic diagram of the skull from above illustrating the different TCD windows and the appearance of the waveforms in the different vessels. ACA, anterior cerebral artery; BA, basilar artery; ICA, internal carotid artery; MCA, middle cerebral artery; OA, ophthalmic artery; PCA, posterior cerebral artery; Pcom, posterior communicating artery; VA, vertebral artery. Reproduced from Warlow CP *et al.* (2008) *Stroke Management*, 3rd edn, Figure 6.31. Oxford, WileyBlackwell.

Other uses of TCD

Assessment of cerebral reactivity

- This allows study of the haemodynamic consequences of a stenosis or occlusion
- If collateral supply, primarily by the circle of Willis, is good, a carotid stenosis may result in no haemodynamic compromise in the ipsilateral MCA. In contrast, if collateral supply is poor, then haemodynamics may be severely affected
- Only limited information can be obtained from resting MCA velocity measurements, owing to cerebral autoregulation preserving resting flow. Therefore the circulation needs to be 'stressed'
- MCA flow velocity is measured at rest and then during a vasodilatory stimulus
- The commonly used vasodilatory stimuli are increased inspired carbon dioxide gas (5–8%) in air, or an intravenous injection of the carbonic anhydrase inhibitor acetazolamide
- In the presence of impaired haemodynamics, the vessels are already vasodilated to preserve flow. Therefore they cannot vasodilate much further and reactivity (the percentage increase in flow velocity) is reduced
- If submaximal dilatory concentrations of carbon dioxide are used, the percentage increase in flow velocity needs to be divided by the increase in blood CO_2; this is estimated by the change in end-tidal CO_2
- In patients with carotid occlusion, a severely impaired reactivity predicts future stroke and TIA
- Reactivity is used by some clinicians to determine when to revascularize patients with carotid occlusion with extracranial–intracranial (EC–IC) bypass and when to treat asymptomatic carotid stenosis with carotid endarterectomy, although there is no trial data to support, or contradict, this approach.

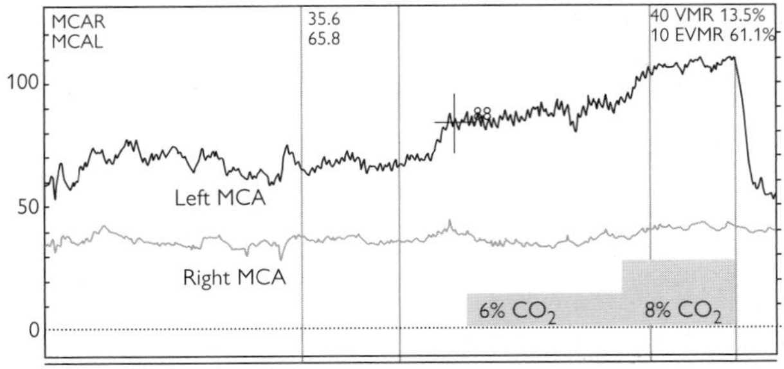

Fig. 7.22 Cerebrovascular reactivity measurement using transcranial Doppler. Increased inspired carbon dioxide (first 6% in air and then 8% in air) is given, which results in a marked increase in MCA flow in normal individuals. In a patient with a haemodynamically significant carotid stenosis this reactivity may be reduced or absent. In this patient with a right carotid occlusion, reactivity is normal in the left MCA but absent in the right MCA. Severely impaired reactivity has been associated with an increased future stroke risk, particularly in patients with carotid artery occlusion. © Hugh Markus.

Further reading

Markus H, Cullinane M (2001) Severely impaired cerebrovascular reactivity predicts stroke and TIA risk in patients with carotid artery stenosis and occlusion. *Brain* **124**, 457–67.

Emboli detection

- TCD is the only technique which can detect circulating cerebral emboli
- Emboli reflect and back-scatter more ultrasound red blood cells and therefore result in high intensity signals in the Doppler spectrum. As they are travelling rapidly through the insonated field these increases are short duration. This is why they are called HITS (High InTensity short duration Signals) although most authorities use the simpler term 'embolic signals'
- They have been detected in patients with a wide variety of potential embolic sources
- Most work has been done in carotid artery stenosis
- In recently symptomatic carotid stenosis they can be detected in about 40% of individuals during an hour long recording from the ipsilateral MCA
- In this setting they predict future stroke risk, and have been used to evaluate antiplatelet efficacy. For example, in the CARESS trial clopidogrel and aspirin were better than aspirin alone in preventing embolization in actively embolizing patients with symptomatic carotid stenosis
- Some surgeons use the technique to monitor for embolic signals in the immediate post-carotid endarterectomy period. A high embolic signal count predicts early postoperative stroke rate. If this is detected, options are to check for technical problems with the operation and/or to give an additional antiplatelet agent (IV dextran has been commonly used).

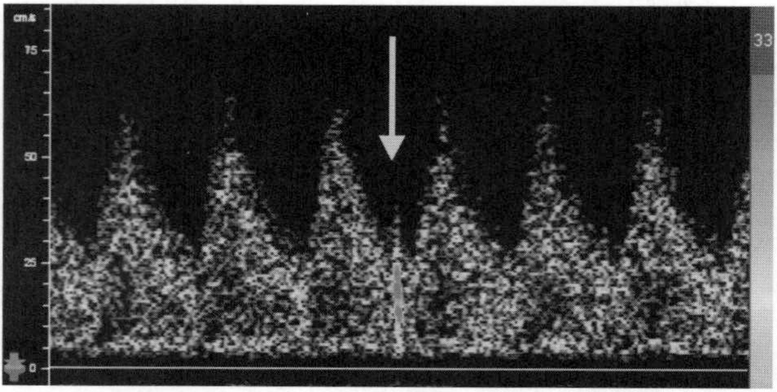

Fig. 7.23 An embolic signal (arrowed), seen as a short duration intensity increase, recorded from the MCA of a patient with carotid stenosis. © Hugh Markus.

Further reading

Markus HS, Droste DW, Kaps M *et al.* (2005) Dual antiplatelet therapy with clopidogrel and aspirin in symptomatic carotid stenosis evaluated using Doppler embolic signal detection; the CARESS Trial. *Circulation* **111**, 2233–40.

Markus HS, MacKinnon A (2005) Asymptomatic embolisation, detected by Doppler ultrasound, predicts stroke risk in symptomatic carotid artery stenosis. *Stroke* **36**, 971–5.

CT angiography (CTA)

This uses CT and intravenous contrast to image the blood vessels in the neck and brain. The technique can be used to investigate the arteries (CTA) and the veins (CTV).

- Good quality images require modern machines with spiral CT
- Here the patient is moved through the rotating X-ray beam
- This allows a faster scanning time and imaging while the bolus of contrast passes through the arteries
- The higher the number of slices (e.g. 16 versus 32 versus 64), the quicker the acquisition and the better the quality.

Advantages

- In contrast to ultrasound, CTA can visualize stenoses in the whole carotid and vertebral tree, and also the intracranial circulation. Therefore it allows detection of vertebral and basilar stenosis and distal carotid stenoses
- Quick acquisition
- Can detect intracranial aneurysms.

Disadvantages

- Reconstructed images may be suboptimal if heavy calcification is present, as is often the case for carotid stenosis. However, examination of the axial source data at appropriate window settings usually enables estimation of the degree of carotid bifurcation stenosis. This is more difficult at the vertebral origins if they are very calcified
- Requires a contrast injection
- The contrast can exacerbate renal impairment in those with pre-existing kidney disease. Prior optimization of hydration and using approprate contrast agents can help to reduce the risk
- Involves a large dose of ionizing radiation.

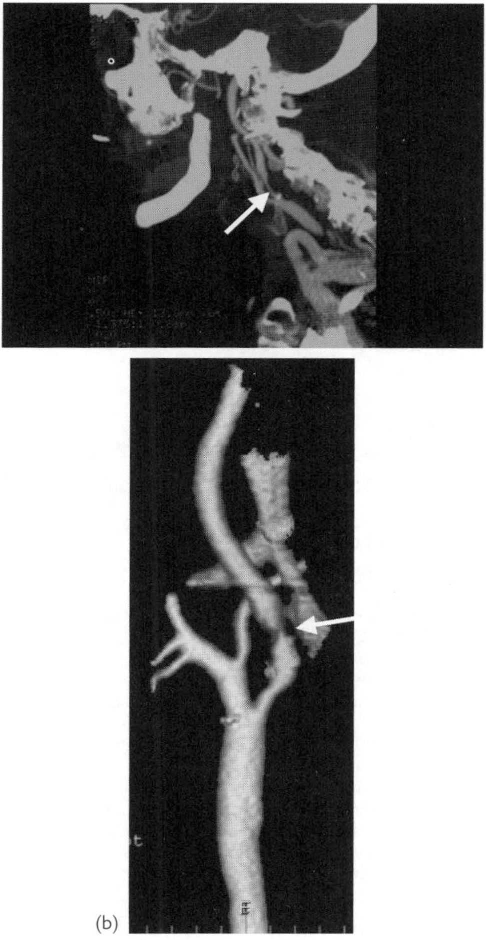

(a) (b)

Fig. 7.24 CTA imaging of carotid stenosis. **(a)** On the upper image there is a proximal ICA stenosis with a speck of calcium visible in the plaque as high signal. **(b)** The lower image shows a reconstructed 3D image from another patient with carotid stenosis. In both cases the stenosis is arrowed. © Hugh Markus.

Magnetic resonance angiography (MRA)

- This uses MR with or without intravenous contrast to image the blood vessels in the brain. The technique investigates:
  - The arteries (MRA)
  - The veins (MRV)
- MRA is very sensitive to flow and is based on the difference in signal between moving blood and stationary brain tissue
- MRA is particularly good for looking at the blood vessels at the carotid and vertebral circulation
- It is also very useful for looking at the intracranial circulation but is susceptible to small movements so if a patient moves slightly it can severely degrade the quality of the images. CTA is equally susceptible to movement but the scan time is shorter so it is less likely to happen.

Methods

Non-contrast
- Time of flight
- Phase contrast.

Contrast
- Contrast-enhanced MRA.

Increasingly, contrast-enhanced MRI is used because of the better signal to noise.

Time of flight (TOF)

- Depends on the relative contrast between flowing blood and stationary tissue
- Images correlate well with carotid angiography for analysing cervical bifurcation disease
- Flow signal dropout secondary to turbulent flow in tortuous and stenotic vascular segments makes interpretation of stenosis in these areas difficult. (These are common predilection sites for atherosclerosis)
- In regions of slow flow, the spin saturation of the scan causes overestimation of stenosis
- MRA is flow-dependent; absence of flow signal does not mean complete occlusion but rather that flow is below a critical value
- This means that stenosis is often overestimated and tight stenosis often appears as a flow gap. Such possible occlusions may then need further investigation to determine whether there is indeed stenosis or it is occluded

Phase contrast (PC-MRA)

- A technique that is helpful specifically in differentiating slow and absent flow from normal flow; it captures only truly patent vessels
- Other imaging sequences (e.g. spin-echo sequence or gradient-echo sequence) should be used with PC-MRA to avoid missing lesions such as paravascular haematomas, which are not captured by PC-MRA

- PC-MRA also has the disadvantage of signal loss because of turbulent flow in tortuous vessels
- Phase contrast is much less used now.

Contrast-enhanced MRA (CE-MRA)

- MRA can also be obtained by giving an intravenous contrast infusion: a paramagnetic contrast agent, based on gadolinium chelates, is given
- Images are rapidly acquired as the bolus passes through the cerebral vessels
- The agent reduces the T1 relaxation times of the fluid in the blood vessels relative to surrounding tissues
- These images have higher signal to noise than non-contrast MRA methods
- The high quality of images from contrast-enhanced MRA has made it the MRA modality of choice
- It overestimates degree of stenosis less than time of flight MRA. In particular, it is better at detecting vertebral origin stenosis, and at differentiating between tight stenosis and occlusion. However, it can still overestimate the degree of stenosis
- Gadolinium has recently been recognized as a likely risk factor for nephrogenic systemic fibrosis (NSF) in patients with acute or chronic severe renal insufficiency (glomerular filtration rate <30 mL/min/1.73m^2) and patients with renal dysfunction due to the hepatorenal syndrome or in the perioperative liver transplantation period. NSF leads to excessive formation of connective tissue in the skin and internal organs, including kidneys, and may be debilitating or fatal. Virtually every case has occurred following a high dose gadolinium contrast MRI in a patient with pre-existing severe renal impairment. Dialysis is thought not to be protective. Therefore, gadolinium-based contrast media are avoided in all MRI scans in patients with significant renal impairment. Time of flight MRA or ultrasound should be used in these patients. Guidelines may change as more knowledge is acquired.

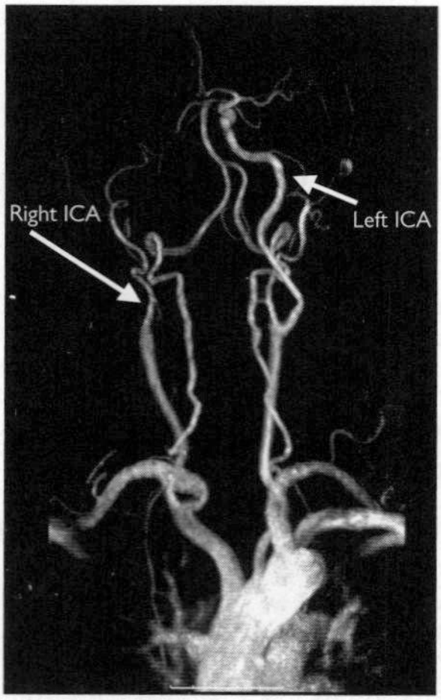

Fig. 7.25 A contrast-enhanced MRA showing a right carotid occlusion (arrowed). The right ICA is missing from its origin along its whole length. This can be appreciated when one looks at the normal left ICA (arrowed). © Hugh Markus.

Assessment of impaired cerebral haemodynamics

When perfusion pressure falls, a series of compensatory events occur to try to preserve perfusion. These can be demonstrated by PET studies.

Perfusion pressure can fall owing to a local occlusion or a systemic reduction (e.g. when the systemic blood pressure falls or after cardiac arrest).

Initially, CBV rises to maintain CBF. This maintains adequate oxygen delivery. When this vasodilatory reserve is exhausted (i.e. the cerebal vessels are fully vasodilated), CBF starts to fall and oxygen extraction per unit volume of blood (the oxygen extraction fraction) rises to maintain adequate oxygenation. As CBF falls further, this compensatory mechanism fails and adequate oxygenation cannot occur, resulting in infarction.

This compensatory mechanism, with vasodilatation and increased CBF, is also seen in patients with cerebral vessel occlusion (e.g. ICA occlusion) if they have inadequate collateral blood supply. The presence of this haemodynamic compromise can be assessed using a vasodilatory stimulus —see 📖 p. 198).

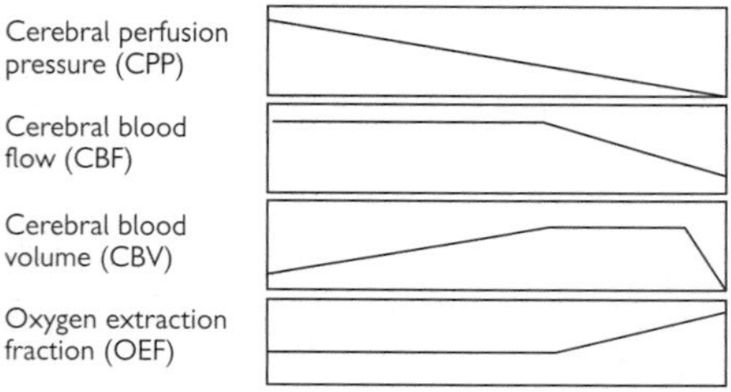

Fig. 7.26 Diagram showing how, as cerebral perfusion reserve falls, initially CBF is preserved owing to an increase in CBV until a critical point after which it falls. At this stage, oxygen extraction fraction starts to rise. © Hugh Markus.

Perfusion–diffusion mismatch

- An estimate of the ischaemic penumbra can be obtained by combining DWI and PWI
- Simplistically:
  - The DWI deficit represents already infarcted tissue (core)
  - The PWI deficit represents tissue at risk (as well as the core) (i.e. hypoperfused)
- The mismatch between the two represents tissue which is not infarcted but hypoperfused, i.e. which could recover if revascularized but could die if not reperfused
- Several recent randomized clinical trials are selecting patients with diffusion–perfusion mismatch to test thrombolytic treatment alternatives beyond the standard 3-hour time window used for IV tPA
- This concept is a bit simplistic:
  - DWI lesions can recover or reduce in size—they don't always represent irreversibly infarcted tissue
  - PWI deficits can represent oligaemia as well as critical hypoperfusion
- Nevertheless, it may prove to be a useful concept in selecting patients for thrombolysis, particularly beyond the 3-hour time window
- CT perfusion can also be used to estimate mismatch. This provides a map of CBV. CBV, although measuring perfusion deficit rather than cytotoxic oedema, in practice is similarly extensive to DWI and can be used on CT to predict initial infarct volume. Therefore mismatch can be estimated using CT.

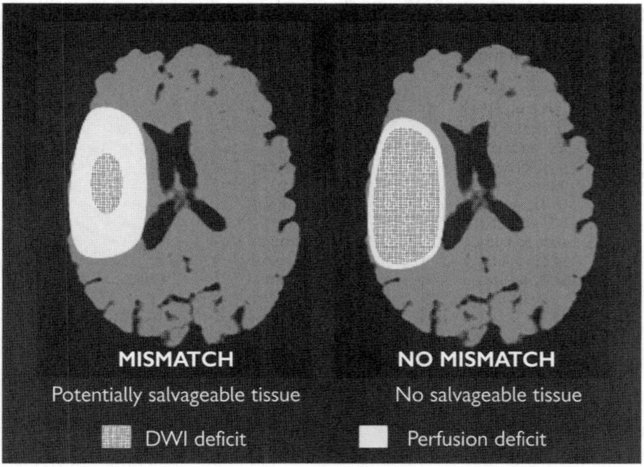

Fig. 7.27 Schematic diagram of the mismatch concept. © Hugh Markus.

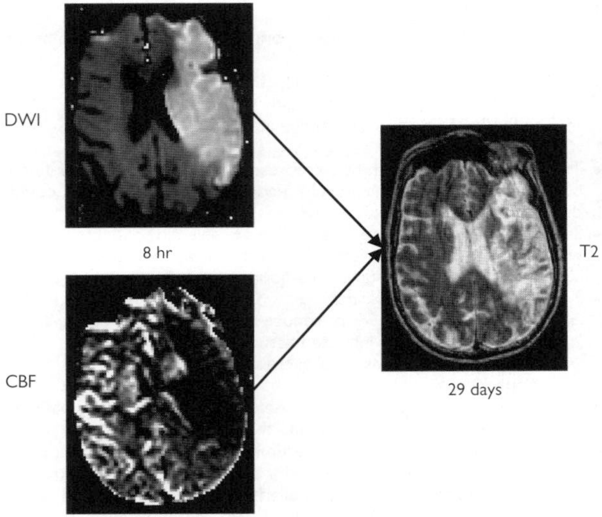

Fig. 7.28 On early MRI at 8 hours there was both a large DWI deficit involving the whole of the left MCA territory and a similar sized perfusion deficit on the perfusion (CBF) map. As these two are matched there is no mismatch. As predicted by the mismatch concept the final infarct size at 29 days was similar to the initial DWI deficit. © Hugh Markus.

Chapter 8

Ischaemic stroke—common causes

Introduction

A large number of different pathologies can cause ischaemic stroke. This chapter covers the common causes. Rare causes of ischaemic stroke are covered in 📖 Chapter 11.

A full list of causes of ischaemic stroke is shown below.

The major mechanisms of ischaemic stroke are:

- Thromboembolism from atherosclerosis in the aorta, extracerebral, and intracerebral arteries
- Cardioembolism
- Small-vessel disease or lacunar stroke.

List of causes of ischaemic stroke

Common

- Thromboembolism
  - Atherosclerosis
  - Aorta
  - Carotid artery
  - Vertebral artery
  - Intracranial atherosclerosis
- Cardiac disease
  - Atrial fibrillation
  - Valvular heart disease
  - Left ventricular thrombus
  - Other cardioembolic sources
- Small-vessel disease.

Less common

- Carotid and vertebral artery dissection
- Connective tissue disorders and cerebral vasculitis
- Infections
- Trauma
- Drug-related
  - Illicit drug abuse
  - Oral contraceptives and hormone replacement therapy
  - Other drug-related
- Moyamoya disease
- Haematological disorders, including prothrombotic states
- Migraine
- Genetic disorders.

Atheroma and large-vessel disease

- Atheroma is by far the most common disorder leading to narrowing of the larger arteries supplying the brain and subsequent stroke
- It affects mainly large and medium-sized arteries, especially at points of arterial bifurcation or curvature. Common sites are shown in Fig 8.1.

Extracranial atheroma causing stroke

- The most common sites are:
  - Aortic arch
  - Carotid bifurcation
  - Vertebral artery origin
  - Proximal subclavian artery
- In addition, atheroma not infrequently affects more distal portions of the carotid and vertebral arteries.

Intracranial atheroma

- The intracranial arteries are structurally different from the extracranial arteries, having no elastic lamina, fewer elastic fibres in the media and adventitia, and a thinner intima
- Atheroma may occur at multiple intracranial sites, including:
  - Carotid siphon
  - Middle cerebral artery
  - Anterior cerebral artery
  - Distal vertebral artery
  - Basilar artery.

Ethnic differences in distribution of atheroma

There are important ethnic differences in the distribution of atheroma. Knowledge of these differences can be useful when managing patients and deciding on optimal imaging approaches.

- In white individuals, extracranial atheroma, particularly of the carotid bifurcation and vertebral origin, is most common. Intracranial atheroma is much less common. Atheroma in the coronary arteries and aorta is also common
- In black and Asian individuals, intracranial atheroma is relatively much more common, and extracranial carotid stenosis is less common
- The nature of these differences remains uncertain, including the relative contribution of genetic and environmental factors
- Table 8.1 shows comparative frequencies between ethnic groups.

Table 8.1 Comparative frequency of intracranial stenosis in patients presenting with stroke from different ethnic groups

Ethnic group	Frequency (%)
Chinese	33–50
Thai	47
Korean	56
South Asians	54
US whites	1
UK whites	3
US blacks	6
UK blacks	18
US Hispanics	11

Adapted from Gorelick PB, Wong KS, Bae HJ, Pandey DK (2008) Large artery intracranial occlusive disease: a large worldwide burden but a relatively neglected frontier. *Stroke* **39**, 2396–9. With additional data from Markus HS, Khan U, Birns J *et al.* (2007) Differences in stroke subtypes between black and white patients with stroke: the South London Ethnicity and Stroke Study. *Circulation* **116**, 2157–64.

Pathophysiology of atheroma

- The early stages of atherosclerosis begin in childhood or early adulthood
- Figure 8.1 shows a schematic diagram of the stages of atherosclerosis
- A key early event is believed to be endothelial damage or dysfunction which is followed by deposition of fat within the arterial wall resulting in a fatty streak
- Inflammation is another central process. Circulating monocyte-derived macrophages invade the arterial wall. There is an inflammatory response within the arterial wall with T lymphocyte activation and cytokine production
- Cholesterol and other lipids are deposited, particularly within the intramural macrophages which convert to foam cells
- Arterial smooth muscle cells migrate into the lesion and proliferate, fibrosis occurs, and fibrous plaques are formed. These plaques have a lipid core and a fibrous cap and begin to encroach into the vessel lumen. Calcification in the vessel wall and plaque is frequent
- For reasons not fully understood, these well developed plaques may remain quiescent for many years but can become 'unstable' or 'active'. In particular, this may lead to plaque ulceration and erosion and secondary thrombosis on the plaque surface. Platelet aggregation is believed to be particularly important in this process
- Embolism can then occur from the adherent thrombus. Embolism is believed to be the primary mechanism by which atherosclerotic plaques cause stroke. It is much less common for them to cause stroke by haemodynamic compromise
- However, embolic and haemodynamic factors may interact, i.e. if perfusion pressure is lower, the effect of emboli may be greater and they may be less likely to fragment and break up, leading to vessel recanalization
- After becoming active, plaques can heal up. This has important clinical implications. Following a stroke or TIA secondary to a carotid stenosis, the risk of subsequent stroke is markedly increased for the next 2–3 years (particularly in the first month), after which it returns to that of an asymptomatic carotid stenosis.

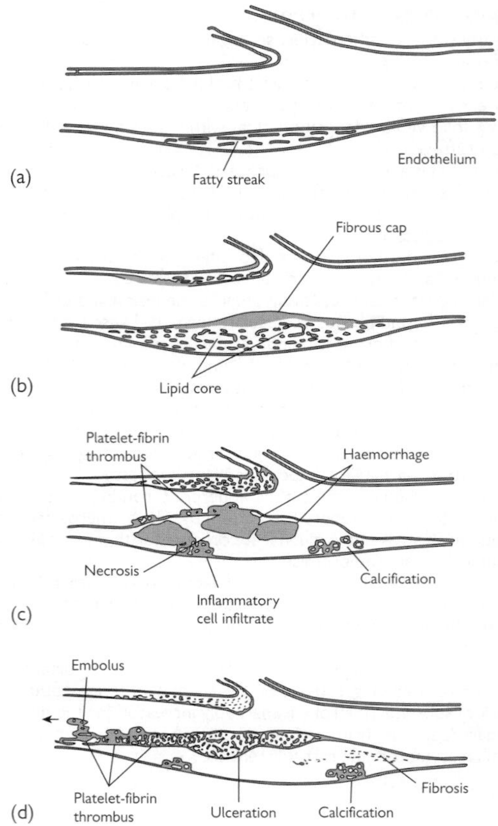

Fig. 8.1 Schematic diagram of the stages of carotid atherosclerosis. **a** Deposition of lipid in the vessel wall as a fatty streak; **b**, increased deposition of lipid and formation of fibrous material occurs; **c**, a more advanced plaque with inflammatory cell infiltration, calcification, necrosis, and new vessel formation; **d**, ulceration occurring on the plaque surface with secondary platelet aggregation on the luminal wall. This final stage is called an unstable plaque and is associated with thromboembolism. Reproduced from Warlow CP *et al.* (2008) *Stroke Management.* Oxford, WileyBlackwell.

Importance of embolism

- It was initially thought that large artery stenosis usually caused stroke by haemodynamic compromise secondary to vessel obstruction
- We now know embolism is the predominant process. Evidence for this includes:
  - Emboli can be directly visualized in the retina
  - Embolic signals, representing circulating emboli, can be detected using TCD in the MCA of patients with carotid stenosis. They are more common in symptomatic stenosis, more frequent after a recent event, and predict future stroke risk independent of the degree of stenosis
  - Emboli occluding vessels can be seen on cerebral angiography
  - The risk of stroke is transiently, but markedly, increased after TIA or stroke in patients with carotid stenosis. This suggests the degree of stenosis, which does not change rapidly over time, is not the most important process
- Emboli may be platelet–thrombus aggregates, or less commonly cholesterol crystal. The latter can lodge in retinal vessels and be visible for a prolonged period.

The role of haemodynamic factors

- Although embolism is more important than haemodynamic compromise, haemodynamic factors can be important
- They can sometimes be a direct cause of stroke. During a reduction in perfusion pressure (e.g. severe hypotension), infarction may occur distal to the stenosis particularly in the watershed areas (see 📖 p. 94)
- Carotid occlusion is associated with an increased risk of stroke, although not as great as that seen in tight carotid stenosis
- Collateral supply, in particular the patency of the circle of Willis, plays a crucial role in determining the outcome of carotid stenosis and occlusion. For example, in a patient with a complete circle of Willis, internal carotid occlusion may be asymptomatic. In contrast, in a patient without either an anterior communicating artery or posterior communicating artery ipsilateral to the symptomatic carotid, carotid occlusion is likely to result in a large infarct.

Dolichoectasia

- This describes dilatation and tortuosity seen in the basal intracerebral vessels, particularly the basilar artery
- Atheroma is believed to be the major cause but other causes include congenital defects in the vessel wall, connective tissue disorders, and Fabry disease
- This appearance is particularly common in the elderly
- It is frequently an asymptomatic finding seen on structural MRI (as dilated signal voids in vessels, or on MRA)
- It most commonly causes symptoms in the basilar artery
- Symptoms may be caused by:
  - Thromboembolism—thrombus within the dolichoectatic vessel
  - Brainstem compression leading to cranial nerve and other brainstem dysfunction.

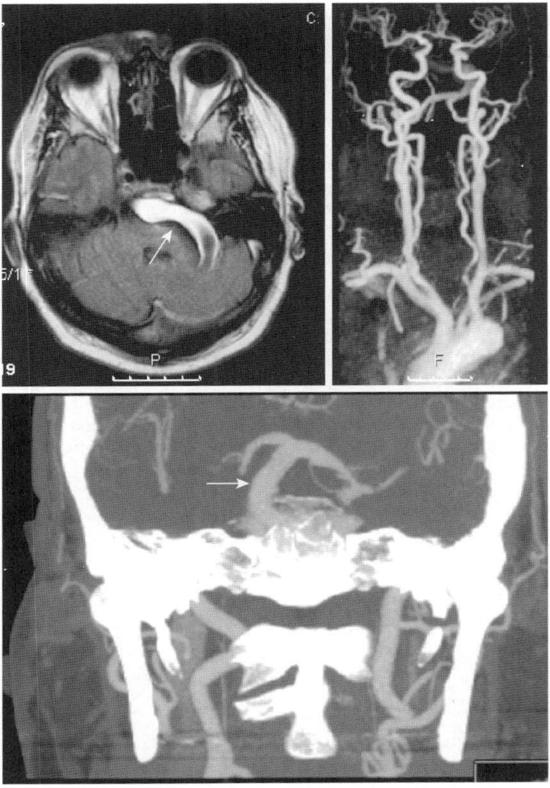

(a) (b) (c)

Fig. 8.2 Pictures of dolichoectatic basilar artery. **(a)** On the MRI there is a dilated and tortuous basilar artery. This is confirmed on the contrast enhanced MRA **(b)** and on the CTA **(c)**. The abnormality is arrowed.

Cardioembolism

- Embolism from the heart causes 20–25% of ischaemic stroke in most populations
- Atrial fibrillation is the most important cardioembolic source on a population basis. It accounts for about 12% of all stroke, and a higher proportion in the elderly
- A large number of cardiac abnormalities can cause embolism
- Some of these are associated with a high risk of embolism. Therefore if one of these is identified in a patient with stroke there is a high probability that they are related to the stroke
- Others are associated with a much lower risk of embolism. Therefore their identification in a patient with stroke does not mean that they are necessarily the cause of stroke. An example of this is a patent foramen ovale (PFO)
- Particularly in elderly patients, potential cardioembolic sources can coexist with other potential causes of stroke, and knowing which is the real cause of stroke can be impossible
- Thrombus emboli are believed to be particularly important in cardiac embolism. This is supported by the much greater reduction in stroke seen with warfarin, compared with antiplatelet agents, in conditions such as atrial fibrillation and valvular heart disease.

A list of cardioembolic sources is shown below. Those with higher rates of embolism are shown in italics.

Left atrium

Thrombus
- *Atrial fibrillation*
- Other atrial arrhythmias
- Atrial septal aneurysm

Atrial myxoma

Left ventricle

Mural thrombus
- *Post-acute myocardial infarction*
- *Left ventricular aneurysm/akinetic segment*
- *Cardiomyopathy*

Myxoma and other cardiac tumours

Mitral valve disease

Rheumatic mitral valve disease
Prosthetic heart valve
Infective endocarditis
Marantic endocarditis
Mitral valve prolapse (📖 p. 223)

Aortic valve

Rheumatic aortic valve disease
Prosthetic heart valve
Infective endocarditis
Marantic endocarditis
Calcific stenosis
Syphilis
Other causes of aortic regurgitation, e.g. Marfan's disease

Right to left shunt

Patent foramen ovale
Atrial septal defect
Ventricular septal defect
Pulmonary arteriovenous fistula
Congenital heart disease

Iatrogenic

Cardiac surgery
Cardiac catheterization
Cardiac angioplasty and stenting
Cardiac valvuloplasty

Specific cardioembolic sources

Atrial fibrillation

- Non-rheumatic AF is by far the most common cause of cardioembolic stroke in developed countries
- Thrombus forms within the left atrium—particularly within the left atrial appendage, and embolizes to the brain
- AF secondary to rheumatic heart diseases is associated with a higher risk of embolism but is rare in developed countries
- In non-rheumatic AF, the absolute risk of stroke is 4% per annum, six times greater than for patients in sinus rhythm. This is an average
- A number of factors are associated with higher or lower risk. Markers of increased risk include:
    - Increasing age
    - Previous embolic event
    - Hypertension
    - Diabetes
    - Left ventricular dysfunction on echocardiography
    - Enlarged left atrium on echocardiography
- Lone AF—this describes AF in the absence of other cardiac disease and with normal echocardiography in younger individuals (<60 years). It is associated with a low stroke risk of approximately 0.5% per annum
- Paroxysmal AF carries the same risk as persistent AF
- All patients with AF and previous stroke or TIAs should be considered for warfarin unless there are contraindications. This is covered in detail on 🕮 p. 298.

Infective endocarditis

- Infection occurs most commonly on already abnormal native valves, or in patients with prosthetic heart valves
- It is also common in intravenous drug abusers
- About 20% of patients with infective endocarditis have stroke or TIAs
- Stroke can be the presenting feature but more often it occurs in an already unwell patient. Mycotic aneurysms may occur which may bleed. Clues to diagnosis include fever, cardiac murmur, raised ESR, mild anaemia, raised WBC, and vegetations on echocardiography. Blood cultures may not always be positive and repeated blood cultures are often required.

Prosthetic heart valves

- Mechanical heart valves are associated with a markedly increased risk of stroke
- Anticoagulation with warfarin is standard treatment to prevent stroke in this group. With anticoagulation the risk of embolism is approximately 2% per annum
- Bioprosthetic heart valves, including porcine valves, have a lower risk of embolism than metallic valves
- Patients with bioprosthetic valves are often treated with antiplatelet agents alone, although some authorities recommend anticoagulation, particularly in the first few months following valve insertion.

Rheumatic valve disease

- This is an important cause of stroke in developing countries
- Rheumatic fever earlier in life results in valvular damage and destruction
- Stroke is most common with mitral valve disease, particularly in patients who also develop AF.

Mitral valve prolapse

- This is a common clinical and echocardiographic finding
- It was thought to be associated with stroke but more recent data suggests this association is absent or very weak
- Therefore it should not be thought of as the cause of stroke in an individual patient unless there are complicating features such as severe mitral regurgitation or infective endocarditis.

Patent foramen ovale and stroke

- PFO is a communication between the left and right atrium. This is present in the fetus and persists into adult life in about 20% of individuals
- Uncertain importance as a cause of stroke
- Case-control studies show PFO prevalence is higher in cryptogenic stroke patients under age 55 years compared with controls
- Possible stroke mechanisms include:
  - Paradoxical embolism from venous thrombosis (most likely)
  - Associated cardiac arrhythmias
  - The abnormality causing stroke is linked to PFO but not pathophysiologically related
- Risk of stroke probably higher with larger PFO and atrial septal aneurysm (ASA)
- PFO can be diagnosed on echocardiography (with contrast agent injection) or by transcranial Doppler ultrasound of the MCA (also with contrast injection). Sensitivity of both tests is increased by a Valsalva manoeuvre which raises right atrial pressure
- Transoesophageal echocardiography is more sensitive than transthoracic echocardiography
- Optimal management remains uncertain
- PFO can be closed percutaneously with a variety of umbrella and other devices with low complication rates (1%)
- Uncontrolled studies suggest closure is associated with a low recurrent stroke rate. Other natural history studies suggest the risk of recurrence is low without closure
- Some authorities recommend anticoagulation with warfarin (at least for 6 months to 1 year), others recommend closure, while others recommend antiplatelet agents
- Randomized trials are comparing closure with medical treatment
- PFO has also been associated with migraine with aura. Whether closing the PFO reduces migraine frequency remains controversial.

Atrial myxoma

- The most common primary cardiac tumour
- Portions of the tumour may embolize to the brain, resulting in stroke and TIA
- Occasionally, neoplastic cerebral aneurysms can form
- Clinical features include:
  - Recurrent stroke
  - Cardiac murmurs which vary from day to day
  - Mitral valve disease, either stenosis from mitral valve during diastole or regurgitation secondary to tumour associated valve trauma
  - Systemic symptoms and signs, including weight loss, malaise, fever, arthralgia, finger clubbing, anaemia, and raised ESR
- Diagnosis is made on echocardiography
- Cardiac catheterization may be necessary
- Surgical excision is the treatment of choice.

Further reading

Messe SR, Silverman IE, Kizer JR *et al.* (2004) Practice parameter: recurrent stroke with patent foramen ovale and atrial septal aneurysm: report of the Quality Standards Subcommittee of the American Academy of Neurology. *Neurology* **62**, 1042–50.

Overell JR, Bone I, Lees KR (2000) Interatrial septal abnormalities and stroke: a meta-analysis of case-control studies. *Neurology* **55**, 1172–9.

Small-vessel disease

This describes disease in the small perforating intracerebral arteries (<800 μm and, mostly, <400 μm).

Clinical importance

Small-vessel disease causes:

- Lacunar stroke—the cause of 20% of ischaemic stroke
- Vascular dementia—small-vessel disease is the most important cause of this
- Gait apraxia
- Non-dopa-responsive Parkinsonian syndrome (less commonly).

Pathology

Damage is seen both in the small arteries and in the brain parenchyma.

Arterial damage

A number of different pathologies may contribute, including:

- Hyaline arteriosclerosis—hyaline wall thickening occurs with smooth muscle cells being replaced with collagen, presumably reducing the ability of the vessels to vasodilate normally
- Lipohyalinosis
- Fibrinoid necrosis—with more aggressive vessel destruction
- Atheroma at or near the origin of the small perforating vessels.

Parenchymal lesions

- Small discrete lacunar infarcts (referred to as 'lacunes' or 'small lakes')
- Diffuse ischaemic injury without frank infarction seen radiologically as leukoaraiosis (low signal on CT, high signal on T2 or FLAIR MRI). Pathologically, axonal loss, ischaemic demyelination, and gliosis are found.

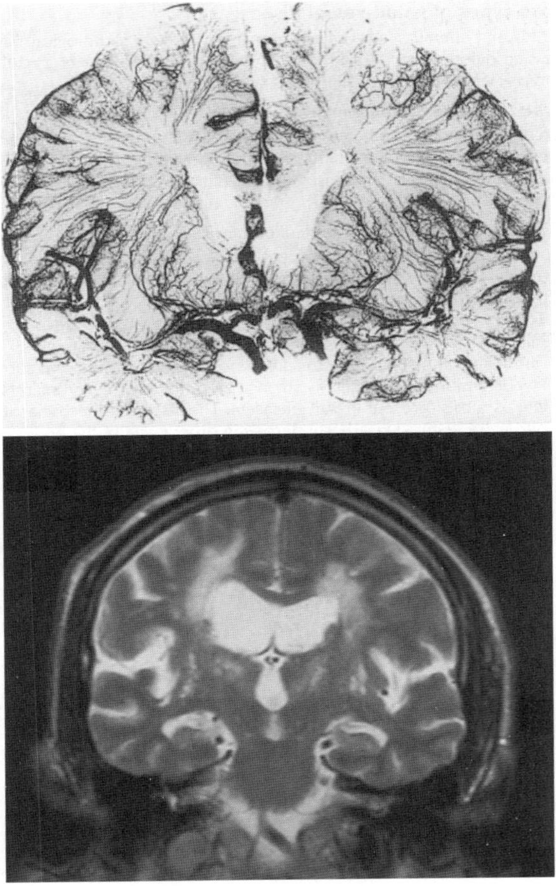

(a)

(b)

Fig. 8.3 Leukoaraiosis first occurs in the regions at the distal end of the perforating arterial supply. **(a)** This is illustrated by the microinjection radiological plate showing the arteriolar supply of the periventricular region. Reproduced from Donnan G, Norrving B, Bamford J, Bogousslarsky J (eds) (2002). *Subcortical stroke*, 2nd edn. Oxford, Oxford University Press. **(b)** An MRI scan of a similar coronal view is also shown. The high signal on MRI (leukoaraiosis) first develops in those areas furthest from the origin of the perforating arteries, i.e. those which have the lowest perfusion pressure. Reproduced with permission from Markus H (ed.) (2003) *Stroke Genetics*. Oxford, Oxford University Press.

Two types of small-vessel disease

C. Miller Fisher first suggested there may be two pathological patterns causing different sorts of lesions. This is now supported by radiological and risk factor data.

Type 1—isolated lacunar infarction

Microatheroma in the larger vessels from which the perforating arteries arise, or in the larger proximal perforating arteries (200–800 μm diameter), causes larger, often isolated, lacunar infarcts in the absence of leukoaraiosis.

Type 2—lacunar infarcts with leukoaraiosis

Lipohyalinosis or other similar pathologies in the smaller perforating arteries (<400 μm diameter) cause multiple smaller lacunar infarcts and often also leukoaraiosis.

- These two patterns can be distinguished radiologically, particularly on MRI
- There appear to be risk factor differences between these two subtypes. Hypertension is a particularly strong risk factor for lacunar infarcts with leukoaraiosis (present in 90% of cases). The classical atherosclerotic risk factors (smoking, atherosclerosis in other parts of the body) are commoner for the isolated lacunar infarct subtype
- How the small-vessel disease pathology causes the type 2 subtype is uncertain. An important factor may be impaired vessel reactivity and autoregulation, leading to hypoperfusion and inability to cope with fluctuations in blood pressure. It has also been suggested that increased blood–brain barrier permeability may occur, resulting in exudation of plasma constituents into the vessel wall and parenchyma
- Embolism is not thought to play a major role in either subtype of small-vessel disease, although there is no doubt emboli can occasionally cause small deep lesions.

(a)

(b)

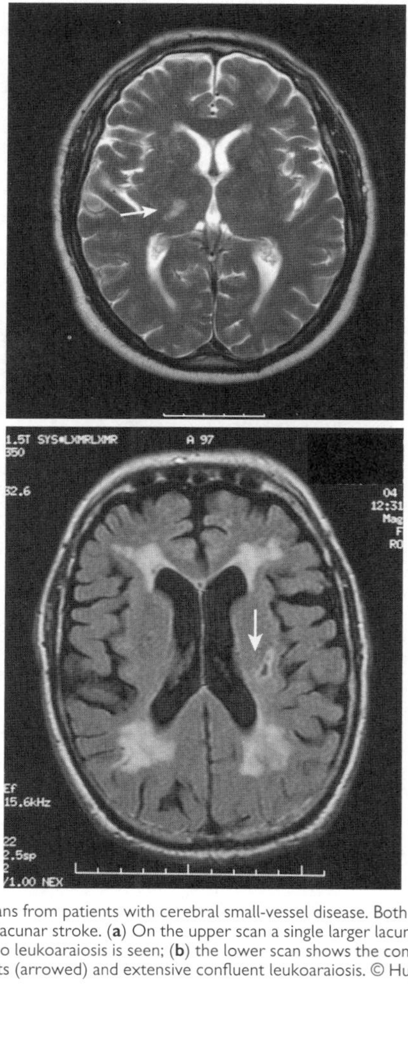

Fig. 8.4 MRI scans from patients with cerebral small-vessel disease. Both have presented with lacunar stroke. (**a**) On the upper scan a single larger lacunar infarct (arrowed) and no leukoaraiosis is seen; (**b**) the lower scan shows the combination of lacunar infarcts (arrowed) and extensive confluent leukoaraiosis. © Hugh Markus.

Chapter 9

Acute stroke treatment

Acute treatment of stroke

This chapter will deal mainly with ischaemic stroke, although many of the principles also apply to haemorrhagic stroke; details specific for cerebral haemorrhage are given in 📖 Chapter 13. Following stroke, a series of damaging consequences occur, each of which requires appropriate action to treat and/or prevent.

- Initial ischaemic damage
- Subsequent extension of brain damage into the ischaemic penumbra
- Early recurrent stroke
- Secondary deterioration owing to a number of causes, including:
    - Brain oedema
    - Raised intracranial pressure
    - Epilepsy
    - Secondary complications
- Secondary complications, including:
    - Aspiration and pneumonia
    - Epilepsy
    - DVT and pulmonary embolus
- Organ systems may fail
    - Heart failure, arrhythmia, myocardial infarction
    - Respiratory distress
    - Renal failure
    - Liver compromise from drug treatment
    - Skin breakdown
    - Muscle and bone changes
    - Dehydration
    - Decreased nutrition but increased catabolism
    - Psychological difficulties
- Physiological variables may become deranged
    - Blood pressure
    - Diabetes
    - Fever.

In addition, most stroke patients are elderly and commonly have other comorbidities. Therefore, acute treatment of the stroke patient requires consideration of many different aspects.

Key principles of stroke care

Care of the acute stroke patient requires:

- A systematic approach
- Attention to detail
- Concentration on doing the simple things well.

This is greatly aided by having agreed protocols and for some areas (e.g. thrombolysis) having standard proformas.

Scheme of treatment

Treatment of acute stroke may be split into several components:

- General emergency treatment of the patient
- Acute treatment of the cerebral ischaemia/haemorrhage itself
    - Thrombolysis or other reperfusion strategies
    - For haemorrhage, reversing coagulation disorders
- Treatment of specific causes of stroke
- Treatment of physiological variables
- Prevention and treatment of complications
- Early secondary prevention.

Key points in acute treatment of stroke

- Consider thrombolysis or acute treatment of haemorrhage
- Treat physiological variables
- Identify and treat problems with systemic organ systems
- Start secondary prevention as soon as possible
- Anticipate and treat complications
- Rehabilitation starts from day 1
- Manage patients on a specialized stroke unit or equivalent.

General emergency treatment

These are the steps taken when any seriously ill patient arrives in hospital.

- Check and protect the airway. Intubate if necessary
- Check breathing
  - Suction the patient if necessary
  - Use a bedside saturation monitor to check the capillary oxygen
- Check the circulation
  - Good pulse?
  - Is there an arrhythmia?
  - Is the blood pressure adequate, or too high or too low?
- Is there fever?
- Check BM/blood glucose in all patients on arrival: occasionally hypoglycaemia will masquerade as stroke
- Check the bladder and bowels
- Set up IV access
- Give IV fluids if drowsy or unsafe swallow
- Treat seizures if needed—however, single seizures during acute stroke are common and do not require treatment unless recurrent.

Pathophysiology of stroke

Treatment of the vascular event

The primary problem in ischaemic stroke is an occlusion of a cerebral artery. This needs to be unblocked as soon as possible if ischaemic neurons are to be saved. Spontaneous reperfuson occurs in a proportion of cases but this can be increased by reperfusion therapies.

There are several methods of achieving this:

- Intravenous thrombolysis
- Intra-arterial thrombolysis
- Mechanical retrieval of the embolus.

In cerebral haemorrhage, the haematoma grows over the first 24 hours, worsening the clinical outcome. Therefore here the specific treatment must be aimed at:

- Stopping the haematoma growth
- Reversing any coagulopathy
- Removing the haematoma.

The rationale for reperfusion: the ischaemic penumbra

- If recovery is to occur, successful reperfusion must take place before neuronal death
- As perfusion pressure in the brain falls, different CBF thresholds which relate to possibility of recovery of function are passed
- Recovery depends on the concept of the ischaemic penumbra, i.e. that there is tissue which is critically hypoperfused but not yet infarcted
- After an acute ischaemic stroke there is:
    - A central core of irreversibly damaged tissue
    - Surrounding this is an ischaemic penumbra
    - Surrounding this is an area of hypoperfusion
- Studies in primates have shown that tissue in the ischaemic penumbra can survive if reperfusion occurs early enough, but will die if no reperfusion occurs
- Duration of ischaemia is important. The longer the ischaemia, the less likely penumbral tissue will survive
- Studes with PET in man have demonstrated the existence of penumbral tissue (identified as tissue with increased oxygen extraction which may progress to recovery or infarction). The extent of this 'penumbral' tissue was very variable: none at 3 hours in some stroke patients whereas in exceptional patients penumbral tissue existed as late as 18 hours. For more details of PET and imaging of penumbral tissue see 🕮 Chapter 7.

>50	Normal
>21	Oligaemia: normal neuronal activity, reduced CBF
11–20	Ischaemic penumbra: functionally silent but viable
6–10	Irreversibly damaged tissue

Fig. 9.1 The relationship between blood flow levels and ischaemic injury, illustrating levels at which the ischaemic penumbra occurs. The data is derived from animal models. CBF, cerebral bloodflow, measured in ml/100 mg/min.

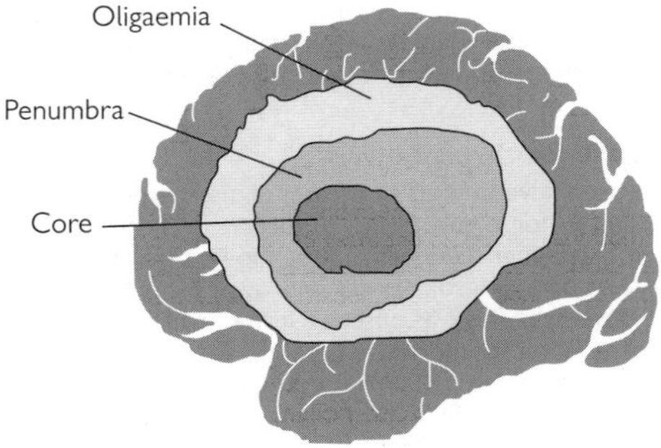

Fig. 9.2 Diagram of the ischaemic penumbra, which surrounds an inner core of irreversibly damaged tissue.

Further reading

Baron JC (1999) Mapping the ischaemic penumbra with PET: implications for acute stroke treatment. *Cerebrovascular Disease* **9**, 193–201.

Markus HS (2003) Cerebral perfusion and stroke. *Journal of Neurology, Neurosurgery and Psychiatry* **75**, 353–61.

Thrombolysis

Thrombolysis is the first treatment that has been shown to be effective in acute stroke. A lytic agent, most commonly recombinant tissue plasminogen activator (rtPA; company name Alteplase) is administered either intravenously (most commonly) or intra-arterially to break down the clot.

- The *in-vivo* target is the enzyme plasmin which breaks down the crosslinked fibrin of the clot and disrupts the thrombus
- Plasmin circulates in inactive form as plasminogen but is activated by thrombolytic agents
- There is trial evidence for two drugs, rtPA and urokinase
- Newer thrombolytics such as desmetoplase are also being evaluated
- In randomized clinical trials, streptokinase given within 6 hours of stroke onset increased haemorrhage and death rates; this is not used in stroke.

The evidence for thrombolysis

There have been several trials of thrombolysis, the pivotal trial being the National Institute for Neurological Disorders and Stroke (NINDS) trial published in December 1995 which first showed that treatment administered within 3 hours of stroke onset improved patient outcome by about one third on average. This was offset against a small but significant increase in the risk of cerebral haemorrhage (6%).

- No other individual trials of IV thrombolysis given within 3 hours have shown a statistical benefit, but meta-analysis of available trials shows a consistent benefit for IV rtPA given within 3 hours (see Figs 9.3 and 9.4)
- The benefit is much greater when rtPA is given even earlier within the initial 3-hour period. The chance of a good outcome is better if the patient is thrombolysed at 60 minutes than at 90 minutes. Therefore, although patients must be treated within 3 hours, do *not* wait for 3 hours to treat; treat as quickly as possible
- The meta-analysis suggested there may be a benefit up to perhaps 4–5 hours. In 2008 the ECASS 3 trial confirmed this benefit—patients were treated between 3 and 4.5 hours (mean 3 hours 59 minutes) post stroke. There was a significant 1.3–1.4 times increase in favourable outcome (modified Rankin score 0 or 1)
- All trials have studied patients under 80 years of age. Therefore the relative benefit in patients over 80 is uncertain.

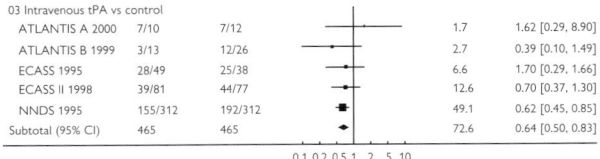

03 Intravenous tPA vs control				
ATLANTIS A 2000	7/10	7/12	1.7	1.62 [0.29, 8.90]
ATLANTIS B 1999	3/13	12/26	2.7	0.39 [0.10, 1.49]
ECASS 1995	28/49	25/38	6.6	1.70 [0.29, 1.66]
ECASS II 1998	39/81	44/77	12.6	0.70 [0.37, 1.30]
NNDS 1995	155/312	192/312	49.1	0.62 [0.45, 0.85]
Subtotal (95% CI)	465	465	72.6	0.64 [0.50, 0.83]

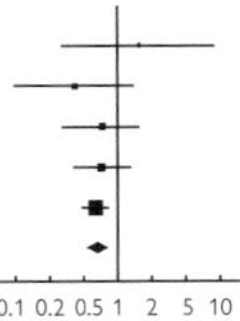

(continued....)

Fig. 9.3 Cochrane review showing meta-analysis of trial data giving rtPA for ischaemic stroke within 3 hours of stroke onset. The outcome of death or dependency at the end of follow up is reduced in the treated group by 36% (odds ratio of 0.64). Reproduced with permission from Wardlaw JM, del Zoppo G, Yamaguchi T, Berge E. Thrombolysis for acute ischaemic stroke. *Cochrane Database of Systematic Reviews* 2003 Issue 2. Art. No.: CD000212. DOI: 10.1002/14651857.CD000212. Copyright © Cochrane Collaboration, reproduced with permission.

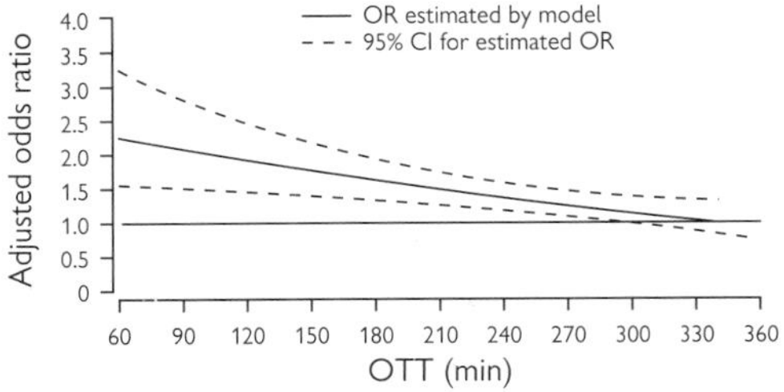

Fig. 9.4 Combined analysis of the data from all of the randomized trials of rtPA in acute ischaemic stroke (excluding ECASS 3). The line indicates the odds ratio of a favourable outcome with thrombolysis plotted against time from stroke onset to rtPA. The solid line shows the odds ratio itself and the dotted lines the 95% confidence intervals. Note how the odds ratio of a good outcome is much higher earlier after stroke. Reproduced from Hacke W, Donnan G. Fieschi C *et al.* (2004) Association of outcome with early stroke treatment: pooled analysis of ATLANTIS, ECASS, and NINDS rt-PA stroke trials. *Lancet* **363**, 768–74, with permission of Elsevier.

Thrombolysis in clinical practice

There has been concern that the results of thrombolysis might be worse in clinical practice than in clinical trials but this does not seem to be the case.

- A very large European audit (The Safe Implementation Thrombolysis Stroke-Monitoring Study; SITS-MOST) looked at the safety of thrombolysis with IV tPA when given within 3 hours of stroke onset in 6483 patients
- Results suggested that outcomes were as good, if not better, than those reported in clinical trials and better than pooled data from placebo-treated patients in the clinical trials
- Other aspects of stroke care have improved during that time since the trials and this may explain why SITS-MOST patients appeared to do better than those patients treated with rtPA in the clinical trials.

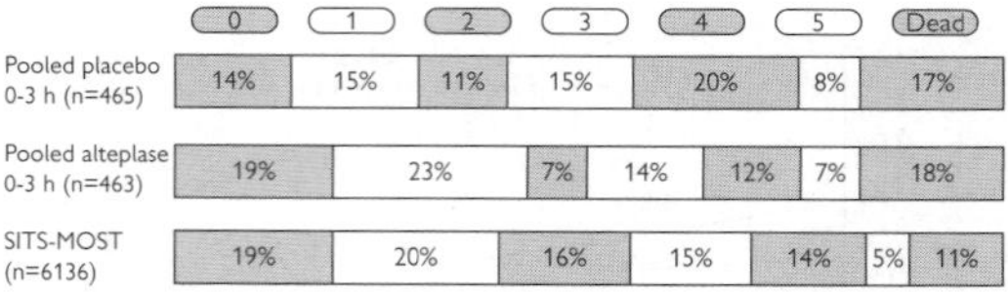

Fig. 9.5 Results from the SITS-MOST register. The figure shows the outcome at 3 months according to Rankin score. Numbers at the top are the Rankin scores. 0 means excellent recovery. The results suggest that 5% more people are Rankin 0 (cured) after thrombolysis and 5% more patients are Rankin 1 (minor symptoms but no disability) after thrombolysis. Reproduced from Wahlgren W, Ahmed N, Dávalos A *et al.* for the SITS-MOST investigators (2007) Thrombolysis with alteplase for acute ischaemic stroke in the Safe Implementation of Thrombolysis in Stroke-Monitoring Study (SITS-MOST): an observational study. *Lancet* **369**, 275–82, with permission from Elsevier.

Thrombolysis-related intracerebral haemorrhage

- This is the major complication of thrombolysis
- The haemorrhage is usally within the area of infarction—haemorrhage at a remote site is rare
- The frequency of haemorrhage and even the presence of symptomatic haemorrhage depends on the definition used. This is illustrated by the frequency of haemorrhage in ECASS 3 which varied from 1.9 to 7.9% in the rtPA-treated group depending on the defintion used (see Table 9.1). For more on definitions, see 📖 Chapter 13
- To screen for haemorrhage, all patients who have been treated with thrombolysis should have repeat brain imaging at 24 hours.

Factors which have been related to an increased risk of haemorrhage include:

- Poorly controlled elevated blood pressure
- Poorly controlled elevated plasma glucose
- Areas of well established hypodensity (i.e. established infarction) on CT imaging
- Recent brain infarction at another site
- Not adhering to the thrombolysis protocol
- Leukoaraiosis on MRI scan.

Risk of symptomatic intracerebral haemorrhage in the two treatment arms in the ECASS 3 trial

Table 9.1 Prespecified Safety End Points and Other Serious Adverse Events

Adverse Events	Alteplase Group (N=418)	Placebo Group (N=403)	Odds Ratio (95% CI)	P Value
Prespecified safety end points	no. (%)			
Any ICH	113 (27.0)	71 (17.6)	1.73 (1.24–2.42)	0.001
Symptomatic ICH				
According to ECASS III definition	10 (2.4)	1 (0.2)	9.85 (1.26–77.32)	0.008
According to ECASS II definition	22 (5.3)	9 (2.2)	2.43 (1.11–5.35)	0.02
According to SITS–MOST definition	8 (1.9)	1 (0.2)	7.84 (0.98–63.00)	0.02
According to NINDS definition	33(7.9)	14 (3.5)	2.38 (1.25–4.52)	0.006
Fatal ICH	3 (0.7)	0	—	—
Symptomatic edema	29 (6.9)	29 (7.2)	0.96	0.89
Death	32 (7.7)	34 (8.4)	0.90 (0.54–1.49)	0.68

Reproduced with permission from Hacke W *et al.* (2008). Thrombolysis with alteplase 3 to 4.5 hours after acute ischemic stroke. *N Engl J Med* **359**: 1317–29.

Administering thrombolysis—the practicalities

- The patient must be seen by a doctor who is competent in diagnosing stroke and be able to distinguish stroke mimics
- The patient must have a clinical diagnosis of a stroke syndrome
- The onset of stroke must be known, or must be deducible, to be definitely within 3 hours (or 4.5 hours for those units using this window following the ECASS results)
  - A patient waking up from sleep with symptoms cannot be considered to be within 3 (or 4.5) hours. Patients waking from sleep should only be thrombolysed if they went to sleep within the last 3 (or 4.5) hours and were well at that time
  - A collateral history from relatives, carers or others is often very helpful in assessing time of onset
- The patient needs a brain scan to exclude contraindications
- It is very important to remember that you do not need to see the infarct or the subtle signs suggesting infarction
- On the scan check that there is no:
  - Haemorrhage
  - Cause for the symptoms other than stroke, e.g. brain tumour
  - Well established infarct—suggesting the time period is longer than 3 hours
- The patient must have no standard contraindication to being given thrombolysis such as a bleeding diathesis or being on anticoagulants
- As long as these very simple rules are obeyed, thrombolysis may be given safely to most patients and will improve outcome overall
- A proforma is very useful in ensuring the protocol is adhered to, and contraindications are identified. When assessing a patient it is helpful to use the proforma as a checklist. The proforma used at St George's Hospital is shown below.

For every 20 patients treated, one extra returns to normal (Rankin 0). For every 20 patients treated, one extra returns almost to normal (Rankin 1). The incidence of symptomatic intracerebral haemorrhage is 6%.

Thrombolysis proforma

Initially the patient needs to be very rapidly screened by the admitting doctor or triage nurse. We used the profroma below for this.

A&E or ward screening for thrombolysis

Does the patient have suspected TIA/stroke?	Yes/No
Does the patient still have *any* of these: arm weakness, face weakness, speech disturbance?	Yes/No
Time since onset of symptoms is less than 3 hours	Yes/No
Patient aged over 18 years	Yes/No

If no *to any of these questions, the patient is* not *suitable for IV thrombolysis.*

Contraindications

Is the patient anticoagulated?	Yes/No
History of stroke or head trauma within 3 months?	Yes/No
History of intracranial haemorrhage ever?	Yes/No
History of any major surgery/trauma within 3 months?	Yes/No
Evidence of active internal bleeding?	Yes/No

History of GI bleeding within 3 months?	Yes/No
History of urinary tract bleeding within 3 months?	Yes/No
Could the patient be pregnant?	Yes/No

If the answer to any of these questions is yes then the patient is not *suitable for IV tPA.*

Triage plan

If the patient has passed the screening for stroke thrombolysis and has no contraindications, refer **immediately.**

The stroke doctor then goes through the following proforma/checklist.

1. Provisional diagnosis

Is this likely to be stroke or TIA?	Yes/No

2. Primary screening

Time since symptom onset less than 4.5 hours	Yes/No
Patient aged 18–80 years	Yes/No
Patient's GCS is greater than 8	Yes/No
Does the patient still have any of these: facial weakness, arm weakness, speech disturbance	Yes/No

If the answer to any of these questions is no, the patient is not *suitable for IV tPA.*

3. Baseline observations

Patient's weight............kg
ECG ....
Pulse.......................bpm
BP..........................mmHg
Respiratory rate..........bpm
BM.........................mmol/L
O_2 sats....................%
GCS......................./15
Continue to monitor BP at 15-minute intervals. Cannulate.
Send urgent FBC, U&E, glucose, clotting, G&S, CRP and amylase.

4. Baseline investigation results

Haemoglobin	>10g/dl	Yes/No
Platelets	>100 x 109/l	Yes/No
Glucose	<20 or >2.7 mmol/l.	Yes/No
INR	<1.7	Yes/No
APTT	22–36 seconds?	Yes/No

The answers to all these should be yes but thrombolysis should not *be delayed if results are unavailable and likely to be normal.*

5. Contraindications

Age under 18 or over 80 years	Yes/No
Symptoms more than 3 hours ago?	Yes/No
Time of symptom onset is unknown?	Yes/No
Neurological deficit minor/rapidly resolving?	Yes/No
Very severe stroke (e.g. NIHS>25)?	Yes/No
Was there any seizure activity at stroke onset?	Yes/No
Is subarachnoid haemorrhage suspected?	Yes/No
Is there any evidence of active internal bleeding?	Yes/No

Stroke or head trauma in the past 3 months?	Yes/No
Prior stroke and concomitant diabetes?	Yes/No
Intracranial haemorrhage ever?	Yes/No
History of CNS damage (neoplasm, aneurysm)?	Yes/No
Any intracranial or spinal surgery ever?	Yes/No
Any major surgery or trauma (3 months)?	Yes/No
Arteriovenous malformation or aneurysm?	Yes/No
Known haemorrhagic diathesis?	Yes/No
GI or urinary tract bleeding (3 months)?	Yes/No
GI ulcer disease (3 months)?	Yes/No
Oesophageal varices?	Yes/No
Severe liver disease (failure, cirrhosis, hepatitis)?	Yes/No
Endocarditis or pericarditis (current)?	Yes/No
Pancreatitis?	Yes/No
Pregnant or recent delivery (10 days)?	Yes/No
Non-compressible vessel puncture (10 days)?	Yes/No
Lumbar puncture in the last 7 days?	Yes/No
Recent CPR (10 days)?	Yes/No
History of haemorrhagic diabetic retinopathy?	Yes/No
Receiving oral anticoagulants, e.g. warfarin?	Yes/No
Heparin within 48 hours and APTT high?	Yes/No
Blood pressure limits >185/110 (either)?	Yes/No
or IV medication needed to reduce BP to these limits?	Yes/No
Platelet count below 100 000/mm^3	Yes/No
Blood glucose <50 or >400 mg/dl?	Yes/No

rtPA must not be given if the answer to any of these questions is yes

6. Assent

There is a 1 in 8 chance of significant recovery and a 1 in 18 chance of symptomatic ICH.

Patient assents to thrombolysis?	Yes/No
or thrombolysis judged in patient's best interest?	Yes/No

7. Neuroradiology ***Time of CT***...............

Contraindications: intracranial haemorrhage?	Yes/No
Alternative pathology?	Yes/No
Caution: more than one-third MCA territory?	Yes/No

Provisional report...
Reviewing doctor:................................ Grade.........

8. Final checklist

Systolic BP...................<185	Yes/No
Diastolic BP...................<110	Yes/No

If IV therapy needed before thrombolysis, rtPA should not be given (EU Licence).

Assent obtained	Yes/No
or judged to be in the patient's best interest	Yes/No
Thrombolysis starting within 4.5 hours of onset?	Yes/No
Decision to thrombolyse agreed by Consultant	Yes/No

9. Administering rtPA

1. Begin infusion as soon as decision to thrombolyse made.
rtPA (Alteplase) dose: 0.9 mg/kg (maximum dose 90 mg).
Give 10% as bolus over 2 minutes followed by 90% infusion over 60 minutes.
Time infusion started: ....
2. Transfer patient to stroke unit
3. Cross aspirin/dipyridamole/heparin/warfarin off drug chart for 24 hours
4. *Do not* catheterize the patient or insert a nasogastric tube for 24 hours.

10. BP monitoring and treatment

BP should be <185/110 mmHg

Pre/during thrombolysis:	every 15 minutes
Post-thrombolysis:	15 minutes for 2 hours
then	30 minutes for 4 hours
then	hourly for 18 hours.

11. FOLLOW UP IMAGING: CT scan in 24 hours.

12. SIGNATURE

Name of person completing form:......................Grade.............
Signature...

APPENDIX

A. Labetalol to treat hypertension during/after infusion of rtPA.
- Diastolic >140 mmHg: IV labetalol 40 mg over 2 min, then infuse 2–8 mg/min
- 230/(121–140): IV labetalol 20 mg over 2 min, then infuse 2–8 mg/min
- If SBP (185–230)/(110–120): IV labetalol 10 mg over 2 min, then 2–8 mg/min
- If patient needs antihypertensive medication, monitor BP every 15 minutes.

B. Suspected ICH during/after infusion of rtPA
- Stop rtPA infusion and assess patient. Inform stroke consultant
- Urgent CT scan. Urgent FBC, APTT, INR and crossmatch
- If appropriate to reverse rtPA, use cryoprecipitate 6–8 units and platelets if count low.

C. Major haemorrhage elsewhere (e.g. GI tract)
- Stop rtPA infusion and assess patient. Inform stroke consultant
- Urgent FBC, APTT, INR and crossmatch
- If appropriate to reverse rtPA, use cryoprecipitate 6–8 units and platelets if count low.

Immediate post-thrombolysis care

- After thrombolysis the current guidelines are that patients should not be given anticoagulants or antiplatelet agents for approximately 24 hours
- By 24 hours the patient may be given antiplatelet agents for secondary prevention and subcutaneous heparin for DVT prophylaxis
- BP should be monitored closely over the first 24 hours and aggressively managed if excessive (e.g. systolic pressure >185 mmHg, diastolic pressure >110 mmHg); a protocol for this is given in the proforma above
- If haemorrhage occurs, neurosurgical consultation is not indicated. However, agents to reverse bleeding (e.g. cryoprecipitate, fresh frozen plasma) should be readily available.

Avoiding and treating complications

- A number of treatment studies show that if the protocol is not adhered to, the risk of complications increases and possibly the efficacy decreases
- The major complication is cerebral haemorrhage within the infarcted region.
  Whether one should try to identify signs of early ischaemia and not thrombolyse if they are present and extensive is controversial:
  - The NINDS trial did not use any such CT cut-off
  - However, later trials used extensive early CT changes as an exclusion criterion: if greater than one-third of the MCA territory has ischaemic changes, then thrombolysis was not administered. Many units use this cut-off today
  - Identifying early CT changes may be difficult and requires training. This is covered in 📖 Chapter 7. A standardized scoring system (e.g. the ASPECTS scale, described on 📖 p. 168) may be helpful to ensure that all brain regions are observed.

Angio-oedema and anaphylaxis is a rare complication of rtPA; it is more common in patients on ACE inhibitors.

- It is life-threatening but rapidly reversible if treated promptly
- Symptoms include bronchospasm, hypotension, laryngeal and facial oedema, and urticaria
- Treat with IV adrenaline (epinephrine), 0.5 mL of a 1:1000 solution (i.e. 0.5 mg) IM. Repeat after 5 minutes if there is no improvement. Giving adrenaline IV is potentially hazardous and should be reserved for patients with immediately life-threatening profound shock
- Give chlorphenamine by IM or slow IV injection in a dose of 20 mg
- For patients with a severe or recurrent reaction, and in all patients with asthma, give hydrocortisone (sodium succinate) in a dose of 100–300 mg (depending on body size) by slow IV or IM injection.

Extending the time window for thrombolysis

IV thrombolysis has now been shown to benefit patients only when given within the first 4.5 hours. However, meta-analysis data suggest there may be some, although less, benefits if given after 4.5 hours. A number of approaches are being used to try to extend the time window.

- Trials are exploring the use of rtPA in all ischaemic stroke up to 6 hours post stroke
- Intra-arterial thrombolysis has been shown to be effective up to 6 hours
- New thrombolytics, (e.g. desmoteplase) may have longer time windows and better risk–benefit ratios; this is being tested in clinical trials
- PET imaging suggests that some patients have remaining ischaemic penumbra beyond 4.5 hours while others do not. The implication is that the former group may benefit from thrombolysis beyond 4.5 hours while the latter group will not (but may get side effects). Selecting these patients with PET is not practical, but MRI and CT offer methods by which the 'ischaemic penumbra' may be estimated
- MRI has been used to identify patients with diffusion–perfusion mismatch (see 📖 p. 178) as a crude indicator of existing penumbral tissue. Simplistically, tissue which is abnormal on DWI is thought to be destined for infarction, while tissue normal on DWI but abnormal on perfusion imaging is potentially salvageable. This has been shown to be a bit simplistic but nevertheless DWI–PWI mismatch does correlate with outcome
- CT perfusion is being used in a similar way. The core defined by the cerebral blood volume threshold matches DWI lesion volume and penumbral plus core on CT perfusion matches the PWI lesion volume
- Trials are selecting whether this method may be used to identify a group who may benefit from IV rtPA beyond 3 hours.

Sonothrombolysis

- *In-vitro* data suggest ultrasound itself may cause clot lysis
- It may act synergistically with rtPA
- One phase 2 trial, CLOTBUST, found standard TCD monitoring with a 2 MHz transducer increased recanalization rates in patients undergoing IV thrombolysis
- Another trial using low frequency ultrasound, which can deliver more energy through the skull, was associated with increased cerebral haemorrhage
- The addition of an ultrasound contrast agent (such as microbubbles) may increase recanalization rates further
- Further trials are required.

Intra-arterial thrombolysis

Intravenous thrombolysis will recanalize about one-third of vessels.

- The advantages of intra-arterial thrombolysis are that:
  - It is given in a very controlled fashion
  - It uses a lower dose of rtPA
  - It can establish whether the artery is still occluded
  - tPA is given directly into the clot
  - It may be combined with mechanical recanalization techniques
  - The success of recanalization may be assessed immediately
  - Further treatment may be applied until successful or the maximum dose of rtPA is exceeded.
- The disadvantages of intra-arterial thrombolysis are:
  - It is very time-consuming. While it takes only minutes to set up an infusion of thrombolysis, it may take up to an hour to set up the angiography suite to work and to catheterize the patient
  - This leads to a delay in delivery of thrombolysis
  - It may be technically difficult to identify and place a catheter within the artery, e.g. in acute carotid occlusion or in tortuous vessels
  - It requires a trained radiologist
- The PROACT trials used pro-urokinase which is metabolized to the active drug urokinase *in vivo*
- Pro-urokinase is also known as recombinant pro-urokinase or r-proUK
- The trial was small (180 subjects randomized to receive 9 mg of intra-arterial pro-urokinase with or without heparin within 6 hours of stroke onset) but provides evidence of potential benefit up to 6 hours
- The absolute increase in patients with slight or no disability at 3 months was 15% in the pro-urokinase group compared with the placebo group
- Therefore, seven patients need to be treated for one to achieve benefit
- The haemorrhage rate in the pro-urokinase group was 10%, versus 2% in subjects who received placebo
- However, no difference was noted in mortality (25% for pro-urokinase versus 27% for placebo).

In those units in which it is practised, intra-arterial thrombolysis is used as:

- A therapy for patients who arrive >3 hours from symptom onset and who have less than one-third involvement of the MCA territory on initial scans
- As a rescue therapy—some units give IV rtPA immediately and then if clinical recovery does not occur, and/or recanalization does not occur as determined on TCD, progress to intra-arterial therapy
- In cases where IV rtPA is throught to have less benefit, e.g. carotid T occlusions.

Mechanical clot lysis and retrieval

A number of devices have been developed to mechanically disrupt or retrieve the clot. The most studied is the Mechanical Embolus Removal in Cerebral Ischemia (MERCI) retrieval device. This is a catheter with a cork-screw on the end which is inserted into the artery and then corkscrewed into the clot and then pulled out. Again, this will unplug the artery and revascularize the brain.

- The recanalization rates are about 40–50%
- The results may be dramatic given the device is so dainty
- There is not enough evidence of general benefit to recommend its use outside a clinical trial
- Initial results were encouraging and the USA FDA licensed the device. However, there is insufficient data to be sure of its benefit and further randomized trial data is required.

Further reading

Evidence for thrombolysis

Hacke W, Kaste M, Bluhmki E *et al.* ECASS Investigators. (2008) Thrombolysis with alteplase 3 to 4.5 hours after acute ischemic stroke. *New England Journal of Medicine* **359**, 1317–29.

The National Institute of Neurological Disorders and Stroke rt-PA Stroke Study Group (1995) Tissue plasminogen activator for acute ischemic stroke. *New England Journal of Medicine* **333**, 1581–7.

Sonothrombolysis

Alexandrov AV, Molina CA, Grotta JC *et al.* for the CLOTBUST Investigators (2004) Ultrasound-enhanced systemic thrombolysis for acute ischemic stroke. *New England Journal of Medicine* **351**, 2170–8.

Intra-arterial thrombolysis

Furlan A, Higashida R, Wechsler L *et al.* (1999) Intra-arterial prourokinase for acute ischemic stroke. The PROACT II study: a randomized controlled trial. Prolyse in acute cerebral thromboembolism. *Journal of the American Medical Association* **282**, 2003–11.

Mechanical clot lysis and retrieval

Smith WS, Sung G, Starkman S *et al.* (2005) Safety and efficacy of mechanical embolectomy in acute ischemic stroke: results of the MERCI trial. *Stroke* **36**, 1432–8.

Neuroprotection

Following brain ischaemia a sequence of events occurs that results in brain damage.

- Brain ischaemia rapidly depletes intracellular ATP
- This leads to failure of membrane-bound ion channels
- This metabolic aberration results in accumulation of intracellular ions (especially calcium) and water by osmosis: cytotoxic oedema
- The falling blood flow means the cells cannot maintain their ionic balance and depolarize
- Calcium floods into the cells, triggering cell death mechanisms.

Several hours after the onset of ischaemia, the blood–brain barrier starts to break down and become permeable, allowing large plasma proteins to enter the extracellular space. Water follows when reperfusion occurs, causing vasogenic oedema. This process starts within a few hours of stroke and peaks at 5 days. It may result in leakage of blood into the brain tissues and haemorrhagic transformation.

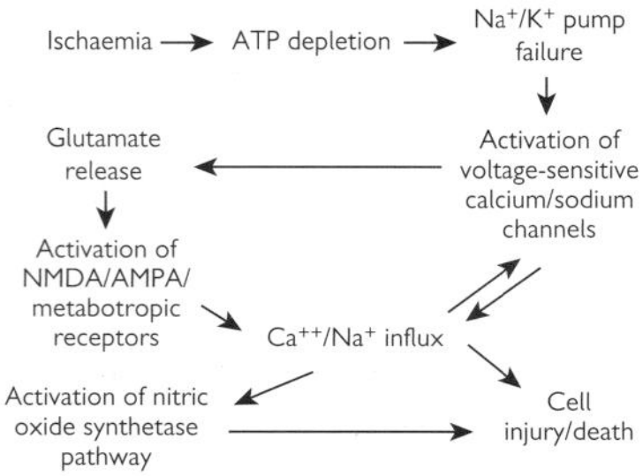

Fig. 9.6 A simplified diagram of events in the early part of the ischaemic cascade.

Trials of neuroprotection in stroke

It has been hoped that drug therapy can intervene in this ischaemic cascade and this is the rationale behind neuroprotection. Many agents have worked in animal models, but none have had replicable positive results in man.

Drugs have been developed which target many aspects of the ischaemic cascade.

Agents tested include:

- Calcium channel antagonists
  - After SAH, nimodipine reduces vasospasm and therefore subsequent stroke but it has no effect in acute ischaemic stroke
- Potassium channel openers
- Glutamate antagonists
- Anti-adhesion molecules
- N-methyl-D-aspartate (NMDA) receptor antagonists and modulators
  - NMDA receptors control the entrance of calcium into cells
  - They are therefore a logical therapeutic target
  - Unfortunately, no drug has been shown to be effective
  - The simplest agent, magnesium, which is a voltage-dependent channel blocker, showed some promise but a large trial (IMAGES) has not confirmed this
- Alpha-amino-3-hydroxy-5-methyl-4-isoxazolepropionic acid (AMPA) receptor antagonists
- Membrane stabilizers
  - Citicholine is a compound involving the synthesis of cell membranes
  - A small study showed that it may help stroke patients recover
  - However, no large scale trials have confirmed this
- Growth factors
  - Experiments have been done on fibroblast grown factor and transforming growth factor and these have not been successful
- Glycine-site antagonists
- Free radical scavengers
  - The free radical scavenger NXY-059 appeared to show benefit in The Stroke Acute Ischemic NXY-059 Treatment (SAINT-I) study but this was not replicated in the SAINT-2 trial.

Possible reasons for negative neuroprotection trials despite positive animal studies include:

- They really don't work
- Poor experimental methods in animal studies
- Animal models are not representative for human stroke
- They were tested in animal models when given before or just after stroke; in human stroke they cannot be given as quickly
- Treating one aspect of the ischaemic cascade is too simplistic and cocktails of a number of drugs may be more effective.

Further reading

Savitz SI, Fisher M (2007) Future of neuroprotection for acute stroke: in the aftermath of the SAINT trials. *Annals of Neurology* **61**, 396–402.

Antiplatelet therapy

Aspirin

- Most trials of antiplatelet agents in stroke have been in long-term secondary prevention rather than the acute phase
- In this setting, aspirin, clopidogrel, and the combination of aspirin and dipyridamole have been shown to be effective
- The risk–benefit ratio could be different in acute stroke owing to the risk of promoting haemorrhagic transformation within an infarct
- The International Stroke Trial (IST) and Chinese Aspirin Stroke Trial (CAST) showed in 40 000 patients that aspirin, given within 48 hours of stroke onset, has a small benefit in improving acute stroke outcome
- Both trials showed a small but significant reduction in recurrent ischaemic stroke risk of about 1 in 100 patients treated
- This was not accompanied by a significant risk of haemorrhagic stroke
- In each trial individually there was no significant reduction in death or dependency, but when both trials were combined in a meta-analysis there was a significant reduction in both endpoints
- As soon as haemorrhage has been excluded on brain imaging, aspirin should be started. A loading dose of 300 mg is usually given, followed by 75–150 mg OD. If the patient cannot swallow, it may be given rectally
- This reduces the risk of recurrent stroke by about one-third.

Table 9.2 Summary of results of the IST and CAST trials. Outcomes were assessed at 28 days in CAST and at 14 days and 6 months in IST

	CAST		IST	
	Aspirin	No aspirin	Aspirin	No aspirin
Number randomized	10 335	10 320	9719	9714
Early death (%)	3.3*	3.9*	9.0	9.4
Recurrent ischaemic stroke (%)	1.6**	2.1 **	2.8***	3.9 ***
Haemorrhagic stroke (%)	1.1	9	9	8
Recurrent stroke or death (%)	5.3*	5.9*	11.3*	12.4*
Dead or dependent at 28 days/6 months (%)	30.5	31.6	61.2	63.5

All the figures except the numbers randomized are percentages. *$P<0.05$; **$P<0.01$; ***$P<0.001$. IST, The International Stroke Trial (1997) Lancet **349**, 1569–81. CAST, randomized placebo-controlled trial of early aspirin use in 20,000 patients with acute ischaemic stroke. CAST (Chinese Acute Stroke Trial) Collaborative Group (1997) Lancet **349**, 1641–9.

Alternative antiplatelet agents in acute stroke

Dipyridamole

- The combination of dipyridamole and aspirin has been shown to be more effective than aspirin alone, and of similar effectiveness to clopidogrel alone, in the long-term secondary prevention of stroke (see 📖 Chapter 10)
- However, there is almost no data on the use of dipyridamole in acute stroke (i.e. being given within the first 48 hours)
- Nevertheless, many clinicians start aspirin and dipyridamole as soon as cerebral haemorrhage has been excluded.

Clopidogrel

- Clopidogrel has been shown to be slightly more effective than aspirin alone, and to have similar efficacy to the combination of aspirin and dipyridamole in the long-term secondary prevention of stroke (see 📖 Antiplatelet agents, p. 292)
- However, there is much less data on the use of clopidogrel in acute stroke
- Nevertheless, if patients cannot tolerate aspirin we give clopidogrel during the acute phase
- If clopidogrel is given acutely, a loading dose of 300 mg is recommended to achieve therapeutic plasma levels rapidly
- In patients with TIA and minor stroke, recent data has demonstrated a high early risk of recurrent stroke, which is much higher than previously appreciated. This is as high as 10–12% in the first week
- This risk appears to be particularly high in large artery disease (carotid and vertebral stenosis)
- This has led to the suggestion that aspirin and clopidogrel should be used in this setting
- Some preliminary data suggest the combination may be of benefit:
  - It reduced the rate of asymptomatic embolization monitored on TCD, compared with aspirin alone in patients with acute carotid stenosis and stroke/TIA (CARESS study)
  - It non-significantly reduced risk of recurrent stroke in patients with TIA and minor stroke in the phase II FASTER trial
- Phase III trials are planned to see if this combination really does help in this setting
- However, in long-term secondary prevention of stroke this combination was no better than clopidogrel alone, primarily because of an increase in bleeding complications (MATCH trial) and therefore it cannot be recommended for all patients until there is more data.

Further reading

Kennedy J, Hill MD, Ryckborst KJ *et al.* (2007) FASTER Investigators. Fast assessment of stroke and transient ischaemic attack to prevent early recurrence (FASTER): a randomised controlled pilot trial. Lancet Neurology **6**, 961–9.

Markus HS, Droste DW, Kaps M *et al.* (2005) Dual antiplatelet therapy with clopidogrel and aspirin in symptomatic carotid stenosis evaluated using Doppler embolic signal detection; the CARESS Trial. *Circulation* **111**, 2233–40.

Anticoagulation

Anticoagulation could be used in a number of settings in acute stroke.
1. At full dose for all patients with ischaemic stroke
2. In patients with cardioembolic sources, particularly atrial fibrillation
3. As proplylaxis for DVT.

Full dose anticoagulation in acute stroke

- Trial data has shown no benefit for full dose anticoagulation in acute phase
- The largest trial, the International Stroke Trial (IST), showed no overall benefit of subcutaneous heparin, with virtually identical death and dependency rates at 6 months (see Table 9.3)
- There was a reduction in recurrent stroke risk of about 1 in 100 (similar to that seen with aspirin), but this was countered by a similar increase in the risk of haemorrhagic stroke (which was not seen with aspirin)
- An early trial of low-molecular weight heparin in Hong Kong showed a benefit, but this could not be confirmed in a subsequent trial
- Therefore heparin should not be routinely used in acute stroke.

Table 9.3 Results from the IST showing that subcutaneous heparin reduced recurrent stroke risk, but increased hameorrhagic stroke risk

	IST	
	Heparin	**No heparin**
Number randomized	9717	9718
Death within 28 days (%)	9.0	9.3
Recurrent ischaemic stroke (%)	2.9*	3.8*
Haemorrhagic stroke (%)	1.2**	0.4**
Recurrent stroke or death (%)	11.7	12.0
Dead or dependent at 6 months (%)	62.9	62.9

All the figures except the numbers randomized are percentages. *$P<0.01$; **$P<0.00001$. IST, The International Stroke Trial (1997) Lancet **349**, 1569–81.

Anticoagulation in acute cardioembolic stroke

- Anticoagulation is a proven treatment for secondary prevention of cardioembolic stroke, primarily with atrial fibrillation (see 🕮 p. 298)
- When to start anticoagulation in patients with acute stroke and atrial fibrillation is controversial; there are no good quality study data
- There is the concern that it may result in haemorrhagic transformation, particularly for larger infarcts
- A reasonable approach is to wait for 2 weeks in patients with larger infarcts, but to start straight away in cases of TIA and minor stroke

- For larger infarcts we perform a CT scan prior to anticoagulation to ensure there is no spontaneous haemorrhagic transformation; if there is, we delay anticoagulation further.

Prophylaxis for DVT and pulmonary embolus

- DVT is very common after stroke, particularly in patients with hemiparesis and may result in pulmonary embolus
- In our experience many unexpected deaths in acute stroke patients turn out to have pulmonary embolus as a contributing cause at post mortem
- There is evidence that low dose heparin reduces pulmonary embolus risk in other settings, such as the postoperative period
- However, in acute stroke there is no trial evidence that the routine use of subcutaneous heparin improves outcome when given to all stroke patients
- In the PREVAIL trial, patients with ischaemic stroke with leg weakness of at least 2 on the NIHSS were randomized to receive either 5000 units unfractionated heparin twice daily or 40 mg of the low molecular weight heparin (LMWH) enoxaparin daily starting within 48 hours of stroke and continued for 10 days. Treatment allocation was not blinded, but the endpoints were objectively defined by routine venography (in 82% of subjects) and/or compression ultrasound in all subjects
- Enoxaparin was associated with a reduced risk of venous thomboembolic events of 43%, representing eight fewer events per 100 patients treated (number needed to treat for benefit: 13). Bleeding complications were rare
- Therefore, if DVT prophylaxis is used, LMWH is the agent of choice
- We tend to use LMWH prophylaxis in acute ischaemic stroke patients with severe hemiparesis, previous history of DVT, and/or new immobility
- Patients with proven pulmonary embolus should receive full anticoagulation with heparin followed by warfarin which is usually given for 3–6 months
- A not uncommon situation is the stroke patient with cerebral haemorrhage or other haemorrhagic complication (e.g. GI bleed) who develops pulmonary embolus. An inferior venous cava (IVC) filter is an option in such cases
- Thigh-length graduated compression stockings do not prevent DVT in acute stroke patients.

Further reading

Sherman DG, Albers GW, Bladin C *et al.* (2007)The efficacy and safety of enoxaparin versus unfractionated heparin for the prevention of venous thromboembolism after acute ischaemic stroke (PREVAIL study): an open-label randomised comparison. *Lancet* **369**, 1347–55.

The CLOTS trial collaboration (2009). *Lancet* **373**, 1958–65.

Acute stroke unit care

Considerable evidence from randomized trials has shown care on a stroke unit reduces mortality. Much of this is from subacute and rehabilitation units (see 📖 Chapter 16). More recently evidence has also become available for acute stroke units.

A large study comparing acute stroke unit care versus conventional care across many hospitals in Italy confirmed this finding. The results are shown is Table 9.4.

Exactly what components of acute stroke unit care improve outcome is uncertain but important factors include:

- Improved control of physiological parameters
  - Glucose
  - Pyrexia
  - Hypoxia
  - Blood pressure
- Prevention of complications
  - DVT and pulmonary embolus
  - Infection
- Hydration and feeding
- Reduced early recurrence
- Attention to detail and standard management protocols.

Thrombolysis is an important aspect of acute stroke care but does not account for the benefit seen in the trials as very few patients were thrombolysed in these studies and most were before widespread tPA use.

Therefore all stroke patients should be managed in a specialized unit.

Further reading

Livia Candelise, Monica Gattinoni, Anna Bersano *et al.*, on the behalf of the PROSIT Study Group (2007) Stroke-unit care for acute stroke patients: an observational follow-up study. *Lancet* **369**, 299–305.

Table 9.4 Two year outcome in patients admitted to acute stroke units compared with non-stroke unit/specialized stroke care

	Stroke unit (n=4936)	**Control (n=6636)**
Follow up (months)	19·7 (6·9)	20·4 (7·2)
Lost to follow up	172 (3%)	175 (3%)
In-hospital case fatality	542 (11%)	1034 (16%)
Death after discharge	821 (17%)	1348 (20%)
Alive at follow up	3401 (69%)	4079 (61%)
Rankin score=0*	735 (22%)	804 (20%)
Rankin score=1*	871 (26%)	941 (23%)
Rankin score=2*	547 (16%)	604 (15%)
Rankin score=3*	590 (17%)	740 (18%)
Rankin score=4*	471 (14%)	713 (17%)
Rankin score=5*	187 (5%)	277 (7%)
Stroke recurrence	195 (4%)	265 (4%)
Rehabilitation programme	1089 (22%)	1381 (21%)
New hospital admissions	835 (17%)	992 (15%)

Data was acquired from a large number of Italian hospitals although the study was observational rather than randomized. Data are mean (SD) or number (%). *Data are numbers (percentage of those alive at follow up).

Controlling physiological parameters

There is only limited evidence from randomized trials as to how intensively to control physiological and biochemical variables in the acute phase of stroke.

Studies comparing stroke outcome between countries have suggested that those units with better outcome control these variables more intensively.

Blood pressure

- Approximately 80% of stroke patients are hypertensive on admission, partly owing to pre-existing hypertension and also as an acute stress response to the stroke itself
- A higher blood pressure after stroke could be:
  - A good thing by increasing cerebral perfusion
  - A bad thing if it extended infarction, and increased the risk of both haemorrhagic transformation and recurrent stroke
- It has been suggested by different authorities that one should:
  - Increase blood pressure after stroke; non-randomized studies have suggested this may improve neurological scores
  - Reduce blood pressure
- Considerable epidemiological evidence suggests that high blood pressure after acute stroke is associated with worse outcome
- Recent evidence from phase 2 randomized controlled trials suggests lowering blood pressure may possibly be beneficial in ischaemic stroke (Control of Hypertension and Hypotension Immediately Post Stroke; (CHIPPS study), and may reduce haemorrhage expansion in cerebral haemorrhage (INTERACT study). Larger phase 3 trials are under way
- A reasonable approach in this currently evidence-free zone is to:
  - Avoid more than a 10% reduction in systolic BP within the first 24 hours unless blood pressure exceeds a high threshold value.
  - Start treatment if systolic pressure exceeds 200 mmHg systolic or diastolic pressure exceeds 110 mmHg
  - If blood pressure is below these limits then wait 48 hours before deciding on treatment
- In most cases blood pressure can be lowered using oral agents. (For choice see 📖 Chapter 10)
- If more rapid reduction is required this can be achieved with intravenous agents such as labetalol or, if less severe, with oral calcium channel blockers such as nifedipine. Sublingual nifedipine administration is not recommended as this may cause the blood pressure to drop excessively
- If rapid reduction of blood pressure is performed it should not be lowered at a rate >15 mmHg/hour, and precipitous falls should be avoided
- In patients with carotid occlusive disease, or other large artery stenoses/occlusions, lowering blood pressure may induce ischaemia and should be done more cautiously.

Hypotension

Hypotension episodes in the acute stroke setting may lead to cerebral hypoperfusion to the penumbra, and stroke extension.

Therefore blood pressure and heart rate should be closely monitored in the first few days post stroke.

The causes of hypotension are:

- Bleeding (e.g. GI haemorrhage on aspirin)
- Myocardial infarction
- Cardiac arrhythmia
- Heart failure
- Dehydration
- Sepsis
- Massive pulmonary embolus.

Treatment includes:

- Treatment of the underlying cause
- Fluid replacement
- Raising the foot of the bed
- Stopping hypotensive drugs
- Sometimes cardiac pressor drugs (e.g. noradrenaline) are necessary.

Hyperglycaemia

- An acute elevation of blood glucose often occurs in stroke
- This may represent:
  - Underlying diabetes mellitus in a known diabetic
  - Underlying diabetes mellitus in a newly diagnosed diabetic
  - A stress response in non-diabetics
- In animal models, elevated glucose is associated with increased infarct size and worse outcome
- Epidemiological data has associated elevated glucose in the acute phase following stroke with poor outcome. However, whether this is a consequence of the elevated glucose, or the elevated glucose is merely associated with some other parameter that worsens outcome, is not known
- It makes sense that better glycaemic control might improve outcome after stroke. However, this hypothesis as yet is unproven
- One randomized trial (GIST) failed to show a benefit. However, it was stopped early before the full sample size was obtained, and the glucose reduction seen in patients treated with insulin was modest
- Further data is required
- In the interim, it is reasonable to treat excessively raised glucose although the cut-off at which treatment should be instituted is controversial
- In our unit, we try to keep blood sugar below 10 mmol/L and use insulin to treat higher blood sugar concentrations. Our protocol is shown in Table 9.5.

Table 9.5 Sliding scale protocol for insulin administration post stroke

Blood glucose (mmol/L)	Units of insulin/hour	IV fluid
<3.0	0	40 ml 10% dextrose STAT, then 40 ml/hour
3.1–4.0	0	Dextrose 10% 40 ml/hour
If, after 2 hours, blood glucose is still <3mmol/L, call diabetic team		
4.1–6.9	1	Dextrose 10% 40 ml/hour
7–8.9	2	Dextrose 10% 40 ml/hour
9–11.9	3	Dextrose 10% 40 ml/hour
12–14.9	4	Dextrose 10% 40 ml/hour
15–17	6	Normal saline (0.9%) 40 ml/hour
>17	8	Normal saline (0.9%) 40 ml/hour and *seek urgent advice from diabetes team*

Fever

- Pyrexia is associated with worse outcome following stroke in animal models
- Pyrexia appears to be associated with worse outcome in stroke in man; however, whether this is a causal relationship is uncertain
- Fever may be central in origin but is often indicative of infection somewhere
- Common sites are:
  - Pneumonia
  - Urinary tract infection (especially if catheterized)
- And, less commonly:
  - Biliary
  - Large bowel diverticuli
  - Cellulitis
  - Joints
- Stroke itself may be associated with mild pyrexia.

Any patient with a fever should be carefully evaluated to identify a source of infection.

Appropriate other investigations may help, such as:

- FBC looking at the white cell count
- C-reactive protein
- Chest X-ray
- Urinalysis and culture
- Blood culture.

It has been suggested that fever should be treated with antipyretics (e.g. paracetamol). In 2008 the Paracetamol in Stroke study (PAIS) randomized stroke patients to high-dose paracetamol (6 g/day) or placebo started in the first 12 hours after symptom onset and continued for 3 days. Patients were included if they had a body temperature of between 36°C and 39°C at baseline. The planned sample size was 2500, but the trial was stopped after inclusion of 1368 patients for 'logistical reasons'. The primary analysis showed that 37% (260/697) of patients improved beyond expectation in the paracetamol group, and 33% (232/703) improved beyond expectation in the placebo, a difference that was not statistically significant (OR 1.21, 95% CI 0.97–1.51, $P=0.09$). There was a suggestion that there might be benefit in patients with a higher baseline temperature (>37°C)(OR 1.43, 95% CI 1.02–1.97).

Do not forget other causes of fever such as DVT or comorbidities, e.g. inflammation owing to flare-ups of arthritis (crystal arthropy or other forms of acute but non-infective arthritis can cause fever and be simply treated by joint aspiration and injection).

Hypothermia as a treatment

- Hypothermia is effective in stroke treatment in animal models
- A 2–3°C drop in temperature may be associated with a reduction in infarct volume of as much as 80%
- Cooling appears to delay a number of deleterious phenomena, including intracerebral acidosis, changes in blood–brain barrier permeability, impaired cerebral energy metabolism, and changes in the release of excitotoxic amino acids
- In man it has been shown to improve outcome in the treatment of cardiac arrest
- There have been small trials in stroke which are promising
- However, there is no large scale evidence that confirms its utility.

Further reading

Hypotension

Anderson CS, Huang Y, Wang JG *et al.* for the INTERACT Investigators. (2008) Intensive blood pressure reduction in acute cerebral haemorrhage trial (INTERACT): a randomised pilot trial. *Lancet Neurology* **7**, 391–9.

Potter JF, Robinson TG, Ford GA *et al.* (2009) Controlling hypertension and hypotension immediately post-stroke (CHHIPS): a randomised, placebo-controlled, double-blind pilot trial. *Lancet Neurology* **8**, 48–56.

Willmot M, Leonardi-Bee J, Bath PM (2004) High blood pressure in acute stroke and subsequent outcome: a systematic review. *Hypertension* **43**, 18–24.

Hyperglycaemia

Gray CS, Hildreth AJ, Sandercock PA *et al.* (2007) GIST Trialists Collaboration. Glucose-potassium-insulin infusions in the management of post-stroke hyperglycaemia: the UK Glucose Insulin in Stroke Trial (GIST-UK). *Lancet Neurology* **6**, 397–406.

Complications of stroke

Avoiding and treating complications is an important part of acute stroke care.

Common complications include:

- The deteriorating patient
- Cerebral oedema
- Aspiration and pneumonia
- DVT and pulmonary embolus
- Haemorrhagic transformation of an infarct
- Hydrocephalus (with cerebral haemorrhage)
- Epilepsy.

The deteriorating patient

Deterioration occurs in about 40% of patients during the first week after stroke and may present as:

- Worsening neurological scores: GCS or NIHSS
- New neurological signs
- Reduced conscious level.

Causes include:

- Extension of initial stroke
- Recurrent stroke
- Haemorrhagic transformation
- Cerebral oedema
- Hyponatraemia
- Secondary complications:
  - Epilepsy
  - Pneumonia and aspiration
  - Pulmonary embolus.

Risk factors include:

- Infarct already visible on CT
- Large infarct
- High blood pressure
- High glucose.

Management should include:

- Correction of physiological and metabolic derangements (see 🕮 p. 258)
- Treatment of secondary infections
- Treatment of dehydration
- Treatment of hypoxia which may result from aspiration, pneumonia or pulmonary embolism
- Brain imaging to exclude haemorrhagic transformation, cerebral oedema or recurrent stroke.

Cerebral oedema

- Cerebral oedema is an important cause of deterioration after large stroke. It is a greater problem in younger stroke. In older individuals, atrophy may have created space into which the swollen brain may expand

- Transtentorial herniation occurs mainly within 24–48 hours of cerebral haemorrhage and at 4–5 days after cerebral infarction
- The principal cause is supratentorial cerebral oedema resulting in secondary brainstem compression
- It may cause:
  - Drowsiness and reduced conscious level
  - Pupil asymmetry
  - Breathing abnormalities
- There is often a stable period followed by a deterioration with progressive impairment of consciousness, coma, and respiratory failure.

Treatment of cerebral oedema

General measures:

- Elevate the head and upper body 20–30°
- Position the patient to avoid compression of jugular veins
- Avoid glucose-containing intravenous solutions and/or hypotonic solutions
- Normothermia
- Normovolaemia and mean arterial blood pressure >110 mmHg
- Intubation
- Hyperventilation can be used as a supportive measure prior to surgery
- Barbiturates
- Steroids have little or no benefit—they are effective in vasogenic oedema (e.g. associated with brain tumours) but not in the cytotoxic oedema associated with infarction.

Specific measures include:

- Osmotherapy
- Hemicraniectomy.

Osmotherapy

- These agents are often used although this is not supported by trial data
- Options used include:
  - Mannitol
  - Glycerol.

Mannitol

- Start with 0.5–1.0 g/kg
- Then give 0.25–0.5 g/kg every 4 hours
- It is best used as a temporary holding measure before more definitive interventions such as surgical intervention.

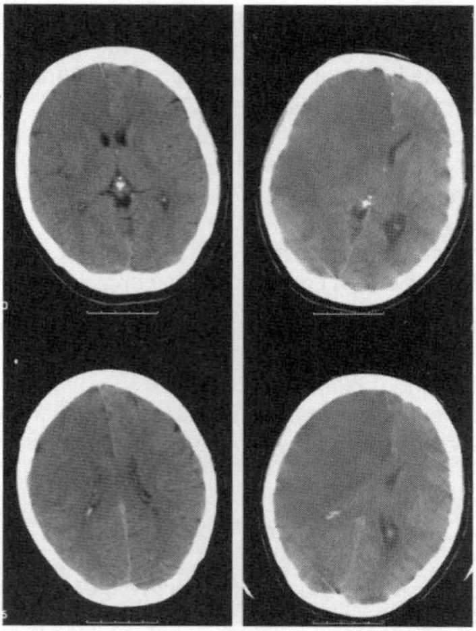

Fig. 9.7 CT scans showing massive right hemisphere swelling. The two images on the left are from a scan at 4 hours post stroke and show early ischaemic changes in the right carotid (both MCA and ACA) territory. The corresponding images on the right are from a scan the following day and show an established infarct with brain swelling into the left hemisphere. © Hugh Markus.

Hemicraniectomy

- First described in 1935
- Recently interest has been rekindled in this operation in patients with large MCA stroke
- A large bone flap is removed on the side of infarction site and the dura opened to reduce the pressure
- The operation is life-saving
- A recent meta-analysis of data from 129 patients from three small randomized controlled trials showed a highly significant reduction in mortality from 71% to 22% (see Fig. 9.8)
- There has been concern that the operation merely saves disabled patients
- Larger trials with quality of life assessments are required
- Results are less good in older patients (>50 years)
- Patients with early signs of large MCA infarcts should probably be identified early and operated upon within 24 hours
- Some clinicians only operate if the stroke affects the non-dominant hemisphere on the premise that quality of life will be poor if the speech areas are affected.

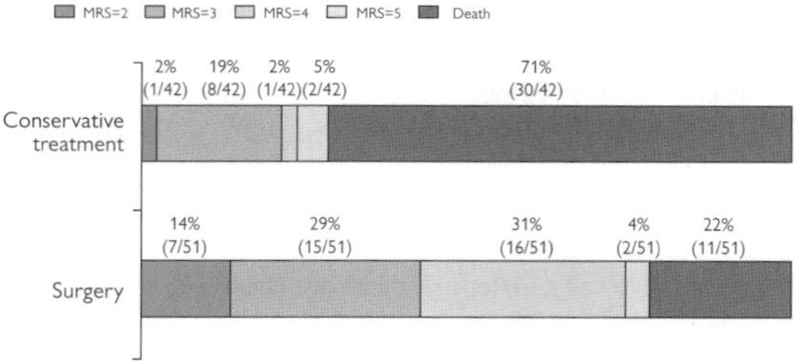

Fig. 9.8 Results of meta-analysis of the DECIMAL, DESTINY, and HAMLET studies showing improved outcome (measured by modified Rankin scale) in operated versus non-operated patients. Reproduced from Katayoun Vahedi K, Hofmeijer J, Juettler E *et al.* for the DECIMAL, DESTINY, and HAMLET investigators (2007) Early decompressive surgery in malignant infarction of the middle cerebral artery: a pooled analysis of three randomised controlled trials. *Lancet Neurology* **6**, 215–22, with permission of Elsevier.

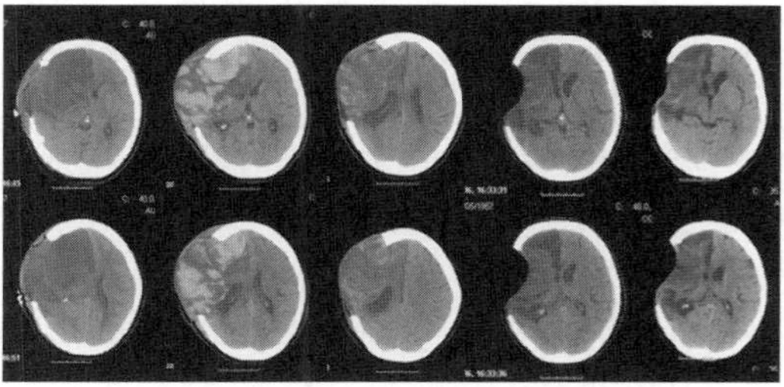

Fig. 9.9 A series of scans from a patient in their 40s with a right MCA infarct who had a hemicraniectomy. On the day 17 scan, secondary haemorrhage into the infarct can be seen. Over time the swelling resolves and has completely resolved by the day 50 scan. © Geoffrey Cloud.

Seizures after stroke

- Seizures complicate about 10% of strokes and are more common if there is cortical involvement
- About a third occur within the first week, and most of these within the first 24 hours
- Late onset seizures, occurring 2 weeks after the acute event, peak within 6–12 months after the stroke; they have a higher recurrence rate than early onset seizures
- One should only call it epilepsy if there are recurrent seizures. This develops in about one-third of early onset and half of late onset seizures
- Single seizures post stroke, particularly in the acute phase, do not need treatment
- If seizures are recurrent, standard anticonvulsants should be used; commonly used options are shown in Table 9.6. Phenytoin is less commonly used now due to its worse side effect profile. However, it can be useful acutely because plasma levels correlate with efficacy, and it can be used in acutely ill patients to guide dosage. If used acutely the patient can be loaded with IV phenytoin at 15 mg/kg (rate not greater than 50 mg/min) with ECG and blood pressure monitoring, followed by 300 mg OD IV (or orally) with dose then guided by plasma levels
- IV benzodiazepines should not be used after a single or couple of seizures in the acute phase. They are associated with respiratory depression and are sometimes used inappropriately, particularly in emergency departments. These seizures are usually self-terminating. Status epilepticus complicating acute stroke is very uncommon.

Table 9.6 Anticonvulsants commonly used to treat post-stroke seizures

Drug	Seizure types for which it is indicated	Pharmacokinetics	Side effects	Plasma therapeutic ranges
Carbamazepine	Focal	Enzyme inducer	Rash, diplopia, headache, dizziness, conduction block	Unhelpful
Sodium valproate	Any	No enzyme induction	Tremor, weight gain	Unhelpful
Lamotrigine	Any	No enzyme induction	Rash	Unhelpful
Phenytoin	Any	Enzyme inducer	Narrow therapeutic range, ataxia, nystagmus, gum hypertrophy, megaloblastic anaemia	10–20 mg/l (40–80 μmol/l)

Myint K, Staufenberg EFA, Sabanathan K (2006) Post-stroke seizure and post-stroke epilepsy. *Postgraduate Medical Journal* **82**, 568–72.

Dysphagia, swallowing, and aspiration

Dysphagia is common following stroke, particularly in patients with hemiparesis and/or brainstem stroke. The dysphagic patient is:

- Unable to protect their airway and may develop aspiration pneumonia or choke on food
- They cannot take medication and sufficient nutrition orally
- Therefore, it is imperative that swallowing is assessed early in all stroke patients
- The gag reflex is not a good determinant of the competence of swallowing
- The only way to test swallowing is to get the patient to swallow something (e.g. a small amount of water) and watch them do it
- Patients who cannot swallow should have a nasogastric tube placed to facilitate administration of their medication, oral nutrition, and hydration
- There is some debate as to the best timing of this; there is no strong eidence for guidance
- The FOOD trial randomized patients within 7 days of admission between early tube feeding and no tube feeding. A total of 859 patients was enrolled by 83 hospitals in 15 countries into the early versus avoid trial. Early tube feeding was associated with a non-significant reduction in risk of death of 5.8% (95% CI –0.8 to 12.5, P=0.09) and a reduction in death or poor outcome of 1.2% (–4.2 to 6.6, P=0.7)
- In most patients with dysphagia we tend to insert a nasogastric tube soon after stroke (within 48 hours) both to make the patient more comfortable with adequate hydration and to allow medication administration. It also allows intravenous fluids to be avoided which have the risk of precipitating cardiac failure in the predominantly elderly stroke population who often have cardiac comorbidity.

Swallowing assessment

Clues to difficulty swallowing include:

- Impaired conscious level
- Difficulty managing secretions
- A 'wet' sounding voice
- Choking or coughing while eating and/or drinking.

To assess swallowing:

1. With the patient sitting in upright position, place your index and middle fingers over patient's thyroid cartilage
2. Give the patient 60 ml of water in a cup
3. Instruct the patient to first take a small sip of water
4. If a problem is detected, *stop*!
5. If no problem occurs, proceed
6. Ask the patient to drink the remaining water as quickly and comfortably as possible
7. Allow 5 seconds to drink the water
8. Ask the patient to count out loud from 1 to 10.

If the patient fails the swallowing assessment or is too drowsy to swallow, then insert a nasogastric tube.

It is important to remember that swallowing may be normal soon after stroke but become unsafe. This is particularly common in larger infarcts that develop cerebral oedema, and swallowing may deteriorate a few days after stroke. Therefore swallowing needs monitoring over the first few days.

Acute psychiatric problems

Acute psychotic states may develop unexpectedly in acute stroke patients. Causes include:

- Acute organic reactions
- Severe depression
- Acute paranoid psychosis
- Exacerbation of pre-existing schizophrenia or mania.

Clues to the cause and management may be obtained from the history:

- Neurological and endocrine symptoms
- Past psychiatric problems
- Suicide attempts
- Medication history (cimetidine, anticholinergics)
- Drug history, including alcohol, cannabis, cocaine
- Drug withdrawal (e.g. benzodiazepines, barbiturates)
- Underlying systemic disease (cardiac, renal, hepatic or respiratory failure)
- Dementia
- Infection.

Management

- It is important to try to manage patients using a calm approach and a well lit, quiet place
- Management involves treatment of the underlying cause and withdrawal or reduction of as many psychotropic drugs as possible
- Avoid hypnotics
- If sedation is required, small doses of olanzapine (5–10 mg, maximum 20 mg daily) or chlorpromazine (25–50 mg max qds) may be given orally.

Alcohol withdrawal

This is not uncommon. It may need treatment. We use a benzodiazepine in reducing doses.

	Diazepam	**Chlordiazepoxide**
Day 1:	15 mg qds	30 mg qds
Day 2:	10 mg qds	30 mg tds
Day 3:	10 mg tds	20 mg tds
Day 4:	5 mg qds	20 mg bd
Day 5:	5 mg tds	10 mg bd
Day 6:	5 mg bd	10 mg nocte
Day 7:	5 mg nocte	

Also give vitamin B1 (thiamine), 100 mg orally two or three times daily for 3 weeks.

Patients with severe thiamine depletion or Wernicke's should have IV administration of B vitamins (e.g. Pabrinex) for 5 days followed by oral administration.

Further reading

Dysphagia, swallowing, and aspiration

Dennis MS, Lewis SC, Warlow C; FOOD Trial Collaboration (2005) Effect of timing and method of enteral tube feeding for dysphagic stroke patients (FOOD): a multicentre randomised controlled trial. *Lancet* **365**, 764–72.

Early secondary prevention of stroke

- Recent data has suggested that the risk of recurrent stroke after TIA and minor stroke is much higher than was previously appreciated
- In the prospective OXVASC study the risk of recurrent stroke following TIA was 8.0% (95% CI 2.3–13.7) at 7 days and 11.5% (4.8–18.2) at 1 month. Following minor stroke the 7-day and 1-month risks were 11.5% (4.8–11.2) and 15.0% (7.5–22.5). The survival curves are shown in Fig. 9.10. It is clear that the risk is highest very soon (within a couple of days) after the initial event
- The risk seems to be highest in patients with large artery disease (carotid and vertebral stenosis)
- Screening measures (e.g. the ABCD2 score, see 📖 p. 28) have been devised to identify high risk TIA patients
- This means that patients should be assessed urgently for secondary prevention measures
- How much of this early risk we can prevent, and which measures we should use, is uncertain and the subject of clinical trials
- There is some suggestion that more intensive antiplatelet regimens may be useful—the FASTER and CARESS trials suggest that clopidogrel and aspirin may be more effective than aspirin alone. This is now being tested in a large phase 3 trial
- Carotid endarterectomy should be performed as soon as possible in patients with TIA and minor stroke (see 📖 p. 302)
- A package of measures including urgent assessment and early secondary prevention was associated with a dramatic reduction in recurrent stroke risk in the EXPRESS study; 90-day risk was reduced from 10.3% (32/310 patients) in phase 1 to 2.1% (6/281 patients). However, this was an observational study comparing two management strategies, one which followed the other, rather than a randomized trial. Other alterations in care may have also occurred during the period of study which could have impacted on the differences in outcome.

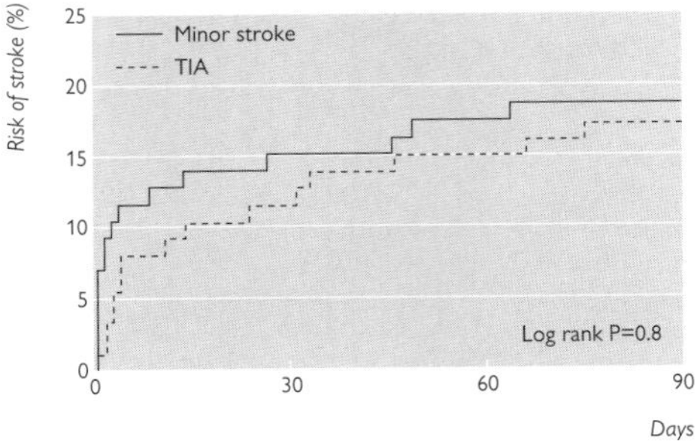

Fig. 9.10 Risk of recurrent stroke following TIA and minor stroke in patients in the prospective OXVASC study. Reproduced from Coull AJ, Lovett JK, Rothwell PM (2004) Population based study of early risk of stroke after transient ischaemic attack or minor stroke: implications for public education and organisation of services. *BMJ* **328**, 326, with permission from BMJ Publishing Group Ltd.

Further reading

Giles MF, Rothwell PM (2007) Risk of stroke early after transient ischaemic attack: a systematic review and meta-analysis. *Lancet Neurology* **6**, 1063–72.

Lovett JK, Coull AJ, Rothwell PM (2004) Early risk of recurrence by subtype of ischemic stroke in population-based incidence studies. *Neurology* **62**, 569–73.

Rothwell PM, Buchan A, Johnston SC (2006) Recent advances in management of transient ischaemic attacks and minor ischaemic strokes. *Lancet Neurology* **5**, 323–31.

Rothwell PM, Giles MF, Chandratheva A *et al.* (2007) Early use of Existing Preventive Strategies for Stroke (EXPRESS) study. Effect of urgent treatment of transient ischaemic attack and minor stroke on early recurrent stroke (EXPRESS study): a prospective population-based sequential comparison. *Lancet* **370**, 1432–42.

Chapter 10

Secondary prevention of stroke

Introducing stroke prevention

Types of stroke prevention

- Primary—in people who have never suffered stroke or TIA
- Secondary—in patients who have suffered stroke or TIA.

Secondary prevention can be usefully considered in two phases:

- Early secondary prevention
- Long-term secondary prevention.

Recent data has shown that the early risk of stroke after minor stroke and TIA is high—about 10–12% in the first week.

- The risk appears highest in stroke due to carotid/vertebral stenosis
- Early carotid endarterectomy is important in appropriate cases
- In this setting, a higher risk of treatment-related complications may be acceptable because of the greater potential benefit: for example, more intensive combination antiplatelet regimens might have a benefit owing to the high risk of stroke, compared with the slightly increased risk of bleeding over a short period of increased risk. More intensive antiplatelet and other preventative regimens may well be appropriate in this setting and are being tested
- For guidance on early secondary prevention see 📖 p. 272.

Most data on secondary prevention is on long-term secondary prevention. Most of these studies have included few patients within the first few days post stroke or TIA.

General considerations in secondary prevention

- The challenge of secondary prevention is to prevent a second stroke
- One in four strokes are second events
- Ischaemic stroke may be considered part of a systemic vascular disease process. As such, patients with symptomatic vascular disease in other vascular beds such as the coronary arteries (angina or myocardial infarction) or leg arteries (claudication) should also be considered for secondary stroke prevention
- The lifestyle advice given to address risk factors for vascular disease and stroke in primary prevention (see 📖 Chapter 1) should always be reinforced. The difference in secondary prevention is that the risk of stroke recurrence is higher. There is no time to lose to address risk factor modification and this generally requires medical intervention and, in some cases, surgery. Lifestyle changes remain important but there is less time for them to take effect
- Secondary prevention is a lifelong commitment involving a close relationship between doctor and patient. At the core is good patient education to ensure compliance
- Compliance is key and all secondary prevention treatment regimens should be tailored to the patient

- In some circles it can be argued that secondary prevention should not be: 'Should I lower this stroke patient's blood pressure?' or 'Should I put this stroke patient with AF on warfarin?' but rather 'How much can I lower this individual's blood pressure to maximize their risk reduction without making them ill?' and 'Why should I not be starting anticoagulation in a person with a stroke episode found to be in AF?'

Non-compliance

- Remember, as the number of medications goes up, the compliance goes down
- If the drugs aren't working (e.g. the blood pressure is still high on four medications), the patient may be treatment-resistant but it is more likely that they are not taking the medication
- You should bear non-compliance in mind but you should never be accusatory to your patient.

Assessing and explaining benefit

Risk:benefit ratios

When considering any preventative measure, one should consider:

- How effective it is at preventing stroke?
- What are the risks of the treatment?

The best way to present data on treatment benefits to a patient is using the number needed to treat (NNT). This is the number of patients needed to treat to prevent one additional bad outcome. It is calculated from the absolute risk reduction. It gives a good idea of the benefit of a treatment and is a simple and honest way to present the potential benefit of a treatment to a patient.

The potential benefit and NNT will depend how high the risk of recurrent stroke is during the period of treatment.

- If the risk of stroke is 2% a year, and treatment prevents 50% of stroke (i.e. relative risk of 50%), treating 100 patients for 1 year will only prevent one stroke; i.e. NNT is 100
- If the risk of stroke is 20% over 1 year, and the treatment prevents 25% of strokes, treating 100 patients for 1 year will prevent five strokes; i.e. NNT is 20
- One can see that the less effective treatments prevent more strokes if applied to a high risk group of patients
- This example shows how using relative risk to explain treatments to patients ('this treatment will half your risk of stroke') can be misleading.

Therefore, to assess benefit one needs to know the risk of stroke in the type of patient being treated.

Some rough estimates of stroke risk at different times post stroke are given in Table 10.1.

Certain conditions present particularly high risk, e.g. symptomatic carotid stenosis and atrial fibrillation, and, for these, specific data on risk is given in the relevant sections.

Effectiveness of secondary prevention after stroke

Table 10.1 Effectiveness of stroke prevention strategies

Strategy	Relative risk (RR) reduction, % (95% CI)	Number needed to treat to prevent 1 stroke a year*
Primary prevention strategies		
Antihypertensive therapy if blood pressure elevated	42 (33–50)	7937
Statins if cholesterol levels elevated	25 (14–35)	13333
Antiplatelet therapy		
Aspirin	RR increase, 7 (RR reduction of 5% to RR increase of 22%)	Not significant
Aspirin after myocardial infarction	36 (15–51)	400†
Angiotensin-converting enzyme inhibitor	30 (15–43)	11111
Carotid endarterectomy for asymptomatic stenosis	RR increase, 423 (127–1107)	Not significant
Secondary prevention strategies‡		
Antihypertensive therapy if blood pressure elevated	28 (15–39)	51 (16.5)§
Statins if cholesterol levels elevated	25 (14–35)	57 (10.2)§
Warfarin for non-rheumatic atrial fibrillation|	62 (48–72)	13 (10.5)§
Smoking cessation	33 (29–38)	43 (10.5)§
Antiplatelet therapy		
Aspirin	28 (19–36)	77 (9.9)§
Thienopyridines (versus aspirin)	13 (3–22)	64 (15.9)§
Carotid endarterectomy for symptomatic moderate/severe stenosis¶	44 (21–60)	26 (3.9)§

*Calculated by assuming that the annual risk of stroke is 0.03% (except where otherwise indicated) and using the best estimates of RR reduction from the literature, assuming constant RR reduction over time. Not that the baseline risk is variable (ranging from <1–80%), and therefore the number needed to treat could vary by more than a thousandfold, depending on this risk.

†Calculated by assuming that the risk of stroke is 0.01% over 2 years.

‡Calculated by assuming that the annual risk of recurrent stroke is 7% (except where otherwise indicated) and using the best estimates of RR reduction from the literature, assuming constant RR reduction over time.

§Numbers in parentheses are the percentage of all recurrent strokes avoided a year, assuming that all eligible patients receive the intervention. The percentage was calculated by factoring the absolute risk reduction from the intervention by the prevalence of the underlying risk factor in the population that has already experienced a stroke or transient ischemic attack.

|Calculated by assuming that the annual risk of recurrent stroke in a patient with non-rheumatic atrial fibrillation is 12%.

¶Calculated by assuming that the annual risk of recurrent stroke in a patient with moderate to severe carotid stenosis is 8.8%.

Reproduced from Straus SE, Majumdar SR, McAlister FA (2002). New evidence for stroke prevention scientific review. *JAMA* **288**(11):1388–1395.

Lifestyle measures

A number of lifestyle measures are associated with increased stroke risk, and addressing them is an important part of secondary prevention. Their association with stroke is described in 📖 Chapter 1. There is less data on the extent to which modifying them reduces recurrent stroke risk, partly because randomized controlled trials in this area are difficult to perform.

Lifestyle measures to address include:
- Healthy eating
- Taking more exercise
- Stopping smoking
- Moderating alcohol consumption
- Losing weight.

In addition to possible benefits on stroke risk, lifestyle modification is worth pursuing if only because it provides a context in which the patient adjusts to the stroke and takes the secondary prevention medication. By giving the patient lifestyle measures to address, it also gives the patient some 'control' and responsibility over their condition.

Healthy eating

A healthy 'cardiovascular diet' is important. This should include:
- Plenty of fruits and vegetables—at least five portions a day
- Low levels of fats, particularly saturated fats
- Low salt levels—avoid processed foods, many of which have large amounts of added salt
- Oily fish may reduce cardiovascular risk.

A cardiovascular diet may reduce risk by multiple mechanisms, including lowering BP, reducing weight, lowering cholesterol, and improving glucose tolerance.

Data from a randomized controlled trial in patients post-myocardial infarction showed a Mediterranean diet was associated with a 50% reduction in recurrent MI, death, and other cardiovascular events. No such trials have been performed in stroke but there are likely to be similar benefits.

Details on many suitable diets and healthy eating advice for patients are widely available on the web. For example:
- British Heart Foundation: http://www.bhf.org.uk/keeping_your_heart_healthy/default.aspx
- The DASH diet is a stringent diet aimed at reducing hypertension. It is rich in whole grain foods, fruit, vegetables, low fat or non-dairy product, lean meat, fish, fowl, nuts, and some fats and sweets. www.dashdiet.org

Physical activity

Physical activity probably improves many stroke risk factors. It may:
- Lower BP
- Lower weight
- Improve glucose tolerance.

Overall, it reduces risk of stroke by about a fifth.

Obesity

- Obesity is defined as a body mass index (BMI) of >30 kg/m^2
- It is an independent risk factor for stroke
- Obesity is related to several major risk factors:
  - Hypertension
  - Diabetes
  - Hyperlipidaemia.

Losing weight:

- Improves blood pressure
- Reduces fasting glucose
- Reduces serum lipids
- Improves physical fitness

Alcohol consumption

- Studies indicate that reduction in alcohol intake is useful for primary prevention in stroke. There is no type of alcohol that is either more beneficial or harmful than another
- Chronic alcohol and heavy drinking are risk factors for all stroke subtypes
- There is a J-shaped relationship between alcohol and cardiovascular disease, including stroke
- Alcohol in moderation (20–30 g per day) appears protective—the relative risk reduction for stroke is in the order of 25–30%
- Alcohol intake of >60 g per day causes an increased relative risk of all stroke of about 1.6, but over 2 for haemorrhagic stroke
- High alcohol may increase hypertension, hypercoagulability, and atrial fibrillation
- In the UK, the recommended alcohol intake is 21 international units for a man and 14 for a woman per week.

Smoking

- Smoking contributes to large-vessel atherosclerosis and cardiac disease and thereby stroke
- The risk of ischaemic stroke in smokers is twice that of non-smokers
- The risk of haemorrhagic stroke in smokers is between two and four times higher than that of non-smokers
- After 2 years of stopping smoking, stroke reduces to about 50% and returns to near baseline by 5 years (Framingham data)
- Patients are unable to smoke while in hospital; later, it is important to give them advice on how to stop and perhaps refer to a smoking cessation clinic. Some patients need patches
- However, these are contraindicated in acute stroke and we do not use them until a month has elapsed
- All stroke patients who smoke should be strongly advised to stop and offered appropriate counselling.

Further reading

de Lorgeril M, Salen P, Martin J-L *et al.* (1999) Mediterranean diet, traditional risk factors, and the rate of cardiovascular complications after myocardial infarction. Final Report of the Lyon Diet Heart Study. *Circulation* **99**, 779–85.

Nicotine products to help stop smoking

Product type	How it works
Nicotine gum	When you chew nicotine gum, the nicotine is absorbed through the lining of your mouth
Nicotine patches	Nicotine patches work well for most regular smokers and can be worn around the clock (24-hour patches) or just during the day (16-hour patches)
Nicotine microtabs	These are small tablets containing nicotine which dissolve quickly under your tongue
Nicotine lozenges	Lozenges are sucked slowly to release the nicotine and take about 20–30 minutes to dissolve
Nicotine inhalators	Inhalators look like a plastic cigarette. The inhalator releases nicotine vapour which gets absorbed through your mouth and throat. If you miss the 'hand to mouth' aspect of smoking, these may suit you
Nicotine nasal spray	The spray delivers a swift and effective dose of nicotine through the lining of your nose

Other stop smoking medicines that can help

Product type	How it works
Bupropion hydrochloride (Zyban®)	Bupropion hydrochloride is a treatment which changes the way that your body responds to nicotine. You start taking Zyban 1–2 weeks before you quit and treatment usually lasts for a couple of months to help you through the withdrawal cravings. It is only available on prescription in the UK and is contraindicated in pregnancy
Varenicline (Champix®)	Varenicline works by reducing your craving for a cigarette and by reducing the effects you feel if you do have a cigarette. You set a date to stop smoking, and start taking tablets 1 or 2 weeks before this date. Treatment normally lasts for 12 weeks. It is only available on prescription in the UK and is contraindicated in pregnancy

Blood pressure

- Lowering blood pressure is the single most important intervention in the secondary prevention of stroke
- Blood pressure is an independent risk factor for recurrent stroke and the higher the BP (systolic or diastolic) the higher the risk
- Antihypertensive treatment has been shown to reduce stroke risk in many trials and is associated with up to 40% stroke risk reduction
- Lifestyle modifications are part of the treatment of blood pressure
- Until recently, most data was from primary prevention trials. Some questioned whether reducing established hypertension in patients with stroke could worsen outcome, owing to reduced cerebral perfusion in patients with impaired cerebral autoregulation
- The Perindopril Protection Against Recurrent Stroke Study (PROGRESS) trial demonstrated that reducing blood pressure was as beneficial in secondary prevention as in primary prevention:
  - In PROGRESS, 6105 patients with stroke or TIA within the previous 5 years were randomized to perindopril or perindopril plus indapamide
  - The risk of both haemorrhagic and ischaemic stroke was reduced from 14% to 10% (a relative risk reduction of 28%)
  - Combination therapy resulted in a greater BP reduction (mean 12/5 mmHg) and greater clinical benefit: 43% reduction in recurrent stroke
  - There was no benefit in giving perindopril alone but the BP drop was much less (5/3 mmHg)
  - A similar relative risk reduction was seen in patients with raised or *normal* blood pressure
  - This has led to the suggestion that all patients with stroke should receive antihypertensive agents unless they have low blood pressure
- Most guidelines recommend a target BP of 130/80 mmHg or below and we would aim for this in all stroke patients
- Blood pressure reduction is important for both ischaemic and haemorrhagic stroke
- The overall reduction in stroke and all vascular events is related to the degree of BP lowering achieved
- There is no definite evidence that one class of agent is better—it appears what is most important is the magnitude of the blood pressure drop
- Therefore we usually start a diuretic and ACE inhibitor initially based on the PROGRESS trial evidence
- It is still unclear as to when to start lowering blood pressure in acute stroke (see 🕮 p. 258), but certainly after the first month all stroke patients should be considered to have BP lowered.

For every 1 mmHg blood pressure reduction, recurrent stroke risk is reduced by 3%. Therefore, if BP is reduced by 10 mmHg, stroke risk is reduced by up to 30%.

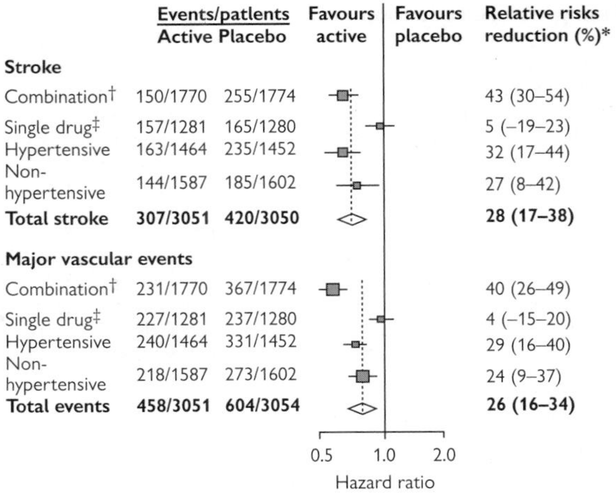

*95% confidence interval in parentheses
†Perindopril plus indapamide
‡Perindopril alone

Fig. 10.1 Rate of stroke during follow up in PROGRESS in the study group as a whole and in the different subgroups. Active treatment was either perindopril or perindopril and indapamide. *95% CI in parentheses; †perindopril plus indapamide; ‡perindopril alone. Reproduced from PROGRESS Collaborative Group (2001) *Lancet* **358**, 1033–41 with permission from Elsevier.

Blood pressure reduction in special groups

- Whilst there is often concern about lowering BP in patients with occlusive or stenotic extracranial disease for fear of reducing the perfusion above the stenosis, this is rarely an issue in clinical practice. In the minority of patients with carotid stenosis/occlusion and impaired haemodynamic reserve, haemodynamic symptoms may well be alleviated by reducing or stopping antihypertensive medication (this may be a useful temporary strategy while revascularization is considered)
- With the recent results of the HYVET study (Beckett *et al.*, 2008) confirming the benefit of primary prevention of BP lowering in those over 80 years, it is reasonable to assume that all stroke patients, regardless of age, should be treated for persistent raised BP after stroke. Frail, older stroke patients are, however, likely to be more susceptible to side effects of antihypertensive drug treatments.

Reference

Beckett NS, Peters R, Fletcher AE *et al.* for the HYVET Study Group (2008) Treatment of hypertension in patients 80 years of age or older. *New England Journal of Medicine* **358**, 1887–98.

Lawes CM, Bennett DA, Feigin VL, Rodgers A (2004) Blood pressure and stroke: an overview of published reviews. *Stroke* **35**, 1024.

PROGRESS Collaborative Group. Randomised trial of a perindopril-based blood-pressure-lowering regimen among 6105 individuals with previous stroke or transient ischaemic attack. *Lancet* **358**, 1033–41.

Cholesterol

- Clinical trials have shown convincingly that reducing cholesterol with statins reduces ischaemic stroke risk
- Most trial data is from studies in patients with coronary heart disease or cardiovascular disease of all types rather than specifically in stroke. For example, the Heart Protection Study (HPS) randomized 20 000 individuals with a history of coronary heart disease, other occlusive arterial disease or diabetes to either simvastatin 40 mg or placebo. Over a mean follow up of 5 years there were highly significant reductions in mortality (13%), major coronary events (27%), and stroke (25%). The reduction in stroke was in ischaemic stroke, with no reduction in cerebral haemorrhage
- Stroke events in these studies were secondary outcomes—the trials were designed to answer the question of reduced myocardial infarct or vascular death
- The Stroke Prevention by Aggressive Reduction in Cholesterol Levels (SPARCL) study was the first trial of statin therapy (atorvastatin 80 mg) to take a group of stroke patients and randomly assigned them to statin or placebo. A total of 4731 patients with previous TIA or stroke were randomized
- The statin group showed a significant reduction in recurrent stroke (absolute risk reduction of 2.2% over 5 years, hazard ratio risk reduction of 16%, NNT to save one recurrent stroke 45)
- Whilst SPARCL has reinforced what is already becoming usual practice of treating all stroke patients with statin therapy, the trial did not include any patients with cardioembolic stroke (e.g. those in AF) and did not address the contentious area of whether to prescribe statin therapy for haemorrhagic stroke. Also, only just over one-fifth of the patients enrolled were female
- In SPARCL there was a slightly increased risk of recurrent haemorrhagic stroke in the treatment group, supporting the suggestion that high-dose statin therapy probably does not benefit such patients
- The benefit seen in SPARCL is thought to be mediated through LDL reduction and, interestingly, subgroup analysis showed that those patients with large-vessel carotid disease stroke benefited most
- The current UK RCP guidelines recommend lipid-lowering treatment in all patients with ischaemic stroke and TIA if total (fasted) cholesterol is 3.5 mmol/L or more
- Our current practice is to prescribe all ischaemic stroke patients statins—on the basis of the results of the HPS trial (and cost considerations) we use 40 mg of simvastatin, except in diabetic patients who are preferentially prescribed atorvostatin 40–80 mg. If simvastatin does not control cholesterol levels, we switch to an alternative agent such as atorvastatin
- We would not routinely prescribe statins for haemorrhagic stroke unless patients had other established atherosclerotic disease, such as symptomatic coronary artery disease
- For patients with both ischaemic and haemorrhagic cerebrovascular disease we generally do prescribe statins

- Statins are thought to act primarily by cholesterol/LDL reduction, and the magnitude of benefit correlates with the degree of cholesterol reduction in clinical trials. It has also been suggested they may have other beneficial 'pleiotropic' effects, including:
  - Plaque stabilization
  - Improved endothelial function
- Unlike BP lowering, the evidence for aggressive lipid-lowering in older patients, especially over the age of 80 years, is sparse.

Other medications also used to treat hyperlipidaemia include:
- Niacin
- Fibrates
- Cholesterol absorption inhibitors.

Table 10.2 Effect of cholesterol reduction of 1 mmol/L of LDL on all stroke, by risk factors and stroke type (any type of lipid lowering medication)

Category	Trials	Events	Percent change in risk (95% CI)
All stroke	41	3319	–20 (–14 to –26)
All stroke in people with known vascular disease	32	2311	–22 (–28 to –16)
All stroke in people without known vascular disease	7	752	–6 (–22 to 14)
Thromboembolic stroke	8	1204	–28 (–35 to –20)
Haemorrhagic stroke	8	149	–3 (–35 to 47)
Fatal stroke	56	678	–2 (–17 to 16)
Non-fatal stroke	40	2519	–23 (–29 to –16)

Reproduced from Prospective Studies Collaboration (2007) Blood cholesterol and vascular mortality by age, sex and blood pressure: a meta-analysis of individual data from 61 prospective studies with 55 000 vascular deaths. *Lancet* **370**, 1829–39, with permission of Elsevier.

Further reading

Law MR, Wald NJ, Rudnicka AR (2003) Quantifying effect of statins on low density lipoprotein cholesterol, ischaemic heart disease, and stroke: systematic review and meta-analysis. *BMJ* **326**, 1423–9.

The Stroke Prevention by Aggressive Reduction in Cholesterol Levels (SPARCL) investigators (2006) High-dose atorvastatin after stroke or transient ischaemic attack. *New England Journal of Medicine* **355**, 549–59.

Diabetes

- Good diabetic control is essential to reduce the risk of further microvascular and macrovascular disease
- Most of the available data on stroke prevention in patients with diabetes are on primary rather than secondary prevention of stroke. Intensive treatment addressing multiple risk factors, including control of hyperglycaemia, hypertension, and dyslipidaemia, have demonstrated reductions in the risk of cardiovascular events
- Tighter glycaemic control has been shown to reduce the occurrence of microvascular complications (nephropathy, retinopathy, and peripheral neuropathy) in several clinical trials, and is recommended in multiple guidelines of both primary and secondary prevention of stroke and cardiovascular disease. Data on the efficacy of glycaemic control on macrovascular complications, including stroke, are more limited
- Analysis of data from randomized trials suggests a continual reduction in vascular events with the progressive control of glucose to normal levels
- Normal fasting glucose is defined as glucose <5.6 mmol/L (100 mg/dL), impaired fasting glucose has been defined as levels between 5.6 and 6.9 mmol/L (100–126 mg/dL). Diabetes is defined by a fasting plasma glucose level >7.0 mmol/L (126 mg/dL) or a non-fasting plasma glucose >11.1 mmol/L (200 mg/dL)
- The glycosylated haemoglobin A_{1c} level is useful in monitoring diabetes control. A level >7% is considered as inadequate control of hyperglycaemia. Therefore one should look for levels of haemoglobin A_{1c} of <7%
- There is good evidence that vigorous control of blood pressure in patients with diabetes mellitus reduces stroke risk. For example, in patients with diabetes randomized into the Hypertension Optimal Treatment trial (HOT), there was a 51% reduction in major cardiovascular events in patients allocated to a target blood pressure of 80 mmHg diastolic compared with those aiming for 90 mmHg
- Although all major classes of antihypertensives are suitable for BP control in patients with diabetes, most patients will require more than one agent. ACE inhibitors and angiotensin receptor blockers are more effective in reducing the progression of renal disease and are recommended as first-choice medications for patients with diabetes mellitus
- Trial evidence also supports reducing cholesterol in this patient group. The HPS demonstrated the beneficial effect of simvastatin use in diabetic patients. A total of 5963 people >40 years of age with diabetes were randomized to simvastatin 40 mg daily or placebo. Simvastatin was associated with a 28% (95% CI, 8–44) reduction in ischaemic strokes (3.4% simvastatin versus 4.7% placebo; P=0.01)
- More rigorous control of blood pressure and lipids should be considered in all diabetic stroke patients.

Homocysteine

- Homocysteine is an independent risk factor for cardiovascular disease and stroke (see 📖 p. 34)
- Homocysteine levels can be reduced by vitamin B complex and folic acid treatment
- However, whether reducing levels in stroke patients reduces risk of recurrent stroke is uncertain
- The Vitamin Intervention for Stroke Prevention (VISP) study randomized patients with a stroke and mild to moderate hyperhomocysteinaemia (>9.5 µmol/L for men, 8.5 µmol/L for women) to receive either a high- or low-dose vitamin therapy (e.g. folate, B6, or B12) for 2 years.The mean reduction in homocysteine was greater in the high-dose group. However, there was no reduction in stroke rates in the patients given high-dose vitamin, with 2-year stroke rates of 9.2% in the high-dose and 8.8% in the low-dose arm. A possible confounding effect was that fortification of bread with folic acid was commenced during the study
- Further trials (e.g. VITATOPS) are examining this question
- Until more data become available, whether to treat elevated homocysteine is a matter of individual choice. In patients in whom we wish to lower it we give daily folic acid 5 mg and 250 mg vitamin B6 (as part of strong vitamin B mixed tablet) supplements.

Further reading

Spence JD (2007) Homocysteine-lowering therapy: a role in stroke prevention? *Lancet Neurology* **6**, 830–8.

Spence JD, Bang H, Chambless LE, Stampfer MJ (2005) Vitamin intervention for stroke prevention trial: an efficacy analysis. *Stroke* **36**, 2404–9.

Antiplatelet agents

- After an ischaemic stroke, all patients should be considered for antiplatelet therapy
- There are three options for long-term secondary prevention:
  - Aspirin
  - Aspirin and dipyridamole
  - Clopidogrel
- All three drugs inhibit platelet activation and aggregation, but by different mechanisms:
  - Aspirin by inhibiting cyclo-oygenase and thromboxane A2
  - Dipyridamole by increasing plasma adenosine and inhibiting platelet phosphodiesterase
  - Clopidogrel by blocking ADP receptors.

Aspirin

- In an Antithrombotic Trialists' Collaboration, meta-analysis of results of 21 randomized trials comparing antiplatelet therapy with placebo in 18 270 patients with prior stroke or TIA, antiplatelet therapy was associated with a 28% relative odds reduction in non-fatal strokes and a 16% reduction in fatal strokes
- Aspirin in doses ranging from 50 to 1300 mg/day appears to prevent recurrent ischaemic stroke
- Higher (1200 mg/day) or lower (75–300 mg/day) have similar effects on stroke prevention
- However, higher doses produce more side effects
- Therefore a dose in the range 75–300 mg daily is recommended.

Ticlopidine

- This is a thienopyridine with a similar mechanism of action to clopidogrel
- It has been evaluated in three randomized trials of patients with stroke. It seems as effective as aspirin but causes neutropenia in 2% of patients. Therefore if used, follow up blood count monitoring is required. However, clopidogrel has similar efficacy without this side effect and is now used instead.

Clopidogrel

- Clopidogrel monotherapy (75 mg od) appears to be as good, or slightly more effective, than aspirin
- If required, to rapidly achieve plasma levels a 300 mg loading dose od is used.

CAPRIE

- The efficacy of clopidogrel monotherapy was compared with that of aspirin in the Clopidogrel versus Aspirin in Patients at Risk of Ischemic Events (CAPRIE) trial
- More than 19 000 patients with stroke, MI, or peripheral vascular disease were randomized to aspirin 325 mg/day or clopidogrel 75 mg/day

- The primary endpoint, a composite outcome of ischaemic stroke, MI, or vascular death, occurred in 8.7% fewer patients treated with clopidogrel compared with aspirin (*P*=0.043)
- However, in a subgroup analysis of those patients with prior stroke, the risk reduction with clopidogrel was slightly smaller and was not significant.

MATCH

- The Management of Atherothrombosis With Clopidogrel in High-Risk Patients With TIA or Stroke (MATCH) trial showed the combination of clopidogrel and aspirin had no benefit over clopidogrel alone
- Patients with prior stroke or TIA plus additional risk factors (*n*=7599) were allocated to clopidogrel 75 mg or clopidogrel plus aspirin 75 mg od
- The primary outcome was the composite of ischaemic stroke, MI, vascular death, or rehospitalization secondary to ischaemic events
- There was no significant benefit of combination therapy compared with clopidogrel on the primary outcome or any of the secondary outcomes
- The risk of major haemorrhage was increased in the combination group compared with clopidogrel alone, with a 1.3% absolute increase in life-threatening bleeding. Although clopidogrel plus aspirin is recommended over aspirin for acute coronary syndromes, the results of MATCH do not suggest a similar risk:benefit ratio for long-term secondary prevention in stroke and TIA survivors.

Dipyridamole

- Limited data suggest that dipyridamole monotherapy is probably about as effective as aspirin. Considerable evidence suggests that the combination of aspirin and dipyridamole is better than aspirin alone
- The European Stroke Prevention Study 2 (ESPS-2) randomized 6602 patients with prior stroke or TIA in a factorial design using a different dipyridamole formulation and aspirin dose compared with ESPS-1. The treatment groups were:
  - Aspirin 50 mg/day plus extended-release dipyridamole 400 mg/day
  - Aspirin alone
  - Extended-release dipyridamole alone
  - Placebo
- The risk of stroke was significantly reduced, by 18% on aspirin alone, 16% with dipyridamole alone, and 37% with a combination of aspirin plus dipyridamole

The ESPIRIT study confirmed this:

- Patients within 6 months of a transient ischaemic attack or minor stroke of presumed arterial origin were randomized to aspirin (30–325 mg daily) with (*n*=1363) or without (*n*=1376) dipyridamole (200 mg twice daily)
- Treatment was open, but auditing of outcome events was blinded
- Mean follow up was 3.5 years (SD 2.0)

- Primary outcome events (the composite of death from all vascular causes, non-fatal stroke, non-fatal MI, or major bleeding complication, whichever happened first) occurred in 13% of patients on aspirin and dipyridamole and in 16% on aspirin alone (hazard ratio 0.80, 95% CI 0.66–0.98; absolute risk reduction 1.0% per year, 95% CI 0.1–1.8)
- Patients on aspirin and dipyridamole discontinued medication more often than those on aspirin alone (470 versus 184), mainly because of headache
  - If dipyridamole is used, the modified release preparation (200 mg bd) should be given as this was the formulation shown to be beneficial in trials
  - If the patient is being NG fed, or in those countries where the slow release preparation is not available, the standard preparation (100 mg tds) can be given. It is available as a liquid
  - Headache is the most common side effect of dipyridamole. If it occurs, reduce the dose to 200 mg od and it may pass after a few days, when the dose can be increased. In 10–20% of cases, headache prevents continued use.

Clopidogrel versus aspirin + dipyridamole

- The recent PRoFESS results randomized stroke patients between 25 mg of aspirin plus 200 mg extended-release dipyridamole bd or clopidogrel 75 mg od
- A total of 20 332 patients was followed for a mean of 2.5 years
- Recurrent stroke occurred in 916 (9.0%) receiving ASA-ERDP and in 898 (8.8%) receiving clopidogrel (hazard ratio, 1.01; 95% CI 0.92–1.11)
- There were more major haemorrhagic events in the aspirin +dipyridamole group (4.1 versus 3.6%, hazard ratio, 1.15; 95% CI, 1.00– 1.32), including intracranial haemorrhage (hazard ratio, 1.42; 95% CI, 1.11–1.83)
- The net risk of recurrent stroke or major haemorrhagic event was similar in the two groups (aspirin+dipyridamole 11.7% versus 11.4% with clopidogrel, hazard ratio, 1.03; 95% CI, 0.95–1.11).

Which regimen should you use?

- Current European and NICE guidance on the basis of the ESPRIT and ESPS-2 studies recommends the combination of dipyridamole modified release as being more effective than aspirin alone
- In patients who cannot tolerate aspirin, clopidogrel is recommended
- The PRoFESS trial suggests aspirin and dipyridamole and clopidogrel are equally effective regimens. The former is cheaper in most countries but the latter means patients have to take only one tablet a day
- Our current practice is to use aspirin and dipyridamole in combination as first line therapy for all new stroke episodes
- For patients with no discernible risk factors, e.g. cryptogenic stroke in young patients under 45 years, we may use aspirin alone at low dose 75 mg on the basis they have a low risk of recurrence with no comorbidity
- For polyvascular patients (i.e. patients with symptomatic atherosclerotic disease outside of the brain) and those with symptomatic coronary disease, we use clopidogrel 75 mg alone
- For patients who are truly aspirin-intolerant or patients having recurrent events on aspirin we use clopidogrel 75 mg alone.

Special situations

In certain situations the combination of aspirin and clopidogrel is often used.

Carotid stenting

Most clinicians use clopidogrel and aspirin therapy perioperatively and usually for a period of 1–3 months post-stenting. This is based on trials in coronary stenting although there are no trial data for carotid stenting.

Large-artery disease during the acute phase

Patients with large-artery disease (e.g. carotid stenosis, MCA stenosis) have a very high risk of early recurrent stroke. In this setting some clinicians use the combination of clopidogrel and aspirin. In the CARESS study in recently symptomatic carotid stenosis it was more effective than aspirin alone in reducing asymptomatic cerebral emboli detected on transcranial Doppler and there appeared to be a reduction in recurrent clinical events (although the study was not powered for this). The combination may be used for:

- Symptomatic high grade carotid stenosis not amenable to intervention
- Symptomatic intracranial stenosis
- While waiting for carotid endarterectomy.

In such cases we use the combination of aspirin 75 mg and clopidogrel 75 mg for 3 months only. During the acute phase, when the risk of recurrent stroke is very high, the additional bleeding risk may be warranted; after 3 months, as the risk of stroke reduces, the risk of bleeding becomes relatively more important.

Lacunar stroke/cerebral small-vessel disease

There are no data addressing what is the best combination in this type of stroke. There is potential concern that, particularly in patients with leukoaraiosis who we know have a markedly increased risk of stroke when on anticoagulant, combination therapy may increase intracerebral haemorrhage risk.

Trials are currently examining this.

Further reading

Aspirin

Antithrombotic Trialists' Collaboration (2002) Collaborative meta-analysis of randomised trials of antiplatelet therapy for prevention of death, myocardial infarction, and stroke in high risk patients. *BMJ* **324**, 71–86.

CAPRIE Steering Committee (1996) A randomised, blinded, trial of clopidogrel versus aspirin in patients at risk of ischaemic events (CAPRIE). *Lancet* **348**, 1329–39.

Clopidogrel versus aspirin+dipyridamole

Diener HC, Bogousslavsky J, Brass LM *et al.* MATCH investigators (2004) Aspirin and clopidogrel compared with clopidogrel alone after recent ischaemic stroke or transient ischaemic attack in high-risk patients (MATCH): randomised, double-blind, placebo-controlled trial. *Lancet* **364**, 331–7.

Sacco RL, Diener HC, Yusuf S *et al.* PRoFESS Study Group (2008) Aspirin and extended-release dipyridamole versus clopidogrel for recurrent stroke. *New England Journal of Medicine* **359**, 1238–51.

The ESPRIT Study Group, Algra A (2007) Medium intensity oral anticoagulants versus aspirin after cerebral ischaemia of arterial origin (ESPRIT): a randomised controlled trial. *Lancet Neurology* **6**, 115–24.

Anticoagulation

Anticoagulation used to be widely used in stroke secondary prevention. However, trials have shown that antiplatelet agents are the better choice except for certain specific situations:

- Atrial fibrillation
- Mechanical prosthetic heart valves
- Certain other high risk cardioembolic sources of embolism
- Some hypercoagulable states.

Anticoagulation in prevention of all ischaemic stroke

- A number of trials have shown that anticoagulation has less or similar efficacy to antiplatelet agents, but that it has a higher risk. Therefore antiplatelet agents are the treatment of choice except in specific circumstances
- **The Stroke Prevention in Reversible Ischemia Trial (SPIRIT)** was stopped early because of increased bleeding among those treated with high-intensity oral anticoagulation (INR 3.0–4.5) compared with aspirin (30 mg/day) in 1316 patients. Intracerebral bleeding was particularly increased in patients with leukoaraiosis on brain imaging
- This demonstrated that high levels of anticoagulation were not beneficial, but trials with lower INRs were then performed
- **The Warfarin Aspirin Recurrent Stroke Study (WARSS)** compared the efficacy of warfarin (INR 1.4–2.8) with aspirin (325 mg) for the prevention of recurrent ischaemic stroke among 2206 patients with a non-cardioembolic stroke. This randomized, double-blind, multicentre trial found no significant difference between the treatments for the prevention of recurrent stroke or death (warfarin, 17.8%; aspirin, 16.0%)
- Rates of major bleeding were not significantly different between the warfarin and aspirin groups (2.2% and 1.5% per year, respectively)
- **The European–Australian Stroke Prevention in Reversible Ischemia Trial (ESPRIT)** randomly assigned patients within 6 months of TIA or minor stroke of presumed arterial origin to anticoagulants (target INR range 2.0–3.0; n=536) or aspirin (30–325 mg daily; n=532). Mean follow up was 4.6 years (SD 2.2)
- The primary outcome was the composite of death from all vascular causes, non-fatal stroke, non-fatal MI, or major bleeding complication, whichever occurred first
- The mean achieved INR was 2.57 (SD 0.86)
- A primary outcome event occurred in 19% patients on anticoagulants and in 18% patients on aspirin (hazard ratio [HR] 1.02, 95% CI 0.77–1.35)
- The HR for ischaemic events was 0.73 (0.52–1.01) and for major bleeding complications 2.56 (1.48–4.43).

Specific diseases and warfarin

Cardioembolic stroke and atrial fibrillation is dealt with on 📖 p. 298.

Warfarin - Aspirin Symptomatic Intracranial Disease (WASID)

Intracranial stenosis

- The Warfarin - Aspirin Symptomatic Intracranial Disease (WASID) trial was designed to test the efficacy of warfarin with a target INR of 2–3 (mean 2.5) versus aspirin for those with angiographically documented >50% intracranial stenosis
- It was stopped prematurely for safety concerns among those treated with warfarin
- At the time of termination, warfarin was associated with significantly higher rates of adverse events and provided no benefit over aspirin
- During a mean follow up of 1.8 years, adverse events in the two groups were death (aspirin, 4.3%; warfarin, 9.7%; HR, 0.46; 95% CI 0.23–0.90; *P*=0.02), major haemorrhage (aspirin, 3.2%; warfarin, 8.3%; HR, 0.39; 95% CI 0.18–0.84; *P*=0.01), and MI or sudden death (aspirin, 2.9%; warfarin, 7.3%; HR, 0.40; 95% CI 0.18–0.91; *P*=0.02)
- The primary endpoint (ischaemic stroke, brain haemorrhage, and nonstroke vascular death) occurred in 22% of patients in both treatment arms (HR, 1.04; 95% CI 0.73–1.48; *P*=0.83)
- Therefore, antiplatelet agents are the preferred treatment in intracranial stenosis.

Carotid and vertebral dissection

- Many clinicians prescribe warfarin for 3–6 months after acute dissection
- This is on the assumption that anticoagulation will be better at inhibiting thrombus formation at the site of dissection
- However, there is no clinical trial data on which to support this decision, and a meta-analysis of the available data (of poor quality) shows no difference between aspirin and warfarin
- Trials are required to determine the best therapeutic approach.

Further reading

Chimowitz MI, Lynn MJ, Howlett-Smith H *et al.* Warfarin-Aspirin Symptomatic Intracranial Disease Trial Investigators (2005) Comparison of warfarin and aspirin for symptomatic intracranial arterial stenosis. *New England Journal of Medicine* **352**, 1305–16.

ESPRIT Study Group, Halkes PH, van Gijn J, Kappelle LJ, Koudstaal PJ, Algra A (2007) Medium intensity oral anticoagulants versus aspirin after cerebral ischaemia of arterial origin (ESPRIT): a randomised controlled trial. *Lancet Neurology* **6**, 115–24.

Gorter JW (1999) Major bleeding during anticoagulation after cerebral ischemia: patterns and risk factors. Stroke Prevention In Reversible Ischemia Trial (SPIRIT). European Atrial Fibrillation Trial (EAFT) study groups. *Neurology* **53**, 1319–27.

Menon R, Kerry S, Norris JW, Markus HS (2008) Treatment of cervical artery dissection: a systematic review and meta-analysis. *Journal of Neurology, Neurosurgery and Psychiatry* **79**, 1122–7.

SPIRIT (1997) Randomized trial of anticoagulants versus aspirin after cerebral ischemia of presumed arterial origin. The Stroke Prevention in Reversible Ischemia Trial (SPIRIT) Study Group. *Annals of Neurology* **42**, 857–65.

Atrial fibrillation

- Anticoagulation with warfarin should be considered in all patients with atrial fibrillation (AF). It is such an effective treatment that one should only not prescribe it if there is a good reason not to do so
- Multiple clinical trials have demonstrated the superior therapeutic effect of warfarin compared with placebo in the primary prevention of thromboembolic events among patients with non-valvular AF
- These trials did not include patients with cardiac valvular disease and AF because it was felt that withholding warfarin was not ethical in this patient group
- An analysis of pooled data from five primary prevention trials of warfarin versus control showed consistent benefits across studies, with an overall relative risk reduction of 68% (95% CI 50–79) and an absolute reduction in annual stroke rate from 4.5% to 1.4%
- This absolute risk reduction indicates that 31 ischaemic strokes will be prevented each year for every 1000 patients treated
- Overall, warfarin use was relatively safe, with an annual rate of major bleeding of 1.3% for patients on warfarin compared with 1% for patients on placebo or aspirin
- The European Atrial Fibrillation Trial confirmed that there was a similar benefit in the secondary prevention of stroke, i.e. in using warfarin in patients who have already had stroke
- The optimal intensity of oral anticoagulation for stroke prevention in patients with AF appears to be 2.0–3.0
- The efficacy of oral anticoagulation declines significantly below an INR of 2.0
- Both persistent AF and paroxysmal AF are potent predictors of first and recurrent stroke, and both should be treated similarly
- Evidence supporting the efficacy of aspirin is substantially weaker than that for warfarin
- A pooled analysis of data from three trials resulted in an estimated RR reduction of 21% compared with placebo (95% CI 0–38)
- The ACTIVE W trial showed that warfarin was more effective than the combination of aspirin and clopidogrel
- There is no evidence that combining anticoagulation with an antiplatelet agent reduces stroke risk compared with anticoagulant therapy alone.

Therefore, unless a clear contraindication exists, AF patients with a recent stroke or TIA should receive long-term anticoagulation rather than antiplatelet therapy.

Predictors of risk in AF

- Data from the AF clinical trials show that age, recent congestive heart failure, hypertension, diabetes, and prior thromboembolism identify high-risk groups for arterial thromboembolism among patients with AF

Difficult management situations

- No data are available to address the question of when to initiate oral anticoagulation in a patient with AF after a stroke or TIA. In the European Atrial Fibrillation Trial (EAFT), oral anticoagulation was initiated within 14 days of symptom onset in about one-half of the patients. Patients in this trial had minor strokes or TIAs and AF. In general, we recommend initiation of oral anticoagulation within 2 weeks of a minor ischaemic stroke or TIA. However, for patients with large infarcts or uncontrolled hypertension, a longer delay may be appropriate to avoid cerebral haemorrhage in an area of haemorrhagic transformation. In such cases we often anticoagulate after 2–3 weeks and repeat a CT scan before starting warfarin to check there is no haemorrhagic transformation
- For patients with AF who suffer an ischaemic stroke or TIA despite therapeutic anticoagulation, there are no data to indicate that either increasing the intensity of anticoagulation or adding an antiplatelet agent provides additional protection against future ischaemic events. In addition, both strategies are associated with an increase in bleeding risk
- Patients with confluent leukoaraiosis on brain imaging have a markedly increased risk of bleeding on warfarin. In many of these cases microbleeds can be seen on gradient spin echo (GRE) MRI but whether this allows one to identify those who are at high risk of warfarin-related bleeding is uncertain
- If GRE MRI suggested an underlying cerebral amyloid angiopathy pattern—multiple areas of lobar haemosiderin deposition in a patient aged over 65 years, we would not anticoagulate
- About one-third of patients who present with AF and an ischaemic stroke will be found to have other potential causes for the stroke such as carotid stenosis. For these patients, treatment decisions should focus on the presumed most likely stroke origin. In many cases, it will be appropriate to initiate anticoagulation, because of the AF, and additional therapy (such as CEA).

Warfarin in the elderly

- Anticoagulation is often underused in the elderly owing to fears of bleeding complications
- The risk of these is of the order of 2% per annum
- Many physicians have then been deterred from prescribing warfarin in the frail elderly with stroke because of the view that this trial figure, where INRs are closely monitored, is likely to be an underestimate. However, the reality seems to be that anticoagulation is generally well tolerated in older people—exactly the group with the highest incidence of AF and the greatest risk of recurrent stroke
- The key issue is not so much a crystal ball estimate of a perceived falls risk in older patients, but more the practicality of a patient having appropriate INR monitoring and compliance with taking daily warfarin. The therapeutic window is tight with anticoagulation for stroke—INR needs to be between 2 and 3. The SPIRIT trial showed that values below this provided little benefit and values much above this were associated with excess bleeding risk.

Alternative treatments to warfarin

- More recent approaches using novel anticoagulants which inhibit either factor Xa or factor II (thrombin) and that do not require therapeutic monitoring have shown promise in early trials. They are unproven currently in secondary prevention of ischaemic stroke due to AF
- Ximelagatran is a direct thrombin inhibitor that is orally administered, has stable pharmacokinetics independent of the hepatic P450 enzyme system, and has a low potential for food or drug interactions
- Ximelagatran was found to be a promising alternative to warfarin. However, serum alanine aminotransferase levels rose transiently >3 times above normal in 6% of patients with ximelagatran, usually within 6 months
- There are currently several trials exploring the use of endovascularly inserted mechanical devices which close the left atrial appendage and therefore reduce left atrial thrombus formation in AF. To date, none of these are proven but they may be an alternative for those patients with ischaemic stroke and AF in whom anticoagulation is otherwise contraindicated in the future.

Anticoagulation for other cardioembolic sources

Valvular heart disease

- Recurrent embolism occurs in 30–65% of patients with **rheumatic mitral valve** disease who have a history of a previous embolic event—therefore anticoagulation is frequently given, ideally before the onset of AF which is a frequent complication of later stage disease
- The risk of stroke is high in untreated patients with **mechanical heart valve prostheses**, and lifelong anticoagulation is standard therapy
- The risk of stroke is lower with **bioprosthetic cardiac valves** and antiplatelet agents alone are often prescribed in the long term. Some clinicians use anticoagulants just for the first few months post valve insertion although there is no trial data for this approach
- **Mitral valve prolapse** is the most common form of valve disease in adults but its embolic risk is low and it does not usually merit anticoagulation
- Systemic embolism in isolated **aortic valve disease** is increasingly recognized because of thrombi or calcium emboli, but antiplatelet therapy is usually used.

Acute MI and left ventricular thrombus

- Stroke or systemic embolism is less common among uncomplicated MI patients but can occur in up to 12% of patients with acute MI complicated by a LV thrombus
- The incidence of embolism is highest in the first 1–3 months after MI
- Thrombus may persist for 2 years in a quarter of cases but is rarely associated with late embolic events
- For patients with an ischaemic stroke or TIA caused by an acute MI in whom LV mural thrombus is identified by echocardiography or another form of cardiac imaging, oral anticoagulation is reasonable, aiming for an INR of 2.0–3.0 for at least 3 months and up to 1 year

- It is also reasonable to anticoagulate patients with akinetic left ventricular segments on echocardiography although again there is no good trial data on which to base this.

Cardiomyopathy

- The incidence of stroke seems to be inversely proportional to ejection fraction
- Figures from the Survival and Ventricular Enlargement (SAVE) study showed:
  - For an ejection fraction of about 32%, a stroke rate of 0.8% per year
  - For an ejection fraction of about 23%, a stroke rate of 1.7% per year
- Warfarin is sometimes prescribed to prevent cardioembolic events in patients with cardiomyopathy. However, there is no randomized controlled trial to substantiate this.

Further reading

The Atrial Fibrillation Investigators. (1994) Risk factors for stroke and efficacy of antithrombotic therapy in atrial fibrillation: analysis of pooled data from five randomized controlled trials. Archives of Internal Medicine **154**, 1449–57.

ACTIVE Writing Group (2006) Clopidogrel plus aspirin versus oral anticoagulation for atrial fibrillation in the Atrial fibrillation Clopidogrel Trial with Irbesartan for prevention of Vascular Events (ACTIVE W): a randomised controlled trial. *Lancet* **367**, 1903–12.

Carotid endarterectomy

Symptomatic carotid artery stenosis is associated with a high risk of early recurrent stroke. Two large trials, the North American Symptomatic Carotid Endarterectomy Trial (NASCET) and the European Carotid Surgery Trial (ECST), have shown that carotid endarterectomy (CEA) is highly effective at preventing recurrent stroke in patients with severe recently symptomatic carotid stenosis.

Management depends on the degree of stenosis, as indicated below. The degree of stenosis varies according to the method used to measure it (Fig. 10.2), and the following advice is given for measurements made using the NASCET method.

≥70% symptomatic stenosis

- Removing the stenosis by endarterectomy almost abolishes the risk of recurrent ipsilateral stenosis
- This has to be balanced against the risk of surgery—about 5% stroke risk in good units—but the benefits greatly outweigh the risk
- The 2-year (3-year in ECST) risk of all stroke and perioperative death was reduced by CEA from 32.3% to 15.8% in NASCET, and from 21.9% to 12.3% in ECST
- The risk of stroke if untreated, and therefore the benefit, decline markedly in the first weeks after stroke. Therefore, to maximize the benefit the operation needs to be done urgently.

50–69% stenosis

- There is less benefit to operating in this group; the trial showed a marginal benefit for this group as a whole
- However, it is reasonable to treat a patient with this degree of stenosis if they have other indicators of high risk as below, and particularly if they can be operated on within the first 2 weeks of symptoms.

<50% stenosis

For patients with carotid stenosis, the trials showed no benefit and operation should not be performed.

Indicators of high risk

- Age >75 years
- Male gender
- Recent symptoms
- Ulcerated plaque on angiography
- Hemispheric symptoms rather than transient monocular blindness
- Stroke (rather than TIA).

Indicators of lower risk

- Opposite of high risk indicators above
- Distal collapse of ICA.

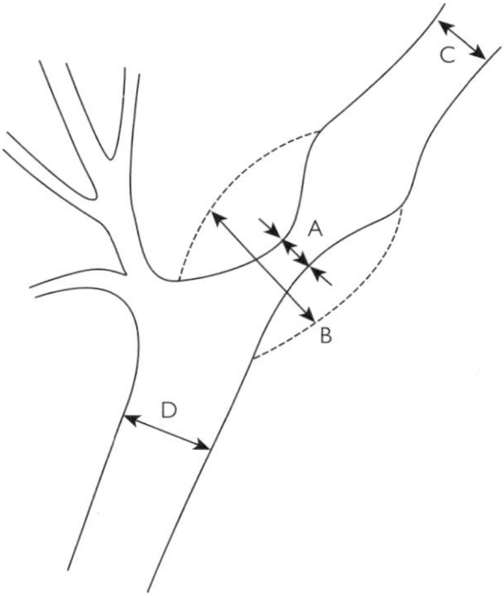

Fig. 10.2 Measurement of carotid stenosis. The degree of stenosis will vary according to the methods used. The advice given here is for measurement using the NASCET method. The ECST method has become less popular because one has to 'guess' where the arterial lumen prior to the stenosis was. The common carotid method (CCM) is simple.
NASCET method, C-A/C x100;
ECST method, B-A/Bx100;
common carotid method (CCM), D-A/D.
NASCET stenosis can be approximately converted to ECST by using the simple formula: ECST = (0.6 x NASCET) + 40.

Timing of CEA

- The chances of recurrent stroke are greatest in the first few weeks after the initial event, and much of the benefit of CEA is lost if surgery is delayed
- A pooled analysis of data from both NASCET and ECST data has made this very clear
- Therefore, for all patients with TIA, operation should be performed urgently
- For patients with stroke, particularly those with larger stroke, some surgeons like to wait 2–4 weeks before operating as the operative risk is higher and there is a risk of reperfusion injury and haemorrhage into the acute infarct after reopening the stenosed carotid artery. There is no good evidence to guide what to do here. We tend to operate urgently when the stroke is small on brain imaging (<1–2 cm maximum dimension) but delay 2–4 weeks if it is larger.

Table 10.3 shows the absolute risk reduction with carotid endarterectomy for symptomatic carotid stenosis from the pooled analysis of randomized controlled trials. It shows that the benefit of operation declines as the time since last symptoms increases, is greater in males, and is greater in the elderly.

Table 10.3 The absolute risk reduction with surgery in 5-year actual risk of ipsilateral carotid ischaemic stroke and any stroke or death within 30 days after trial surgery from the pooled analysis of the RCTs

Factor	All patients
Time since last event (weeks)	**Surgical vs medical (ARR; 95% CI)**
<2	85/627 vs 122/558 (9.2; 4.7 to 13.7)
2 to 4 weeks	63/602 vs 72/452 (6.4; 2.1 to 10.7)
4 to 12 weeks	147/1257 vs 148/1055 (2.9; 0.0 to 5.8)
Gender	
Male	253/2307 vs 301/1868 (6.0; 3.8 to 8.2)
Female	134/929 vs 107/789 (−0.4; −3.8 to 3.0)
Age years	
<65	186/1645 vs 163/1255 (2.2; −0.3 to 4.7)
65–74	169/1303 vs 180/1105 (4.1; 1.2 to 7.1)
≥75	32/288 vs 65/297 (11.9; 5.7 to 18.1)

Rothwell PM, Eliasziw M, Gutnikov SA *et al.* Carotid Endarterectomy Trialists' Collaboration (2003) Analysis of pooled data from the randomised controlled trials of endarterectomy for symptomatic carotid stenosis. *Lancet* **361**, 107–16.

Rothwell PM, Eliasziw M, Gutnikov SA *et al.* Carotid Endarterectomy Trialists Collaboration (2004) Endarterectomy for symptomatic carotid stenosis in relation to clinical subgroups and timing of surgery. *Lancet* **363**, 915–24.

Choosing a patient for CEA

When deciding whether to operate on a patient with symptomatic stenosis a number of considerations are important.

- Does the patient have a severe stenosis (>70%)
- If not, does the patient have a 50–69% stenosis and are they at particularly high risk as indicated by the above markers
- What is the estimated life expectancy of the patient—this needs to be at least 2 years to obtain reasonable benefit from CEA for symptomatic disease (see Interim Life Tables, Table 1.5, 📖 pp. 12–13)
- Can the patient be operated on soon—if there is a delay then any benefit of surgery will be negated
- Does the surgeon have an acceptable operative risk (not more than 5–7%) and do they do enough CEAs to maintain experience? It is important that outcome figures from units are audited, ideally by an independent physician. Outcome is better for patients looked after in larger specialist units
- In patients with larger strokes, one needs to balance the expected life expectancy and whether there is much function left to lose in that ICA territory if further strokes occur. For this reason, we would not operate in large MCA strokes, but limit intervention to patients with TIA or small to moderate sized stroke and moderate disability.

Complications of carotid endarterectomy

Despite having definite benefit, CEA has risks although these are much reduced in specialized units. Causes of stroke include:

- Dislodgement of embolic material during carotid manipulation and dissection
- Haemodynamic ischaemia during clamping of the carotid artery
- Embolism from the site of CEA which is denuded of endothelium and thrombogenic
- Cerebral haemorrhage and seizures owing to reperfusion injury.

Other complications include cranial nerve injuries, particularly hypoglossal nerve injuries.

Carotid stenting

- This offers an alternative to CEA
- Potential advantages are its less invasive nature, with the lack of an incision and potential for cranial nerve palsies
- Initial studies used angioplasty alone, but restenosis rates were very high, and the standard is now to use stenting
- It allows treatment of more distal stenosis inaccessible to surgery.

A number of trials have compared angioplasty and stenting with CEA but as yet no clear benefit for stenting has been shown.

Carotid and vertebral artery transluminal angioplasty study (CAVATAS)

- This randomized trial compared angioplasty with surgical therapy among 504 symptomatic carotid patients, in whom only 26% received stents
- Major outcome events within 30 days did not differ between endovascular treatment and surgery groups, with a 30-day risk of stroke or death of 10.0% and 9.9%, respectively
- Restenosis was significantly more common in the angioplasty arm.

Stent-protected angioplasty versus carotid endarterectomy in symptomatic patients (SPACE)

- A total of 1200 patients with symptomatic carotid artery stenosis was randomly assigned within 180 days of TIA or moderate stroke (to carotid artery stenting (n=605) or CEA (n=595)
- The primary endpoint, the rate of death or ipsilateral ischaemic stroke from randomization to 30 days after the procedure, was 6.84% with carotid artery stenting and 6.34% with CEA (absolute difference 0.51%, 90% CI –1.89–2.91%, P=0.09)
- This trial showed no significant difference but a small trend towards better outocme with CEA.

EVA-3S

- A randomized trial comparing stenting with endarterectomy in patients with a symptomatic carotid stenosis ≥60%
- The trial was stopped prematurely after the inclusion of 527 patients for reasons of both safety and futility
- The 30-day incidence of any stroke or death was 3.9% after endarterectomy (95% CI 2.0–7.2) and 9.6% after stenting (95% CI 6.4–14.0); relative risk of stenting compared with endarterectomy of 2.5 (95% CI 1.2–5.1)
- Why this trial showed such a poor outcome for stenting while SPACE showed no significant difference is uncertain.

International Carotid Stenting Study (ICSS)

- This trial randomized 1700 patients with symptomatic carotid stenosis between carotid endarterectomy and carotid stenting
- The primary endpoint was any stroke, death, or peri-procedural MI
- The 120 day primary endpoint was more common in the stenting group compared with the CEA group: 8.5% versus 5.1%, odds ratio 1.73 (1.18–2.52).

Current recommendations

- Carotid stenting should only be performed in patients who are suitable for CEA
- It may be used in selected patients in whom stenosis is difficult to access surgically, when medical conditions that greatly increase the risk for surgery are present, or other specific circumstances exist such as radiation-induced stenosis or restenosis after CEA
- Initially it was thought that it might be particularly suitable for more elderly patients, but data from SPACE and the run-in phase to the CREST trial has suggested the risk of stenting may be relatively higher in the elderly.

Further trials are ongoing, including the Carotid Revascularization With Endarterectomy or Stent Trial (CREST), and these will provide more information.

Further reading

Mas JL, Chatellier G, Beyssen B *et al.* EVA-3S Investigators (2006) Endarterectomy versus stenting in patients with symptomatic severe carotid stenosis. *New England Journal of Medicine* **355**, 1660–71.

SPACE Collaborative Group (2006) 30 day results from the SPACE trial of stent-protected angioplasty versus carotid endarterectomy in symptomatic patients: a randomised non-inferiority trial. *Lancet* **368**, 1239–47.

Asymptomatic carotid stenosis

- Treatment of asymptomatic carotid stenosis is primary not secondary prevention but is covered here as it is an important area
- The situation differs greatly from symptomatic carotid stenosis because the risk of stroke is much lower—2% per annum compared with 20–30% in the first year for symptomatic stenosis
- Therefore, although trials have shown that CEA results in a large relative risk reduction, the benefit to an individual patient, or absolute risk reduction, is much lower. Essentially, there are many fewer strokes to prevent in this population but CEA carries a similar (or perhaps slightly lower) risk
- The benefit may be even less because, with the widespread use of more effective secondary prevention drugs such as statins, the 2% per annum stroke risk which was estimated from data collected some years ago may be an overestimate.

Two large randomized trials have compared best medical therapy with operation for asymptomatic carotid stenosis.

Asymptomatic Carotid Atherosclerosis Study (ACAS)

- Between 1987 and 1993, 1662 patients with asymptomatic carotid artery stenosis with ≥60% stenosis were randomized to CEA or medical therapy
- After a median follow up of 2.7 years, with 4657 patient-years of observation, the aggregate risk over 5 years for ipsilateral stroke and any perioperative stroke or death was 5.1% for surgical patients and 11.0% for patients treated medically (aggregate risk reduction of 53% [95% CI 22–72%])
- The perioperative risk for CEA was very low (1.5%, excluding risk of angiography) and this made some question how generalizable these results were. However, a similar benefit was found in the larger ACST study.

Asymptomatic Carotid Surgery Trial (ACST)

- Between 1993 and 2003, 3120 asymptomatic patients were randomized between immediate CEA (half underwent CEA by 1 month, 88% by 1 year) and indefinite deferral of any CEA (only 4% per year underwent CEA), and were followed for a mean of 3.4 years
- Including perioperative strokes, the 5-year risk of stroke was 6.4% for CEA versus 11.8% for medical treatment, and 3.5% for CEA versus 6.1% for medical treatment for fatal or disabling strokes
- The absolute risk reduction was similar in ACAS (2.7%) and ACST (2.5%)
- As can be seen, although the relative risk reduction is large the absolute risk reduction is very small, i.e. a lot of operations need to be done to prevent one stroke.

Who should one operate on for asymptomatic stenosis?

- Different clinicians have different views
- It is essential to give patients true information about the potential benefit using data based on the absolute risk reduction or number needed to treat
- We explain to patients that for every 100 patients operated on, over the next 5 years five disabling strokes or deaths will be avoided. This means that 95% will have no benefit over that time period. Many patients feel that this is too small a benefit to warrant intervention
- The trials have suggested that the group who particularly benefit are younger men. In a meta-analysis, no benefit was found in women (see Figure 10.3)
- There is great interest in identifying predictors of stroke risk which would allow a high risk group to be selected. Many have been proposed, including embolic signals on TCD, plaque morphology on ultrasound or MRI, but none are yet proven to be clinically useful.

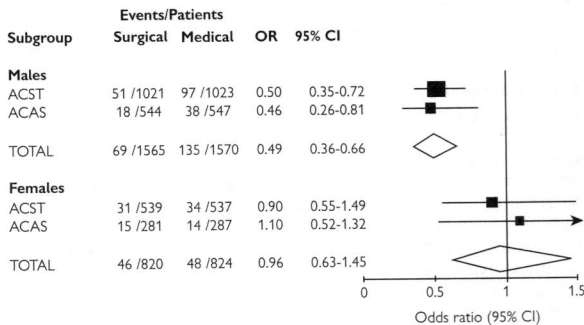

Subgroup	Events/Patients Surgical	Events/Patients Medical	OR	95% CI
Males				
ACST	51 /1021	97 /1023	0.50	0.35-0.72
ACAS	18 /544	38 /547	0.46	0.26-0.81
TOTAL	69 /1565	135 /1570	0.49	0.36-0.66
Females				
ACST	31 /539	34 /537	0.90	0.55-1.49
ACAS	15 /281	14 /287	1.10	0.52-1.32
TOTAL	46 /820	48 /824	0.96	0.63-1.45

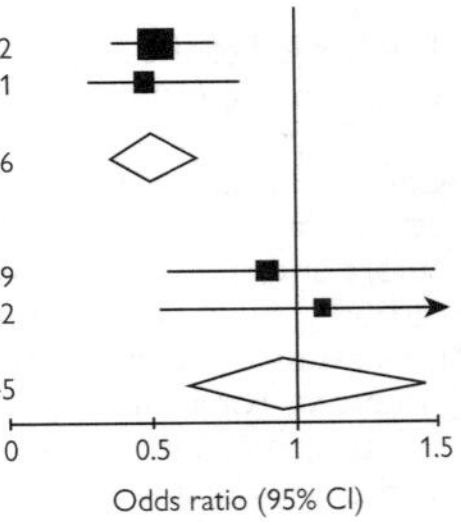

Fig. 10.3 The effect of endarterectomy for asymptomatic carotid stenosis on the risk of any stroke and operative death by sex in ACST and ACAS. Reproduced with permission from Rothwell PM, Goldstein LB (2004) Carotid endarterectomy for asymptomatic carotid stenosis: Asymptomatic Carotid Surgery Trial. *Stroke* **35**, 2425–7.

Further reading

Executive Committee for the Asymptomatic Carotid Atherosclerosis (ACAS) Study (1995) Endarterectomy for asymptomatic carotid artery stenosis. *JAMA* **273**, 1421–8.

Halliday A, Mansfield A, Marro J *et al.* MRC Asymptomatic Carotid Surgery Trial (ACST) Collaborative Group (2004) Prevention of disabling and fatal strokes by successful carotid endarterectomy in patients without recent neurological symptoms: randomised controlled trial. *Lancet* **363**, 1491–502.

Carotid occlusion

- The risk of stroke in carotid occlusion is less than that with tight carotid stenosis but is nevertheless increased
- The risk is highest soon after the occlusion. Presumably with time collaterals occur and/or those high-risk patients with poor collaterals have strokes, leaving a lower risk group
- CEA is not possible in this patient group
- It is possible to bypass the occlusion by an extracranial–intracranial (EC–IC) bypass. In this operation, an anastomosis is made between the superficial temporal branch of the external carotid artery and an intracranial branch of the internal carotid artery through a burr hole in the skull
- However, the EC–IC bypass study showed no benefit for this operation in patients with carotid occlusion, or stenosis or occlusion of the MCA. The perioperative risk of stroke was high
- Therefore EC–IC bypass is not routinely performed
- Studies have shown that only a small proportion of patients with carotid occlusion have impaired cerebral haemodynamics and, in prospective follow up, it is this group that are at high risk of recurrent stroke
- This has led to the suggestion that EC–IC bypass may benefit this subgroup. No estimate of haemodynamic status was performed in the EC–IC bypass
- Cerebral haemodynamics can be measured using PET, or with estimation of cerebral blood flow (with Xenon, CT perfusion or TCD before and after a vasodilatory stimulus such as increased inspired carbon dioxide or IV acetazolamide)
- In occasional patients with carotid occlusion and haemodynamic symptoms some clinicians practise EC–IC bypass but it is important first to demonstrate severely impaired haemodynamics in the MCA territory ipsilateral to the occlusion
- A current trial is trying to determine whether patients with impaired haemodynamics benefit from EC–IC bypass.

Further reading

EC/IC Study group (1985) Failure of extracranial-intracranial bypass to reduce the risk of ischaemic stroke. Results of an international randomized trial. *New England Journal of Medicine* **313**, 1191–200.

Markus H, Cullinane M (2001) Severely impaired cerebrovascular reactivity predicts stroke and TIA risk in patients with carotid artery stenosis and occlusion. *Brain* **124**, 457–67.

Vertebral stenosis

- One in four strokes occur in the posterior circulation and, after stenosis of the internal carotid artery, stenosis of the vertebral artery is the second commonest site of focal atherosclerotic disease in the cerebral circulation
- Within the vertebral artery, the most frequent site for stenosis is the origin of the vessel, and it is thought that such lesions are a cause for embolism into the posterior brain circulation
- Such lesions are now considered to be associated with a high risk of recurrent stroke—comparable to that of high grade symptomatic internal carotid artery stenosis
- Unlike the extracranial internal carotid artery, the vertebral artery is surgically inaccessible and endarterectomy is fraught with complications (to access the vessel the surgeon would have to remove part of the clavicle, and pneumothorax and interruption of the sympathetic chain are common complications). The vessel is, however, easily accessible endovascularly in the majority of cases
- Similarly, the vertebral artery is far more technically challenging to image with duplex ultrasound compared to the internal carotid artery, leading to problems with (under)diagnosis of such lesions. Improvements with non-invasive imaging by CEMRA and CTA show promise for routine screening of all posterior circulation ischaemic stroke patients
- Large case series have shown that endovascular angioplasty of the extracranial vertebral artery is safe and is associated with a high incidence of technical success
- Published experience to date has seen up to a 30% 2-year restenosis rate in patients treated with angioplasty alone and, following both carotid and coronary endovascular experience, expandable vertebral artery specific wall stents have now been developed
- Randomized trials are under way to compare vertebral angioplasty and stenting with best medical therapy
- In centres with the necessary expertise it is reasonable to consider extracranial vertebral artery angioplasty and stenting for patients with posterior circulation stroke and a 50% or greater extracranial vertebral artery stenosis, with no other obvious cause (such as AF or intracranial/tandem stenoses).

Further reading

Flossmann E, Rothwell PM (2003) Prognosis of vertebrobasilar transient ischaemic attack and minor stroke. *Brain* **126**, 1940–54.

Gulli G, Khan S, Markus HS (2009). Vertebrobasilar stenosis predicts high early recurrent stroke risk in posterior circulation stroke and TIA. *Stroke* **40**: 2732–7.

Intracranial stenosis

- Data from prospective studies show that patients with symptomatic intracranial atherosclerosis have a high risk of recurrent stroke
- There is limited data on optimal therapy
- The Warfarin Aspirin Symptomatic Intracranial Disease (WASID) study showed warfarin was no better than aspirin in secondary stroke prevention
- It is possible to stent intracranial stenoses but this has a significant risk and is not yet of proven benefit
- One prospective non-randomized trial has evaluated stenting in a mixed group of patients with intracranial and/or extracranial disease
- The Stenting of Symptomatic Atherosclerotic Lesions in the Vertebral or Intracranial Arteries (SSYLVIA) Trial, a multicentre, non-randomized, prospective feasibility study, evaluated one stent (the NEUROLINK System) for treatment of vertebral or intracranial artery stenosis
- Treatment was carried out on 43 intracranial arteries (70.5%) and 18 extracranial vertebral arteries (29.5%)
- Successful stent placement was achieved in 58 of 61 cases (95%) and 30-day stroke incidence was 6.6%, with no deaths
- Four of 55 patients (7.3%) had strokes later than 30 days, one of which was in the only patient not stented
- Recurrent stenosis >50% within 6 months occurred in 12 of 37 intracranial arteries (32.4%) and six of 14 extracranial vertebral arteries (42.9%). Seven recurrent stenoses (39%) were symptomatic
- However, interpreting benefit requires randomized studies with a non-stented arm and these are taking place.

Further reading

SSYLVIA Study Investigators (2004) Stenting of Symptomatic Atherosclerotic Lesions in the Vertebral or Intracranial Arteries (SSYLVIA): study results. *Stroke* **35**, 1388–92.

Chapter 11

Unusual causes of stroke and their treatment

Introduction

Rare causes of stroke make up a small proportion of stroke cases but it is important that they are recognized because they may require very specific treatment.

Most are more important in younger individuals (in whom conventional risk factors and atherosclerosis are less common). A few (e.g. temporal arteritis) are commoner in the elderly.

In many cases, specialized and specific investigations and a high index of suspicion are required to make the diagnosis.

Rare causes of stroke may be:

- Isolated stroke syndromes
- Part of a more widespread neurological disease
    - Other neurological features, e.g. encephalopathy, seizures, or dementia may occur
- Part of a systemic disease, e.g. systemic vasculitis.

Carotid and vertebral artery dissection

Carotid and vertebral artery dissection are important causes of stroke, particularly in the young.

Epidemiology

- Accounts for up to 10% of young adult stroke (<45 years) and 20–25% (<30 years)
- It has been estimated that one-third of cases of dissection will present with stroke or TIA.

Pathogenesis

- Most carotid and vertebral dissections are extracranial. Intracranial dissections have unique features
- The initial event is usually an intimal tear, allowing blood to track along planes in the arterial wall
- Carotid dissection often tracks upwards as far as the skull base, resulting in a characteristic tapering and angiographic appearance
- Consequences of the dissection include:
    - Thrombus formation at the site of the intimal tear which may result in thromboembolism and stroke
    - Reduction in luminal diameter secondary to extrinsic compression from intramural haemorrhage. This may result in vessel occlusion and haemodynamic compromise
    - Pseudoaneurysm formation—this is common but pseudoaneurysms are usually asymptomatic although occasionally may cause local pressure symptoms. They do not usually rupture
- Most stroke due to dissection is believed to be embolic. This is supported by radiographic patterns suggesting multiple emboli and the detection of asymptomatic emboli using transcranial Doppler ultrasound
- Intracranial dissections are most common in the supraclinoid carotid artery, MCA, fourth segment of the vertebral artery, and the basilar trunk. Intracranial vertebral artery dissection may result in subarachnoid haemorrhage caused by leakage of blood into the CSF.

Causes

- Vertebral and carotid dissection may occur following major penetrating and non-penetrating trauma
- A history of minor trauma is common but whether it relates to the dissection or not is sometimes unclear
- In approximately half of dissections no history of trauma is present
- A number of diseases affecting the arterial wall increase the risk of dissection, including fibromuscular dysplasia and Ehlers–Danlos syndrome type IV
- Minor connective tissue abnormalities on electron microscopy of skin biopsies have been reported in a high proportion of patients with spontaneous dissection.

Classification of causes of cervical artery dissection

Major trauma

- Penetrating trauma
- Blunt trauma.

Carotid dissection

- Basal skull fracture
- Stretching across the lateral processes of C2–3
- Strangulation
- Peritonsillar trauma
- Mandibular fracture.

Vertebral dissection

- Atlanto-axial subluxation
- Cervical spine fracture
- Cervical spine hyperrotation and hyperextension.

Minor trauma

- Chiropractic manipulation
- Neck turning (e.g. during a parade)
- Violent coughing
- Fairground rides
- Sporting activities
- Hyperextension during hairdressing (vertebral dissection).

Iatrogenic trauma

- Endovascular procedures (e.g. angiography, interventional procedures)
- Neck line insertion.

Underlying arterial disease

- Fibromuscular dysplasia
- Ehlers–Danlos syndrome type IV (vascular variant)
- Cystic medial degeneration
- Marfan's syndrome
- Pseudoxanthoma elasticum.

Idiopathic

Clinical features

Extracranial carotid dissection

- Headache—usually ipsilateral and localized to side of dissection in neck, face, orbit, and cheek
- Horner's syndrome—partial ptosis and pupillary constriction resulting from compression and interruption of sympathetic fibres running along the internal carotid artery
- TIA and stroke—TIA and stroke in carotid territory and/or amaurosis fugax or retinal artery infarction. Presenting feature in approximately one-third of carotid dissection. Almost all strokes/TIAs occur within 1 month of dissection onset and the majority within 1 week
- Cranial nerve palsies—most commonly hypoglossal palsy owing to compression of the hypoglossal nerve immediately below its exit through the anterior condylar canal. Glossopharyngeal and vagal nerve palsies occur less commonly.

Extracranial vertebral dissection

- Pain in posterior neck, occipital region, and around the ears
- TIA and stroke in vertebrobasilar territory.

Intracranial dissection

- TIA and stroke in relevant arterial territory
- Subarachnoid haemorrhage, particularly for intracranial vertebrobasilar dissection
- A difficult diagnosis and often only made at post mortem.

Diagnosis

- A high index of suspicion in young stroke patients, even in the absence of history of trauma, is essential
- Duplex carotid ultrasound may show stenosis, occasionally a flap, appearances consistent with occlusion, or high resistance damped Doppler flow signals consistent with distal stenosis. However, ultrasound has a low sensitivity (perhaps only 50%) and MRI-based techniques are better
- MRA may show tapering occlusion or pseudo-occlusion (Fig. 11.1)
- Structural MRI with cross-sectional fat suppressed inversion recovery views through the extracranial carotid or vertebral artery, in combination with MRA, is now the investigation of choice. The axial (cross-sectional) images must go down through the neck. Those available in a normal brain MRI do not go low enough. A hyperintense signal, usually semilunar-shaped, in the wall of the artery in both T1- and T2-weighted imaging is seen in the first week, indicating the presence of mural haematoma
- CT angiography shows similar appearances to MRA
- Digital subtraction angiography is rarely necessary but may show intimal flaps, and appearances of vessel compression and tapering
- Vertebral dissection is more difficult to diagnose than carotid dissection on MRI owing to the smaller vessel lumen. The intramural hyperintense signal is often less clear.

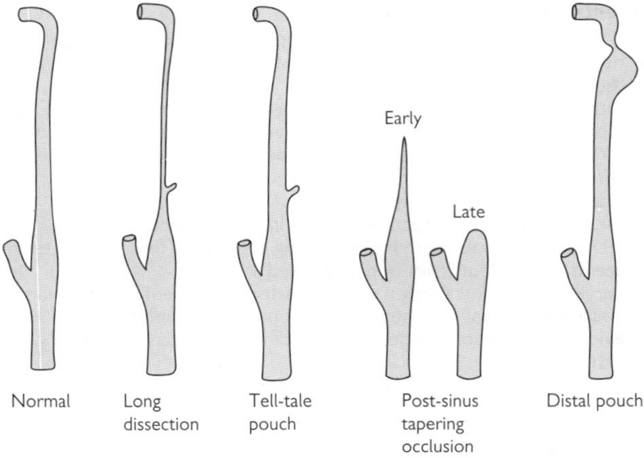

Fig. 11.1 Schematic diagram of different angiographic appearances seen in carotid dissection. Adapted with permission from Brown MM, Markus H, Oppenheimer S (2006) *Stroke Medicine*, Informa Healthcare.

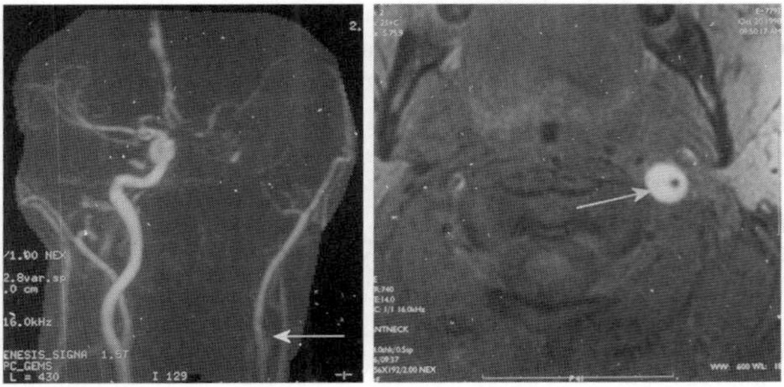

(a) (b)

Fig. 11.2 Carotid artery dissection on MRI and MRA. An MRI sequence from a patient with acute left proximal internal carotid artery dissection. **(a)** MRA demonstrating apparent left internal carotid artery occlusion. This is in fact a pseudo-occlusion caused by compression from thrombus in the false lumen. **(b)** Axial view through the internal carotid artery in the neck demonstrating a high signal within the arterial wall (recent thrombus) surrounding a small residual lumen (low signal). © Hugh Markus.

Treatment

- Anticoagulation—many authorities recommend anticoagulation with heparin and then warfarin to reduce the risk of thromboembolism, usually continued for 3–6 months
- Other authorities suggest antiplatelet agents (e.g. aspirin) are adequate
- No randomized trial data are available. A meta-analysis (Menon *et al*, 2008) found no evidence of difference between anticoagulation and antiplatelet agents
- Trials are examining this question
- MRA is often repeated at 3–6 months. In the presence of residual stenosis or pseudoaneurysm, continuing antiplatelet therapy long term seems sensible but is not evidence-based
- Surgical treatments (tying the carotid artery to prevent embolization) and interventional treatment (stenting) have been used but there is no evidence for these. Arteries usually recanalize spontaneously in any case
- Occasionally, surgical treatment or stenting is required for expanding pseudoaneurysms.

Prognosis

- Limited natural history data suggests risk of recurrent stroke is highest in the first week and very low after 1 month
- Spontaneous recanalization frequently occurs over the first few weeks or months
- Risk of recurrent dissection is very low (<1%) unless there is an underlying disorder (e.g. Ehlers–Danlos)
- Pseudoaneurysms are common and usually persist but require no specific treatment and have a very low risk of complications.

Reference

Menon R, Kerry S, Norris JW, Markus HS (2008) Treatment of cervical artery dissection: a systematic review and meta-analysis. *Journal of Neurology, Neurosurgery and Psychiatry* **79**, 1122–7.

Further reading

Beletsky V, Nadareishvili Z, Lynch J *et al.* (2003) Cervical arterial dissection: time for a therapeutic trial? *Stroke* **34**, 2856–60.

Fibromuscular dysplasia

- Typically affects medium-sized and large arteries in middle-aged and young women
- Distal cervical extracranial internal carotid artery most often affected
- Vertebral artery less commonly involved
- Renal arteries also involved: can cause renal artery stenosis and hypertension
- Most common in middle-aged women
- Often asymptomatic: mild degrees in asymptomatic individuals have been reported in as many as 1% of angiograms
- Can present with carotid dissection which may be recurrent
- Occasionally, stenosis can cause TIA or stroke, stroke without dissection, or present with cervical bruit and tinnitus
- Can be diagnosed on contrast MRA and CTA but sometimes requires formal intra-arterial angiography.

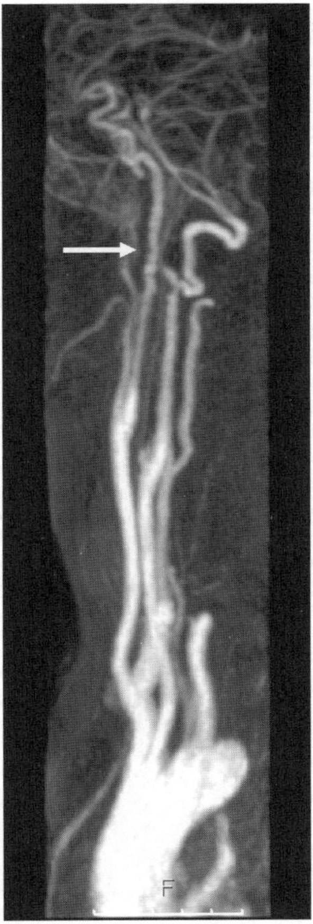

Fig. 11.3 Fibromuscular dysplasia appearances on contrast-enhanced MRA. There is a narrowing of the right ICA shortly after its origin. Distal to this can be seen characteristic beading of the artery (arrowed). © Hugh Markus.

Genetic causes of stroke

Genetic predisposition to stroke may be:
- Monogenic (an abnormality in a single gene results in disease)
- Polygenic (multiple genes contribute to stroke risk and frequently interact with environmental factors).

Monogenic causes of stroke are rare, but important on an individual patient basis. Polygenic/multifactorial contribution to stroke risk is much more important on a population basis but less important for the individual patient.

Diagnosing monogenic causes of stroke can be important because:
- The clinical syndromes can represent difficult diagnostic problems
- Some monogenic causes of stroke have specific treatments
- There are implications for other family members.

Monogenic diseases causing stroke can:
- Cause stroke alone (e.g. CADASIL), sometimes with other neurological features (e.g. migraine)
- Cause stroke as part of a systemic disease (e.g. sickle cell disease).

Diagnosing monogenic causes of stroke

- Always take a family history of stroke and other diseases
- Remember when interpreting family history, diagnoses in other family members may be incorrect (e.g. multiple sclerosis misdiagnosed as CADASIL or vascular dementia diagnosed as Alzheimer's disease)
- Remember a negative family history does not exclude monogenic stroke. Parents may have died young or disease may not be fully penetrant
- Diagnose the stroke subtype and then identify which monogenic diseases cause that subtype
- Look for specific clues (e.g. migraine with aura or MRI evidence of anterior temporal pole involvement for CADASIL).

Monogenic causes of stroke

- Small-vessel disease
  - CADASIL
  - CARASIL
  - Cerebrovascular retinopathy and HERNS
  - COL4A1 small-vessel arteriopathy with haemorrhage
- Large-artery atherosclerosis and other arteriopathies
  - Familial hyperlipidaemias
  - Moyamoya disease
  - Pseudoxanthoma elasticum
  - Neurofibromatosis type I
- Large-artery disease—dissection
  - Ehlers–Danlos syndrome type IV
  - Marfan syndrome
  - Fibromuscular dysplasia
- Disorders affecting both small and large arteries
  - Fabry disease
  - Homocysteinuria
  - Sickle cell disease
- Cardioembolism
  - Familial cardiomyopathies
  - Familial arrhythmias
  - Hereditary haemorrhagic telangiectasia
- Prothrombotic disorders
- Mitochondrial disorders
  - MELAS
- Familial hemiplegic migraine.

CADASIL (cerebral autosomal dominant arteriopathy with subcortical infarcts and leukoencephalopathy)

CADASIL is an autosomal dominant condition causing cerebral small-vessel disease. It is the most common monogenic condition causing stroke without other systemic features.

Pathogenesis

- A systemic arteriopathy with changes in vessels throughout the body (including skin and muscle) but clinical features are only seen in the brain
- Results in lacunar infarction and diffuse regions of ischaemia corresponding to radiological leukoaraiosis (neuronal loss, gliosis, ischaemic demyelination)
- Affects perforating arteries and arterioles within the brain and similarly sized vessels elsewhere in the body
- Results from mutations in *notch3*, a transmembrane protein involved in cell–cell signalling during development
- Arterial smooth muscle cell degeneration occurs, with deposition of granular osmiophilic material (GOM) seen only on electron microscopy. Aberrant extracellular portion of *notch3* is deposited adjacent to GOM
- Mechanisms linking genetic defect to disease are known but mutations do not appear to alter enzyme function. Toxic gain of function or deposition disease most likely
- Impaired cerebral autoregulation has been demonstrated in animal models and man.

Clinical features

- Recurrent lacunar strokes: onset usually 30–50 years but may be much later
- Migraine with aura: onset usually 20–30 years. Ninety per cent of migraine is with aura (in contrast, migraine in the population is 90% without aura)
- Depression: may precede onset of stroke
- Dementia: usually onset 40–60 years but variable
- Encephalopathy: reversible reduction in conscious level usually following migraine with aura attack, fully reversible with conservative treatment. May occur in up to 10%
- Epilepsy may occur in 10%. Variable types
- Premature death: age variable usually 50–75 years.

The clinical phenotype is highly variable even within families. Factors accounting for this variation include:

- Genetic modifiers
- Cardiovascular risk factors including hypertension and smoking.

Diagnosis

- Clinical phenotype with family history
- A family history of young onset stroke, dementia or migraine with aura is often present but is not present in a significant proportion of cases. Remember that a family history of Alzheimer's may in fact be CADASIL vascular dementia, and a family history of multiple sclerosis may be CADASIL

- MRI demonstrates confluent leukoaraiosis with multiple lacunar infarcts. Specific features of CADASIL include anterior temporal pole involvement (sensitivity 90%, specificity 90%), confluent external capsule involvement (sensitivity 90%, specificity 50%). Involvement of the corpus callosum may often occur (remember uncommon in sporadic small-vessel disease but common in multiple sclerosis)
- Anterior temporal pole changes may often be seen on CT if marked. On MRI, these changes are frequent from age 30 onwards and may occur earlier
- Punch skin biopsy can be performed as an outpatient procedure. It must be examined under electron microscopy. Characteristic GOM is seen in 60–80% of cases. Sensitivity 100%
- Genetic testing—there are large numbers of mutations which can occur in any of 22 exons encoding extracellular portions of protein. Almost all are point mutations (few deletions) and all alter a cysteine residue, disrupting cysteine–cysteine bonds in epidermal growth factor-like repeats in the extracellular portion of proteins. Mutations cluster in certain exons: over half are found in exon 4. The distribution of mutations varies in populations. For example, screening exons 3, 4, 5, 6, 8, 11, and 22 in a UK population identifies 90% of CADASIL cases.

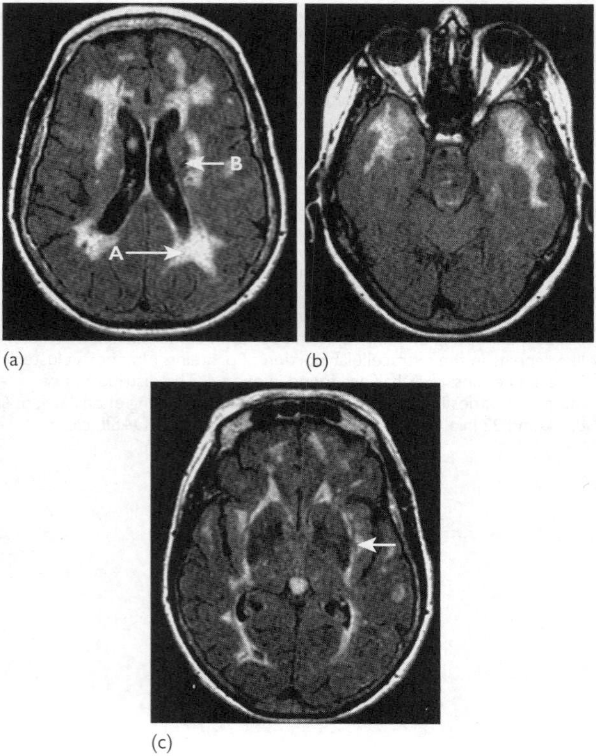

Fig. 11.4 FLAIR MRI appearances of CADASIL: **(a)** showing both leukoaraiosis (arrowed A) and focal lacunar infarction (arrowed B); **(b)** typical involvement of the anterior temporal pole can be seen in a CADASIL patient; **(c)** this scan shows involvement of the external capsule (arrowed). © Hugh Markus.

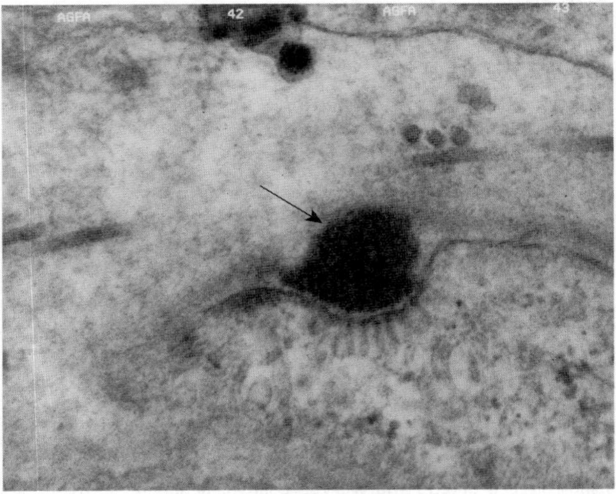

Fig. 11.5 Skin biopsy appearances in CADASIL. Definitive diagnosis of CADASIL is made by demonstrating mutations in the *notch3* gene. However, skin biopsy may also be useful in diagnosis and in over half of individuals shows characteristic granular osmiophilic material (GOM) as arrowed. This appearance can only be seen on electron microscopy; light microscopy appearances are not diagnostic. © Hugh Markus.

Treatment

- There is no specific treatment for the underlying genetic disorder. Symptomatic treatments are effective for many complications
- There is some evidence that cardiovascular risk factors (smoking and hypertension) are associated with earlier onset of stroke and more rapid progression of MRI disease. Therefore, tight cardiovascular risk factor prevention is recommended
- Aspirin or clopidogrel is usually given to patients who have suffered stroke or to older patients (>40 years) even if stroke-free
- Anticoagulation or dual antiplatelet therapy with aspirin and clopidogrel is best avoided owing to the risk of haemorrhage (microbleeds are frequently seen on gradient echo MRI)
- Migraine—attacks are usually infrequent and therefore prophylaxis is usually not necessary. However, usual prophylaxis approaches (e.g. sodium valproate, pizotifen, etc.) are effective if necessary. Triptans may help attacks but there is some concern over their use owing to underlying cerebrovascular disease and the risk of precipitating stroke
- Depression—responds to standard treatment with antidepressants in the same way as non-CADASIL depression
- Epilepsy—responds to normal antiepileptic medication.

Genetic testing

Standardized protocols with genetic counselling should be used, particularly when testing asymptomatic family members or individuals with migraine alone. In such cases, it is recommended that counselling is followed by a period of at least 1 month for reflection and decision-making. Remember an MRI may be considered as a genetic test if it detects specific signs such as anterior temporal pole involvement.

Patient information leaflets are useful to provide information on the disease. One can be obtained from the following web address: http://www.strokecare.co.uk.

Other inherited (non-CADASIL) small-vessel arteriopathies

HERNS/cerebrovascular retinopathy

- Very rare
- Cerebrovascular retinopathy (CRV)—microangiopathy of brain with vascular retinopathy
- Hereditary endotheliopathy with retinopathy, nephropathy, and stroke (HERNS)
- Autosomal dominant inheritance
- Clinical features—progressive visual loss, headache, seizures, focal neurological deficits, progressive cognitive impairment
- Visual disturbance is often the first symptom
- Neurological deficits usually develop later and are sudden onset and 'stroke-like'
- MRI contrast-enhancing lesions with surrounding oedema are usually subcortical—can mimic tumours ('pseudotumours')
- Retinal examination—telangiectatic capillaries and microaneurysms
- C-terminal truncations in human 3'-5' DNA exonuclease TREX1 cause autosomal dominant retinal vasculopathy with cerebral leukodystrophy.

Cerebral autosomal recessive arteriopathy with subcortical infarcts and leukoencephalopathy (CARASIL)

- Described in Japan—very rare
- Cerebral small-vessel arteriopathy in combination with alopecia and orthopaedic problems
- Autosomal recessive
- CARASIL has been associated with mutations in the HtrA1 (HTRA1) gene. HTRA1 is a serine protease that represses signaling by TGF-beta family members.
- Male:female ratio 3:1
- CNS onset usually 20–40 years with stroke (50%) and/or progressive subcortical dementia
- MRI lacunar stroke and leukoaraiosis.

COL4AI small-vessel arteriopathy

- Mutations in gene encoding type IV collagen $\alpha 1$ (COL4A1), a basement membrane protein
- Mutation predisposes mice to cerebral haemorrhage, and risk is increased by trauma
- Mutation identified in families with small-vessel arteriopathy
- Clinical features in human cases:
  - Retinal arteriolar tortuosity
  - Intracerebral haemorrhage
  - Infantile hemiparesis
  - Migraine with aura
  - MRI—leukoaraiosis, dilated perivascular spaces, and microbleeds on gradient echo MRI.

Further reading

CADASIL (cerebral autosomal dominant arteriopathy with subcortical infarcts and leukoencephalopathy)

Dichgans M, Mayer M, Uttner I *et al.* (1998) The phenotypic spectrum of CADASIL: clinical findings in 102 cases. *Annals of Neurology* **4**, 731–9.

Joutel A, Vahedi K, Corpechot C *et al.* (1997) Strong clustering and stereotyped nature of Notch3 mutations in CADASIL patients. *Lancet* **350**, 1511–15.

Markus HS Martin RJ, Simpson MA *et al.* (2002) Diagnostic strategies in CADASIL. *Neurology* **59**, 1134–8.

O'Sullivan M, Jarosz JM, Martin RJ *et al.* (2001) MRI hyperintensities of the temporal lobe and external capsule in patients with CADASIL. *Neurology* **56**, 628–34.

Other inherited (non-CADASIL) small vessel arteriopathies

Gould DB, Phalan FC, van Mil SE *et al.* (2006) Role of COL4A1 in small-vessel disease and haemorrhagic stroke. New England Journal of Medicine **354**, 1489–96.

Hara K, Shiga A, Fukutake T *et al.* (2009) Association of HTRA1 mutations and familial ischemic cerebral small-vessel disease. *N Engl J Med* **360**, 1729–39.

Richards A, van den Maagdenberg AM, Jen JC *et al.* (2007) C-terminal truncations in human 3'–5' DNA exonuclease TREX1 cause autosomal dominant retinal vasculopathy with cerebral leukodystrophy. *Nature Genetics* **39**, 1068–70.

Sickle cell disease

Stroke is a frequent complication of homozygous sickle cell disease (HbSS), particularly in children.

Pathogenesis

- Monogenic disease resulting in substitution of valine for glutamic acid at position 6 of the globin β chain
- Secondary to this, polymerization of the abnormal HbS haemoglobin occurs in regions of low oxygen saturation
- Polymerized haemoglobin deforms red cells, reducing their resilience and impairing their ability to pass through capillaries without becoming impacted
- Patients with full disease are homozygous. Heterozygous HbS individuals have 'sickle cell trait' and are not usually at increased risk of stroke
- Stroke may also complicate haemoglobin C sickle cell disease (HbSC)
- Sickle crises occur
- Haematological crises (sudden exacerbation of anaemia)
- Infectious crises (defective immunity owing to dysfunctional spleen)
- Vaso-occlusive crises (organ ischaemia owing to vessel occlusion).

Cerebrovascular complications in sickle cell disease

- Asymptomatic small-vessel disease
- Stenoses of large extracranial or intracranial vessels, particularly the MCA, secondary to fibrous proliferation of the intima
- Formation of aneurysms
- Moyamoya-like syndrome secondary to basal intracerebral vessel occlusion.

Clinical features

Cerebrovascular

- Ischaemic stroke
- Intracerebral haemorrhage and subarachnoid secondary to new vessel formation (in patients with moyamoya-like syndrome)
- Cognitive impairment.

Non-cerebrovascular

- Haematological crises (sudden exacerbation of anaemia)
- Infectious crises (defective immunity owing to dysfunctional spleen)
- Vaso-occlusive crises(organ ischaemia owing to vessel occlusion).

Diagnosis

- Brain imaging (CT and MRI) may show territorial infarcts and/or small-vessel disease
- Extracranial and intracranial stenoses may be detected by transcranial Doppler ultrasound, MRA, CTA, or angiography
- Full blood count—anaemia with a high reticulocyte count. On a peripheral blood film, one can observe features of hyposplenism, i.e. target cells and Howell–Jolly bodies
- Haemoglobin electrophoresis shows HbS.

Treatment

- Exchange transfusion together with hydration and oxygen therapy for acute episodes
- Prophylactic exchange transfusion has been shown to reduce recurrent stroke risk in patients with MCA stenosis due to sickle cell disease detected using TCD
- Hydroxyurea is used to increase fetal haemoglobin (HbF) which reduces HbS polymerization.

Further reading

Adams RJ, McKie VC, Hsu L *et al.* (1998) Prevention of first stroke by transfusions in children with sickle cell anaemia and abnormal results on transcranial Doppler ultrasonography. *New England Journal of Medicine* **339**, 5–11.

Switzer JA, Hess DC, Nichols FT *et al.* (2006) Pathophysiology and treatment of stroke in sickle cell disease: present and future. *Lancet Neurology* **5**, 501–12.

Fabry disease

- Fabry disease is a rare sex-linked recessive lysosomal storage disease caused by deficiency of α-galactosidase A
- It results in accumulation of glycosphingolipids in vascular endothelial smooth muscle cells and other cell types, including renal glomerular epithelial cells, dorsal root and autonomic neurons, and myocardial cells.

Clinical features

Non-cerebrovascular

- Burning neuropathic limb pain (acroparaesthesia) caused by lipid accumulation in sensory nerves
- Skin angiokeratosis
- Joint pain
- Corneal dystrophy (visible as cloudy streaks in the cornea)
- Renal failure
- Myocardial involvement.

Cerebrovascular involvement

- Small-vessel disease—lacunar infarction and white matter hyperintensities on MRI
- Large-artery disease preferentially affecting vertebrobasilar system with ectatic changes, dilatation, and stenoses
- Stroke often occurs in patients with known Fabry disease. A study in young cryptogenic stroke (18–55 years) found Fabry in 4.9% of men and 2.4% of women. These findings need repeating in different cohorts.

Diagnosis

- α-galactosidase enzyme levels in men and genetic testing if abnormal
- In women, levels may be unhelpful (because sex-linked) and genetic testing is necessary.

Treatment

- Intravenous enzyme replacement therapy is now available
- Very expensive
- Reduces painful symptoms
- No evidence yet that it reduces recurrent stroke risk.

Further reading

Fellgiebel A, Muller MJ, Ginsberg L (2006) CNS manifestations of Fabry's disease. *Lancet Neurology* **5**, 791–5.

Rolfs A, Bottcher T, Zschiesche M *et al.* (2005) Prevalence of Fabry disease in patients with cryptogenic stroke: a prospective study. *Lancet* **366**, 1794–6.

Mitochondrial disorders and MELAS

Mitochondrial DNA mutations result in a variety of systemic syndromes that may include involvement of the neurological system. Some of these cause stroke-like episodes. The archetypical stroke phenotype is MELAS (mitochondrial encephalopathy with lactic acidosis and stroke-like episodes).

Clinical features

- Recurrent stroke-like episodes usually occur in childhood or young adulthood
- Episodes are often accompanied by epilepsy with partial and/or secondary generalized seizures
- Good recovery is often made from initial episodes with marked radiological recovery
- Recurrent episodes are associated with progressive disability and dementia
- Other clinical features include:
  - Sensorineural deafness
  - Migraine
  - Episodic vomiting
  - Other features of mitochondrial disorders, including proximal muscle weakness, cardiomyopathy, external ophthalmoplegia, retinopathy, ataxia
- Overlap may occur with other mitochondrial disorders.

Imaging appearances

- Infarction involves occipital cortex (most commonly) and posterior parietal and posterior temporal regions
- Distribution does not always correspond to cerebral arterial territories
- 'Infarcts' may dramatically improve or disappear over weeks to months
- Increased diffusion (in contrast to restricted diffusion in ischaemic stroke) often seen on DWI
- Magnetic resonance spectroscopy (MRS) may demonstrate lactate both within normal and abnormal appearing brain. (Remember this occurs in any acute ischaemic stroke within lesion)
- White matter hyperintensities and subcortical changes may also occur.

Other diagnostic tests

- Raised CSF lactate on CSF examination
- Mitochondrial DNA analysis may show mutation: this is most common (in 80% of cases it is the A>G3243 mutation) in the transfer RNA *leu* gene
- Genetic analysis on blood may not detect diagnosis caused by unusual mutations or heteroplasmy (genetic abnormality is only present in some cells)
- Muscle biopsy: may show ragged red fibres. DNA analysis on muscle may be positive when negative on blood owing to heteroplasmy.

Treatment

- No proven treatments
- Supportive therapy and treatment of epilepsy during acute episodes

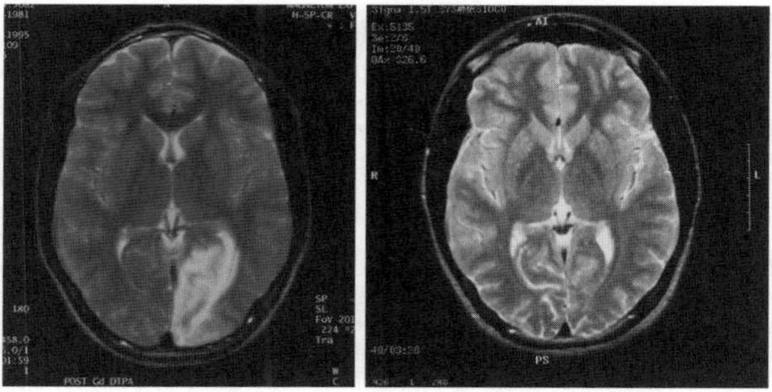

(a) (b)

Fig. 11.6 One pattern seen in MELAS is of 'large infarcts', particularly in the occipitoparietal regions and posterior temporal regions. These may not obey arterial boundaries. A typical example is shown in this boy presenting with right homonymous hemianopia in whom left occipital high signal lesion is seen on T2-weighted MRI **(a)** A characteristic feature of these MELAS 'infarcts' is that remarkable resolution of the MRI abnormalities may occur, as on this repeat scan some months later **(b)** © Hugh Markus.

Moyamoya disease and syndrome

Stenosis and occlusion of the basal intracerebral arteries (terminal ICA, proximal ACA, and MCA) occurs, usually in childhood. These occlusions result in ischaemia and secondary new vessel formation with many small collateral lenticulostriate arteries forming to bypass the occlusion. This pattern looks like a puff of smoke on angiogram: hence its name Moyamoya, meaning 'puff of smoke' in Japanese.

Moyamoya disease is an idiopathic condition, most frequent in Japan and the Far East, but rare in the western hemisphere (although it can occur). Intimal thickening in walls occurs. There is a familial pattern in some cases. It has an autosomal dominant inheritance and incomplete penetrance has been suggested, but the underlying genes(s) are unknown.

Moyamoya syndrome can result from any condition that occludes basal intracerebral arteries in childhood or early adulthood with secondary vessel formation.

Clinical features

- In childhood with stroke secondary to vessel occlusion
- Cognitive problems owing to additional silent infarction may occur
- In adulthood, subarachnoid or intracerebral haemorrhage is caused by bleeding from collateral vessels (the most common presentation)
- In idiopathic Moyamoya, involvement of the posterior circulation is rare
- The incidence is approximately 1 per million in Japan
- Diseases causing secondary Moyamoya syndrome include sickle cell disease, basal meningeal infection, and vasculitis.

Treatment

- Uncertain with no randomized controlled trials
- Extracranial-to-intracranial (EC–IC) bypass recommended by some authorities on the assumption that it improves collateral supply and reduces secondary new vessel formation, particularly for younger patients
- In adults with well developed neovascularization, treatment options are uncertain
- Prior to new vessel formation, antithrombotic agents are frequently given. Following new vessel formation, their use is uncertain and could potentially increase haemorrhage risk
- Control of blood pressure to reduce haemorrhage risk is necessary at all stages of disease.

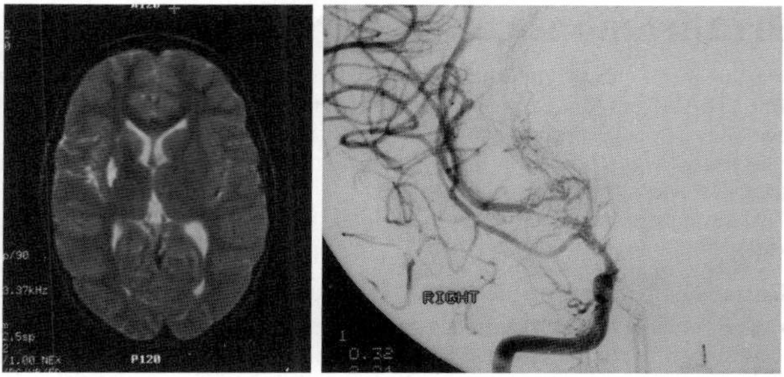

(a) (b)

Fig. 11.7 A case of Moyamoya presenting with a left hemiparesis. **(a)** A right-sided subcortical infarct can be seen on T2-weighted MRI. **(b)** On the intra-arterial angiogram, a tight middle artery stenosis can be seen with new vessel formation bypassing it. © Hugh Markus.

Prothrombotic disorders in stroke

'Prothrombotic state' and 'thrombophilia' are both terms used to describe an increased tendency to clinical thrombosis associated with laboratory evidence of coagulation pathway abnormalities.

Frequently tested for in young stroke, the evidence linking them to sporadic arterial stroke is weak.

They appear to be more important in childhood stroke and stroke in young adults (aged <40 years).

Causes of thrombophilia

- Deficiencies of natural anticoagulant proteins (proteins C and S and antithrombin III)
- Activated protein C resistance which is usually associated with the factor V Leiden polymorphism
- Lupus anticoagulant and antiphospholipid syndrome.

Protein C and S deficiency

- Protein C and S are synthesized by the liver before being released into the general circulation; involved in degradation of factors V and VIII, which play roles in the thrombotic cascade
- Deficiency may be inherited or acquired
- Inherited protein C and S deficiency occurs in approximately 0.4% of the population
- Larger studies in sporadic stroke have found no association with ischaemic stroke. Smaller studies in young stroke (<40 years) have suggested an association; some families in which deficiencies have been reported show an association with stroke
- Overdiagnosis often occurs because:
  - Levels may fall post stroke and during systemic illness. Therefore, repeat 3 months after acute episode to confirm
  - Ethnic differences in levels—for example, the normal levels are lower in black, compared with white, individuals
  - Levels fall on warfarin therapy
- If association with stroke is suspected, treatment is anticoagulation with warfarin. Warfarin should *not* be started without additional heparin cover for at least the first week because it reduces protein C and S concentrations before other vitamin K-dependent coagulation factors
- Warfarin-induced skin necrosis appears to be more common in individuals with protein C deficiency.

Activated protein C resistance

- This is the most common inherited prothrombotic state
- There is functional resistance to the anticoagulation effects of activated protein C, resulting from a point mutation in factor V at the site (Arg 506) where activated protein C cleaves and inactivates the Va procoagulant. The genetic polymorphism is called the Leiden factor V mutation
- Small studies have suggested an association with sporadic stroke but larger studies have not confirmed this

- Possibly stronger associations have been reported in younger patients (<40 years) and specific families
- Heterozygote form (associated with activated protein C resistance) is present in 5% of the normal population; therefore, in clinical practice association may occur by chance
- It is the most common inherited predisposing factor to venous thrombosis (including cerebral venous thrombosis)
- If found in stroke, look for possible paradoxical embolism from venous thrombosis (via PFO)
- Treatment is anticoagulation with warfarin.

Lupus anticoagulant and anticardiolipin antibodies

These are closely related antibodies which react with proteins associated with phospholipids, including the phospholipid moieties of DNA or RNA.

They are most common in patients with SLE but may also occur without SLE and be associated with both arterial and venous thrombosis.

Features of the antiphospholipid antibody syndrome occurring in the absence of SLE include:

- Stroke and other arterial thrombosis
- Venous thrombosis, including cerebral venous thrombosis
- Pulmonary embolism
- Livedo reticularis skin appearance
- Cardiac valve vegetations
- Thrombocytopenia
- Amaurosis fugax in absence of carotid stenosis
- Ischaemic anterior optic neuropathy, probably caused by *in-situ* thrombosis of the posterior ciliary artery
- Other CNS involvement.
- Recurrent miscarriage

Diagnosis

- Lupus anticoagulant is detected in the blood by prolongation of clotting time, probably as a result of interference with procoagulant effects of membrane phospholipids interacting with platelets and clotting
- Prolongation of kaolin cephalin time (KCT) and Russell viper venom test. Adding normal plasma to the blood fails to correct this prolongation
- Anticardiolipin antibody detected by ELISA
- Remember anticardiolipin antibodies can occur secondary to other conditions, e.g. malignancy, HIV infection, and are sometimes transiently associated with stroke. If elevated antibodies are found, repeat level in the convalescent phase.

Treatment

- For full blown syndrome, anticoagulation with heparin and warfarin is usually recommended
- For stroke alone or where association is less certain, antiplatelet agents are usually used
- Subcutaneous heparin during pregnancy may prevent recurrent miscarriage.

Further reading

Prothrombotic disorders in stroke

Haywood S, Liesner R, Pindora S, Ganesan V (2005) Thrombophilia and first arterial ischaemic stroke: a systematic review. *Archives of Disease in Childhood* **90**, 402–5.

Markus HS, Hambley H (1998) Haematological disorders and ischaemic cerebrovascular disease. *Journal of Neurology, Neurosurgery and Psychiatry* **64**, 150–9.

Cerebral vasculitis

Stroke can occur as part of many vasculitic connective tissue disorders, including polyarteritis nodosa (PAN), SLE, rheumatoid arthritis, and Behcet's disease. In these diseases, stroke usually occurs in patients with already diagnosed systemic disease although occasionally they can present with stroke. In contrast, stroke is often the presenting feature in giant cell arteritis (temporal arteritis) and Takayasu's arteritis.

Cerebral vasculitis can be classified by the size of the vessel involved and/or mode of clinical presentation.

Classical presentations of cerebral vasculitis
Acute or subacute encephalopathy
Headache
Acute confusional state—may progress to drowsiness and coma
Intracranial mass lesion
Headache
Drowsiness
Focal signs
Sometimes raised intracranial pressure
Superficially resembling atypical multiple sclerosis
Relapsing–remitting course
Features such as optic neuropathy, brainstem episodes, seizures, headaches, and stroke episodes
Stroke
May be recurrent
May be (but not always) associated with systemic disease and raised inflammatory markers

Modified from Scolding NJ, Jayne DR, Zajicek JP *et al.* (1997) Cerebral vasculitis—recognition, diagnosis and management. *Quarterly Journal of Medicine* **90**, 61–73.

Classification of cerebral vasculitis by size of vessel involved
Large-vessel vasculitis
Takayasu's arteritis
Giant cell (temporal) arteritis
Medium-vessel vasculitis
Polyarteritis nodosa
Wegener's granulomatosis
Isolated CNS vasculitis
Small-vessel vasculitis
Churg–Strauss arteritis
Essential cryoglobulinaemic vasculitis
Vasculitis secondary to connective tissue disorders: SLE, rheumatoid arthritis, relapsing polychondritis, Behcet's disease, and other connective tissue disorders
Vasculitis secondary to viral infection—usually due to hepatitis B and C, HIV, cytomegalovirus, Epstein–Barr virus, and parvo B19 virus

Giant cell arteritis (temporal arteritis)

Pathophysiology

- Affects any medium sized or large artery but by far most commonly involves ophthalmic artery and branches of external carotid artery
- On biopsy, characteristic giant cells are seen (hence its name) accompanied by other changes of vasculitis
- Posterior circulation may be involved
- Pathological studies show vasculitis only involves extracranial vessels up to the level of the dura, suggesting intracranial vascular symptoms result from embolism.

Clinical features

- A disease of the elderly, usually over age 60 years
- Most commonly presents with headache—throbbing or boring and affecting predominantly a temporal location
- May present with uniocular visual loss. This is usually permanent (in contrast to amaurosis fugax secondary to carotid atherosclerosis), but initially may be transient
- Facial pain and scalp tenderness from external carotid artery involvement
- Occasionally there is jaw claudication (pain on exercizing the jaw, i.e. eating)
- On examination, there is tenderness and nodularity or absent pulses on palpation of temporal arteries
- Overlap with polymyalgia rheumatica which presents with malaise and myalgia, particularly affecting the shoulder and hip girdles
- Stroke may occur and the posterior circulation is more involved.

Diagnosis

- ESR usually markedly raised
- All elderly patients presenting with temporal headache or visual loss should have urgent ESR
- Liver function tests, particularly alkaline phosphatase, may be elevated
- Chronic normocytic anaemia may occur
- Definitive diagnosis is on temporal artery biopsy. Lesions may be skip lesions—therefore at least a 2-cm length of artery must be biopsied. There is vasculitis with mononuclear cell infiltrate or granulomatous inflammation, usually with multinucleated giant cells.

Treatment

- To prevent permanent blindness, urgent confirmation of diagnosis and treatment is required
- Start high-dose steroids (prednisolone 40–80 mg/day) as soon as diagnosis is suspected, and before biopsy (which can be delayed by a couple of days and still give diagnostic information). Remember to give osteoporosis protection with steroids
- Symptoms of headache, facial pain, and polymyalgia rapidly resolve
- Slowly reduce prednisolone over next few months, but low-dose treatment is often need for 1–2 years
- Self-limiting disease which usually lasts 1–2 years, although it has a variable duration
- In some cases, additional immunosuppressive agents (e.g. azathioprine) are required
- Serial ESRs can be used to monitor asymptomatic relapse during steroid withdrawal, although occasionally symptomatic relapses have been reported with a normal ESR.

Other cerebral vasculitides

Isolated CNS angiitis

- By definition this is a vasculitis or angiitis affecting only the CNS
- Histology may show granuloma in the arteriolar walls—this led to the older name for the disease, granulomatous angiitis
- Small intracranial vessels are most commonly involved
- It presents with progressive dementia, multiple strokes affecting small arteries, and encephalopathy
- By definition, systemic involvement does not occur although there is an overlap with systemic vasculitis
- ESR may be increased or normal
- CT or MRI scanning shows multiple areas of infarction, particularly in the white matter
- CSF may show increase in protein concentration and slight increase in lymphocyte count
- Angiography is often normal because small vessels are involved beyond the resolution of the technique
- Diagnosis is often only made at brain biopsy or post mortem
- There are no treatment trials or good data on optimal treatment approaches
- Case reports suggest immunosuppressive agents, particularly cyclophosphamide, may be beneficial.

Behçet's disease
- Systemic disorder which may involve the brain
- Most common in individuals from Turkey and Mediterranean regions
- Systemic features include arthritis, urogenital ulceration, uveitis, and recurrent phlebitis
- Neurological involvement includes:
  - Stroke due to vasculopathy affecting medium size and small vessels, particularly in the brainstem
  - Chronic aseptic meningitis
  - Cerebral venous thrombosis
- MRI appearances show preferential brainstem involvement
- Treatment with steroids and immunosuppressive agents
- Frequency of HLA-B51 increased.

Takayasu's arteritis
- Large-vessel arteritis predominantly affecting aorta and its branches at their origin
- Results in regions of vessel irregularity, focal stenosis, and occlusion in these vessels
- Most commonly affects young women, especially from the Far East
- Common features include systemic illness with fever, weight loss, arthralgias, night sweats, malaise, and raised ESR
- Stenoses in vessels arising from the aortic arch may result in brain ischaemia, arm ischaemia (claudication), and occasionally ischaemia in the kidneys and lower limbs
- Aortic regurgitation and coronary artery ischaemia may occur
- Clues on examination include reduced or absent radial pulses or reduced blood pressure which may be asymmetrical
- The type of stroke will depend upon the vessels involved, but both carotid and vertebral territories can be affected
- Diagnosis is usually made on the pattern of involvement of aortic arch vessels seen on CTA, MRA, or intra-arterial angiography
- Treatment is with corticosteroids. This is usually required for a few years
- Prognosis is good with treatment: 5-year survival is 80%.

Diagnostic criteria for Takayasu's

At least three out of six criteria are reported to yield sensitivity and specificity of 90.5% and 97.8%:
- Onset <40 years
- Claudication of extremities
- Decreased pulsation of one or both brachial arteries
- At least 10 mmHg systolic difference in both arms
- Bruit over one or both carotid arteries or abdominal aorta
- Arteriographic narrowing of aorta, its primary branches, or large arteries in upper or lower extremities.

Polyarteritis nodosa (PAN)
- Systemic necrotizing vasculitides includes three related disorders: PAN, Wegener's granulomatosis, and Churg–Strauss syndrome. PAN is a systemic necrotizing vasculitis and aneurysm formation affecting both medium and small arteries. If only small vessels are affected, it is called

microscopic polyangiitis, although it is more associated with Wegener's granulomatosis than classic PAN
- Vasculitis affects medium sized vessels. Involvement of cerebral circulation can occur and cause stroke, TIA, or vascular dementia
- Occasionally disease presents with stroke
- Other features include mononeuropathy or polyneuropathy (mononeuritis multiplex), livedo reticularis, renal involvement, myalgias, weakness, weight loss
- Eosinophilia is often present
- Arteriographic abnormalities and arterial biopsy (if performed) shows polymorphonuclear cells
- Antineutrophil cytoplasmic antibody (pANCA) is often elevated
- Treatment is with steroid and immunosuppressive therapy.

Wegener's granulomatosis
- Systemic vasculitis of medium and small arteries, including venules and arterioles. It produces granulomatous inflammation of the respiratory tracts and necrotizing, pauci-immune glomerulonephritis
- There is nasal or oral inflammation (oral ulcers or purulent/bloody nasal discharge) which may be painful. There may be saddle nose deformity (nose flattened because of destruction of nasal septum by granulomatous inflammation)
- Abnormal CXR showing nodules, infiltrates, cavities
- Microscopic haematuria or RBC casts
- Vessel biopsy shows granulomatous inflammation
- Almost all patients with Wegener's granulomatosis have c-ANCA, but not vice versa
- The current treatment of choice is cyclophosphamide.

Systemic lupus erythematosus
- A systemic disorder which can involve both central and peripheral nervous systems
- Stroke may occur because of:
  - Vasculitis/vasculopathy involving the small vessels
  - Associated lupus anticoagulant syndrome causing thrombosis in large and medium sized vessels
  - Aseptic endocarditis (Liebman–Sacks) causing cerebral embolization
  - Hypertension due to renal disease
  - Cerebral venous thrombosis
- Other involvement of the CNS includes headache, psychiatric presentations, seizures, and encephalopathy
- Systemic involvement includes rashes (photosensitive butterfly facial and discoid), arthralgia and arthritis, renal disease, pleuritis and pericarditis, Raynaud's, and leukopenia
- ESR is raised, complement may be reduced
- Diagnosis is on antibody testing: dsDNA (antibodies to genetic material in cells) and anti-Sm antibody (Sm is a protein found in the cell nucleus)
- Anticardiolipin antibody and lupus anticoagulant may be present.

Illicit drug use

- An important cause of stroke, particularly in younger individuals
- The strongest association appears to be with cocaine but there are also reports with amphetamines and sympathomimetic agents and occasionally other illicit drugs
- In some communities, as many as 10% of young strokes may be associated with drug abuse. How much of this is causal and how much merely innocent association is unclear
- Drug screening should be performed in young stroke patients in whom illicit drug abuse is suspected.

Cocaine

- Associated with both ischaemic and haemorrhagic stroke
- Proposed mechanisms causing stroke include hypertension, vasospasm, vasculitis, cardiac arrhythmias, MI, and increased platelet aggregation
- Stroke appears more common with crack cocaine.

Amphetamines

- Intracerebral and subarachnoid haemorrhage have been associated. Ischaemic stroke is less common but may occur
- Pathological animal studies show small haemorrhages, infarctions, microaneurysms, and perivascular cuffing in small to medium sized vessels following repeated amphetamine injection
- Cerebral angiography may show segmental narrowing and dilatations ('beading') of medium sized intracerebral arteries consistent with vasculitis.

Heroin

- Associated particularly with ischaemic stroke
- Possible mechanisms include infective endocarditis with septic embolism, HIV infection, emboli from contaminants introduced during intravenous injection, hypotension, and possibly a vasculitis.

Infection and stroke

Associations between infection and stroke include:

- Specific infections which can cause stroke
- Non-specific association between recent infection and stroke—many studies have found recent infection is associated with increased ischaemic stroke risk
- Chronic inflammation and infection (particularly with *Chlamydia pneumoniae*) with accelerated atherosclerosis. Trials of antibiotic therapy have failed to reduce cardiovascular event risk after MI
- Infection frequently complicates stroke and may worsen outcome.

Specific infections causing stroke:

- A list is shown in Table 11.1
- Infective endocarditis is an important cause of stroke. Embolism can cause ischaemic stroke, while septic emboli can result in mycotic aneurysm and cerebral haemorrhage (see 🕮 p. 220)
- Meningeal infection can cause secondary vasculitis and thrombosis in basal cerebral arteries as they pass through the meninges. Important causes include tuberculosis, syphilis, and fungi. Contrast-enhanced MRI may show basal meningeal enhancement, and CSF examination is often diagnostic. Acute bacterial meningitis less commonly causes stroke by similar mechanisms
- Some viruses are associated with cerebral vasculitis occurring following acute infection, particularly herpes zoster and, less frequently, chicken pox (especially in children)
- HIV is associated with increased stroke risk by a variety of mechanisms (see 🕮 p. 354)
- Rarely, inflammation of the internal carotid artery in the neck can cause secondary thrombosis and stroke. This can occur because of infections in the neck, including pharyngitis and tonsillitis, especially in children.

Table 11.1 Infection and stroke

Infections directly causing stroke
Infective endocarditis
Meningitis
Chronic
Tuberculosis
Syphilis
Fungal (*Cryptococcus*, *Candida*, *Aspergillus*, mucormycosis)
Acute bacterial
Viral infections
Herpes zoster vasculitis
Chicken pox (*Varicella*)
HIV
Carotid inflammation
Tonsillitis
Pharyngitis
Lymphadenitis
Other associations of infection with stroke
Chronic inflammation/infection associated with atherosclerosis
Recent acute infection associated with increased stroke risk

HIV and stroke

- Stroke incidence is increased in individuals with HIV
- The risk of ischaemic stroke appears to be particularly increased. Cerebral haemorrhage risk may also be increased to a lesser extent (see Table 11.2)
- Many different stroke mechanisms are responsible, making a full diagnostic work-up essential
- Cardioembolism, particularly cardiomyopathy, may account for as much as 20% of HIV ischaemic stroke
- Vasculitis is a more common cause than in non-HIV stroke. Potential mechanisms include basal cerebral artery involvement due to basal meningitis (e.g. tuberculosis), neurosyphilis, and herpes zoster
- The role of hypercoagulability is controversial. Protein S deficiency and lupus anticoagulant are both more common, but recent studies have suggested these abnormalities are as common in HIV patients without stroke. They may be non-specific markers of illness
- With increased survival, an increased incidence of atherosclerotic stroke is becoming evident. Possible mechanisms include direct HIV effects on endothelial cells, secondary lipid abnormalities, and anti-retroviral therapy. Treatment with combination anti-retroviral therapies (CART), particularly those containing protease inhibitors, has been associated with severe premature atherosclerosis, including MI and stroke
- Associated drug abuse is common and may contribute to stroke. Cocaine use is a particular risk
- Causes of cerebral haemorrhage in HIV include thrombocytopenia, hypertension, and mycotic aneurysm secondary to infective endocarditis
- Diagnostic work-up for HIV stroke should include a full young stroke work-up and often lumbar puncture for CSF examination. Prothrombotic disorders should be tested for but if abnormalities are found it should not be assumed that these have caused stroke, and other potential causes should also be sought.

Further reading

Mochan A, Modi M, Modi G (2005) Protein S deficiency in HIV associated ischaemic stroke: an epiphenomenon of HIV infection. *Journal of Neurology Neurosurgery and Psychiatry* **76**, 1455–6.

Ortiz G, Koch S, Romano JG, Forteza AM, Rabinstein AA (2007) Mechanisms of ischemic stroke in HIV-infected patients. *Neurology* **68**, 1257–61.

Table 11.2 Mechanisms of stroke in HIV-positive patients

A. Ischaemic stroke
Cardioembolism
Cardiomyopathy
Endocarditis
Vasculitis
Tuberculosis meningitis
Neurosyphilis
Herpes zoster
Fungal
Accelerated atherosclerosis
Proinflammatory effect on endothelial cells
Indirect induction of lipid abnormalities
Anti-retroviral therapy
Hypercoagulability
Protein S deficiency
Lupus anticoagulant/antiphospholipid antibody (?causal)
Associated substance abuse (leading to vasculitis)
Cocaine
Amphetamine
Injection of particulate matter (used to dilute drugs)
B. Cerebral haemorrhage
Vascular
Vasculitis
Mycotic aneurysm secondary to endocarditis
Cocaine
Haematological
Reduced platelets (thrombocytopenia)
Reduced coagulation factors due to liver disease
Cocaine-induced brain haemorrhage

Cancer and stroke

- An increased risk of stroke has been associated with cancer. Both are common diseases and in many patients may be associated by chance. In some, a causal relationship is likely
- Possible mechanisms causing stroke in cancer patients are shown in the table. These include:
  - Associations with specific tumours
  - Hypercoagulability, particularly associated with disseminated carcinoma
  - Complications of therapy: drug, surgical, and radiotherapy
- Radiation vasculopathy is well recognized. Usually in the years after irradiation to the head or neck, vasculopathy may occur. It may involve extracranial cerebral arteries or intracranial vessels (including microvasculature). It presents with stroke (often recurrent) and dementia (particularly for intracranial small-vessel vasculopathy). Progress is often relentless (particularly for intracranial small-vessel vasculopathy) and there is no proven treatment.

Table 11.3 Possible causes of stroke in cancer patients

Cerebral infarction
Hypercoagulable state
Non-bacterial endocarditis (marantic endocarditis)
Embolism of tumour (including atrial myxoma)
Treatment-related:
Radiation vasculopathy
Interventions, including surgery
Drug therapy
Direct compression of extracranial or intracranial arteries
Opportunistic infections
Cerebral haemorrhage
Haemorrhage into primary brain neoplasms
Haemorrhage into metastases
Melanoma
Bronchial carcinoma
Choriocarcinoma
Hypernephroma
Thrombocytopenia and other coagulopathies
Tumour embolization with aneurysm formation and rupture
Cerebral venous thrombosis
Tumour infiltration of venous sinuses
Tumour compression of venous sinuses
Hypercoagulable state

Chapter 12

Cerebral venous thrombosis

Introduction

- An often difficult diagnosis to make but important because heparin therapy is probably associated with improved outcome, and patients in a severe neurological state can make a good outcome
- Variable clinical presentations, including headache, papilloedema, seizures, focal deficits, intracerebral haemorrhage, and coma, make a high index of suspicion important
- Underdiagnosed
- MRI and MRA have greatly improved ease of diagnosis.

Anatomy

- Venous sinuses drain blood from the brain and bones of the skull
- Situated between the two layers of the dura mater
- Lined by endothelium continuous with the veins
- Contain no valves and walls are devoid of muscular tissue
- Connections exist between venous sinuses and veins of face, scalp, spine, and neck. This provides a path by which pathological processes such as infection can spread into cerebral venous sinuses as well as an alternate route for blood to leave the cranial cavity when obstruction occurs
- A diagram of the anatomy of the cerebral venous sinuses is shown in Fig. 12.1.

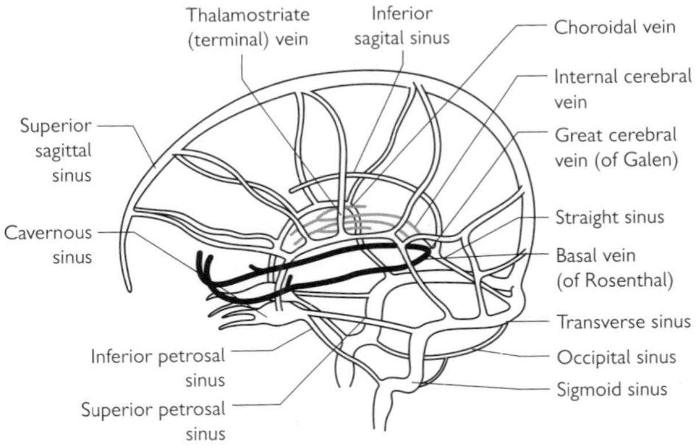

Fig. 12.1 The venous sinuses.

Aetiology

- Causes of cerebral venous thrombosis (CVT) are shown in Table 12.1
- Infection was, and in many parts of the world still is, a major cause of CVT. In developing countries, the proportion caused by infection has fallen from 40% in the 1960s to 10% or less
- Infection is relatively more important for cavernous sinus thrombosis and lateral sinus thrombosis
- Cavernous sinus thrombosis may originate via spread from the medial third of the face, nose, orbit, or paranasal sinuses or by direct spread by ethmoid or sphenoid ear cells or through lateral sinuses from the ear. *Staphylococcus aureus* is the most common pathogen
- Fungal infections may cause CVT, particularly in the cavernous sinus
- Prothrombotic states are an important risk factor. Leiden factor V (causing activated protein C resistance) is the most commonly associated
- Increased risk is associated with pregnancy and particularly puerperium and contraceptive therapy is likely to be mediated via hypercoagulability
- Frequently patients have more than one potential cause of CVT.

Further reading

Ferro JM, Canhão P, Stam J, Bousser MG, Barinagarrementeria F (2004) Prognosis of cerebral vein and dural sinus thrombosis: results of the International Study on Cerebral Vein and Dural Sinus Thrombosis (ISCVT). *Stroke* **35**, 664–70.

Stam J (2005) Thrombosis of the cerebral veins and sinuses. *New England Journal of Medicine* **352**, 1791–8.

Table 12.1 Causes of cerebral venous thrombosis

Infective
Bacterial infections
Fungal infections
Non-infective
Inherited prothrombotic disorders
APC resistance—factor V Leiden polymorphism
Antithrombin III deficiency
Protein C and S deficiency
Prothrombin gene mutation
Hyperhomocysteinaemia
Acquired prothrombotic state
Pregnancy
Puerperium
Lupus anticoagulant/anticardiolipin antibody
Nephrotic syndrome
Dehydration
Inflammatory disorders and vasculitis
Behçet's
Wegener's granulomatosis
SLE
Haematological conditions
Polycythaemia
Anaemia, including paroxysmal nocturnal haemoglobinuria
Thrombocythaemia
Sickle cell anaemia
Mechanical
Head injury
Lumbar puncture
Neurosurgical or other interventional procedures
Neoplasia
Usually haematogenous malignancies
Local compression, e.g. meningioma
Drugs
Oral contraceptives
Asparaginase
Idiopathic

Clinical features

These may arise from:

- Venous infarction which may be haemorrhagic
- Cerebral haemorrhage
- Impaired venous drainage
- Intracranial hypertension

Specific features include:

- Raised intracranial pressure with headache and papilloedema. This manifests particularly when the superior sagittal sinus is occluded owing to impaired absorption of CSF by the arachnoid villae
- Headache owing to raised intracranial pressure or sometimes secondary to haemorrhage
- Focal neurological deficits—these may fluctuate in severity. Hemiplegia is most frequent, and in superior sagittal sinus thrombosis the leg may be more affected than the face and arm
- Seizures—these may occur in the absence of any other deficit although are more common in patients with focal neurological deficits
- Cranial nerve palsy—particularly for cavernous sinus thrombosis.

Common patterns of presentation

Most presentations fall into a number of patterns with different rates of temporal progression.

- Abrupt onset of focal signs mimicking an arterial occlusion
- Subacute onset of focal deficit with or without seizures or elevated intracranial pressure
- Progressive rise in intracranial pressure (clinical picture of normal pressure hydrocephalus). This occurs particularly with superior sagittal sinus thrombosis. MRI and/or MRA is required in such cases to exclude CVT
- Chronic presentations, which can be confused with a brain tumour
- Sudden headache resembling subarachnoid haemorrhage
- Transient focal deficits presenting like TIAs.

Cavernous sinus thrombosis

- This has a unique presentation owing to its anatomy (Fig. 12.2)
- It most commonly occurs secondary to infection in the middle third of the face, sphenoid, ethmoid or maxillary sinuses, and, less commonly, the oropharynx, teeth, neck, and ear
- Presentation is related to venous obstruction, inflammation, and systematic infection
- Headache is common
- Proptosis and oedema of the eyelids and conjunctiva arises secondary to venous obstruction
- Dilatation of facial veins may occur
- Ophthalmoplegia with palsies of III, IV, and VI cranial nerves as they pass through the sinus may occur
- Optic nerve involvement can result in impaired acuity and afferent pupillary deficit
- Papilloedema and retinal vein distension is frequent
- Contralateral cavernous sinus may be affected because of midline communications through circular or intracavernous sinus
- Facial numbness may be confined to the upper two-thirds of the face as the first two divisions of the trigeminal nerve are intracavernous. If the thrombosis or infection spreads into the inferior petrosal sinus, the third division of the trigeminal nerve may also be affected
- The close proximity of the III, IV, and VI cranial nerves and the first two divisions of the trigeminal nerve explains why palsies of these nerves are common in cavernous sinus thrombosis.

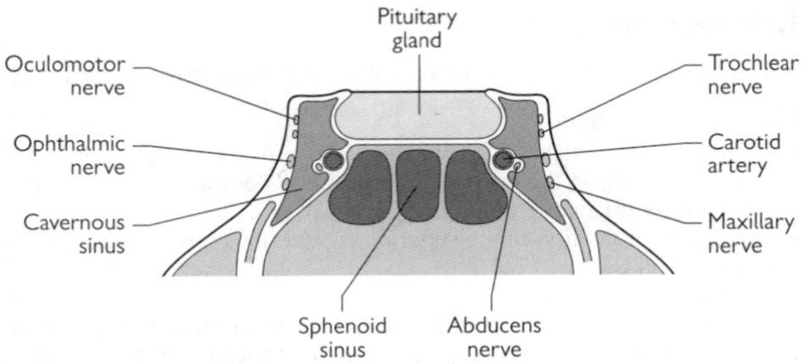

Fig. 12.2 A diagram of a cross-sectional view of cavernous sinus showing close proximity to II, IV, VI, and Va and Vb cranial nerves.

Investigations

MRI is the imaging modality of choice, but CT may show diagnostic features.

CT

- CT may be abnormal in CVT but the findings are often non-specific, particularly early in the disease course. Use of contrast enhancement can improve diagnostic yield
- The posterior portion of the superior sagittal sinus can be directly visualized on CT
- Specific features include:
  - Delta sign—thrombosis of the superior sagittal sinus may appear as a dense triangle at the occiput on an unenhanced scan. Following contrast injection the negative or empty delta sign may be seen (see Fig. 12.3). This is a central lucency ascribed to sluggish or absent blood flow within the superior sagittal sinus surrounded by margin of contrast enhancement
  - Diffuse load density suggestive of oedema
  - Generalized cerebral swelling
  - Haemorrhagic infarcts—mixed hypodensity and increased density corresponding to ischaemia and haemorrhage
  - Intracerebral haemorrhage.
- The occluded venous sinus may be seen on CTV (CT venogram).

MRI and MR venography (MRV)

- The investigation of choice
- Absence of normal 'flow void' in venous sinuses on T2-weighted imaging may be seen
- Intravascular thrombus itself may be seen within sinuses
- MRI will also show similar consequences of venous thrombosis to those seen on CT, namely cerebral swelling, haemorrhagic infarction, and cerebral haemorrhage
- MRV may show absent or reduced venous flow at the site of thrombosis
- MRI and MRV can miss thrombosis in smaller sinuses or in the deep cerebral veins. This may require intra-arterial angiography to detect.

Further reading

Smith R, Hourihan MD (2007) Investigating suspected cerebral venous thrombosis. *BMJ* **334**, 794–5.

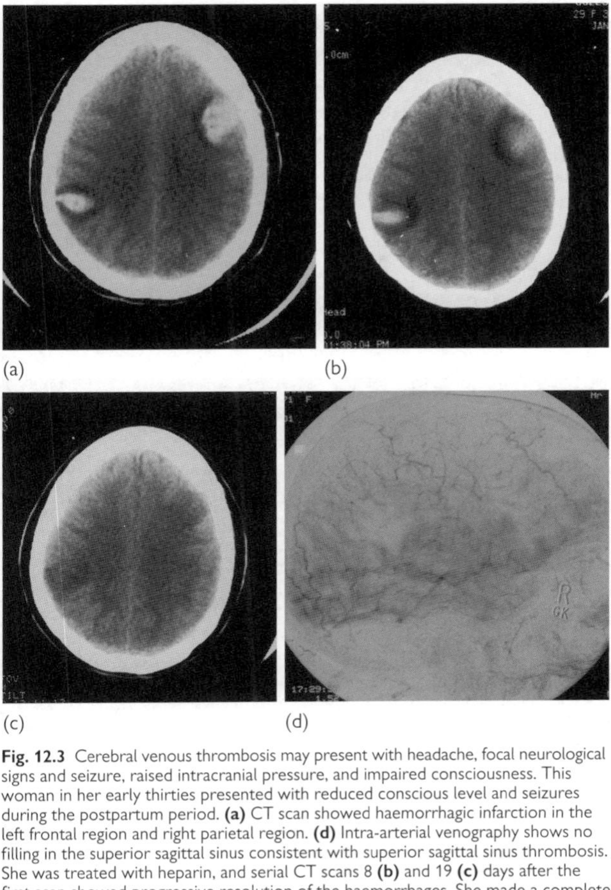

Fig. 12.3 Cerebral venous thrombosis may present with headache, focal neurological signs and seizure, raised intracranial pressure, and impaired consciousness. This woman in her early thirties presented with reduced conscious level and seizures during the postpartum period. **(a)** CT scan showed haemorrhagic infarction in the left frontal region and right parietal region. **(d)** Intra-arterial venography shows no filling in the superior sagittal sinus consistent with superior sagittal sinus thrombosis. She was treated with heparin, and serial CT scans 8 **(b)** and 19 **(c)** days after the first scan showed progressive resolution of the haemorrhages. She made a complete recovery. © Hugh Markus.

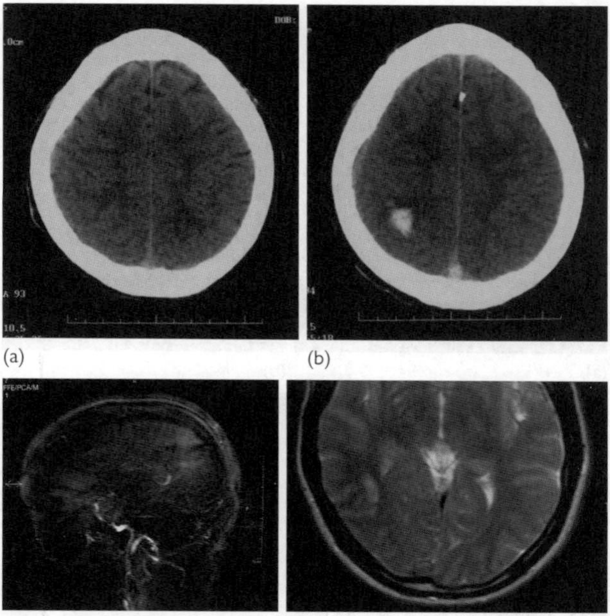

(a) (b) (c) (d)

Fig. 12.4 This patient presented to the acute stroke unit with headache, nausea, and vomiting. **(a)** The initial CT showed no haemorrhage but a 'delta sign' was present, indicating thrombus in the posterior part of the superior sagittal sinus. **(b)** On CT scan at day 5, haemorrhage can now be seen in the right parietal lobe. **(c)** MRA confirmed the diagnosis, showing absence of flow in the superior sagittal sinus. **(d)** On MRI thrombus within the sagittal sinus can be seen. © Hugh Markus.

Treatment

- Most authorities would recommend anticoagulation although there is limited randomized data to support this—one small very underpowered but positive trial. Two further trials have not shown a significant difference but all are too small to derive definitive information. (For meta-analysis showing a non-significant benefit of anticoagulation see Cochrane Database reference below.) Anecdotal experience suggests that even in patients with haemorrhagic infarction and intracerebral haemorrhage, dramatic improvements can occur with anticoagulation. Heparin followed by warfarin for 3–6 months is usually recommended
- If there are underlying abnormalities of coagulation on blood testing or other causes, longer term anticoagulation may be necessary
- Symptomatic treatment for epilepsy, raised intracranial pressure, etc. may be required.

Further reading

Einhäupl K, Bousser MG, de Bruijn SF *et al.* (2006) EFNS guideline on the treatment of cerebral venous and sinus thrombosis. *European Journal of Neurology* **13**, 553–9.

Einhäupl KM, Villringer A. Meister W *et al.* (1991) Heparin treatment in sinus venous thrombosis. *Lancet* **338**, 597–600.

Stam J, De Bruijn SF, DeVeber G (2002) Anticoagulation for cerebral sinus thrombosis. *Cochrane Database Systematic Review* **4**, CD002005.

Prognosis

- Early studies reported poor outcome with high mortality and residual disability. More recent studies show improved outcome, probably because of both better care and diagnosis of milder cases
- With aggressive treatment, prognosis is often good. Dramatic improvement can be seen. Degree of improvement from focal deficits is more rapid and complete than that usually seen for ischaemic stroke.
- In one study of 110 subjects seen between 1975 and 1990, six died from the acute event, and two later from underlying disease. Of the remaining 102, 86% had no neurological sequelae. Four had recurrent seizures. Nine suffered a second cerebral venous thrombosis, usually within the first year (Preter *et al.*, 1996)
- Prognosis is worse for thrombosis of the deep cerebral veins
- High rate of recurrence (as much as 20%) emphasizes the importance of long-term anticoagulation where underlying prothrombotic states can be detected.

Reference

Preter M, Tzourio C, Ameri A *et al.* (1996) Long-term prognosis in cerebral venous thrombosis: follow-up of 77 cases. *Stroke* **27**, 243–6.

Further reading

Ferro JM, Canhão P, Stam J, Bousser MG, Barinagarrementeria F (2004) Prognosis of cerebral vein and dural sinus thrombosis: results of the International Study on Cerebral Vein and Dural Sinus Thrombosis (ISCVT). *Stroke* **35**, 664–70.

Chapter 13

Cerebral haemorrhage

Introduction

Cerebral haemorrhage is classified according to the region into which the haemorrhage occurs:

- Extradural haemorrhage
- Subdural haemorrhage
- Subarachnoid haemorrhage
- Intracerebral haemorrhage.

Cerebral haemorrhage only presents with clinical stroke if there is focal compression in an eloquent brain region, or secondary ischaemic change (e.g. vasospasm in the case of subarachnoid haemorrhage). Intracerebral haemorrhage usually presents with a clinical stroke.

Extradural haemorrhage

- Extradural haemorrhage (EDH) is seldom a cause of a stroke syndrome
- This is when bleeding occurs into the extradural space
- It usually occurs after head injury
- One of the extradural arteries (such as the middle meningeal artery) is ruptured and blood enters the extradural space
- This compresses the brain from the outside, raises ICP acutely and can be fatal
- Ten per cent of extradurals are venous in origin
- It should be suspected in patients with head injury who have a reduced or reducing level of consciousness
- The diagnosis is easily confirmed on brain imaging with CT or MRI
- This is a neurosurgical emergency. These patients need urgent scanning and urgent neurosurgical treatment
- Treatment is by evacuation of the haematoma, either through burr holes or a craniotomy.

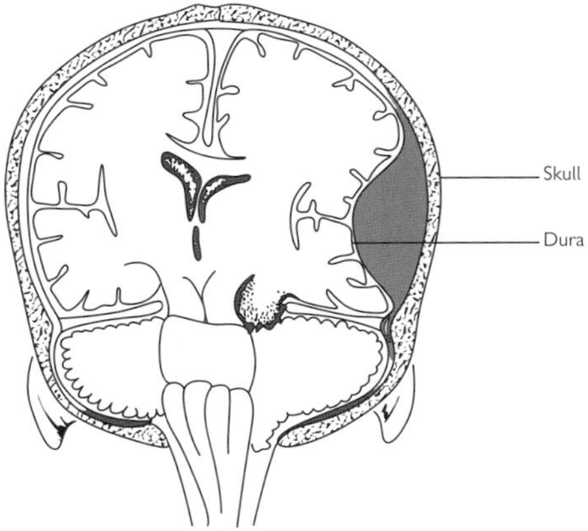

Fig. 13.1 Location of an extradural haemorrhage. Reproduced with permission from www.primary-surgery.org.

Subdural haematoma

- Bleeding occurs into the subdural space
- The fragile veins that bridge the subdural space may tear and blood flows at a low pressure into the subdural space
- It is more common in the presence of brain atrophy, particularly in the elderly and also in chronic alcoholics
- It is normally thought to be caused by trauma, although the actual incident may not be recalled by the patient at the time that the subdural haematoma is diagnosed.

Clinical presentation

- A variety of presentations can occur depending on how acute the subdural haemorrhage is, its size, and its location
- Clinical presentation is often insidious
- It can present as:
  - A stroke with focal symptoms—most commonly hemiparesis but other cortical signs can occur
  - Reduction in conscious level owing to raised ICP
  - Worsening neurological/confusional state, often insidious, particularly in the elderly
- A high index of suspicion should be present in an elderly patient who is having progressive problems such as a deteriorating gait
- Diagnosis is made on brain imaging with CT or MRI. Sometimes the haematoma (if old) is isodense (of a similar density) to brain tissue and can be missed if careful evaluation is not performed. In such cases MRI may be helpful.

Treatment

- A large subdural haematoma (SDH), particularly if there is reduced conscious level or focal neurological signs or neurological progression, is a neurosurgical emergency
- Small subdurals are managed conservatively and usually resolve over time
- Subdurals can be difficult to drain, particularly acutely, as the blood will be partly clotted
- Neurosurgical teams often wait about a week until the haematoma has liquefied
- SDH is drained through a burr hole, otherwise a full craniotomy is required with flushing out the blood clot that remains in the subdural space.

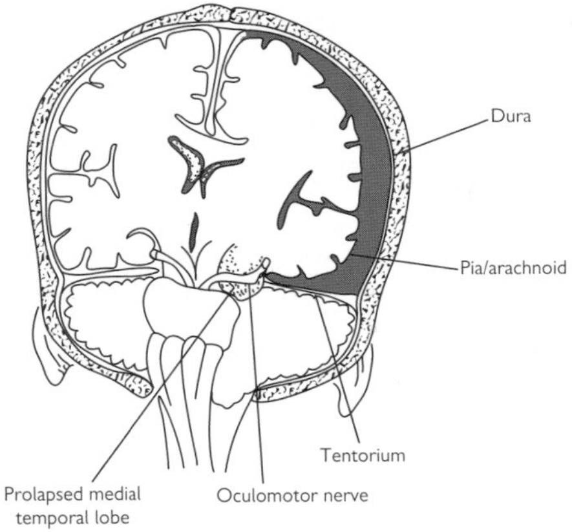

Fig. 13.2 Schematic diagram of the location of a subdural haemorrhage. Reproduced with permission from www.primary-surgery.org.

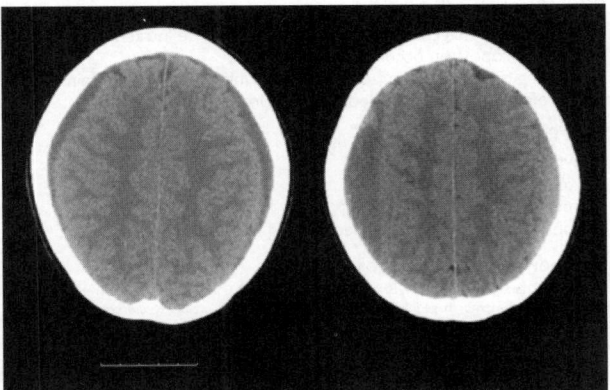

Fig. 13.3 This patient suffered bilateral subdural haemorrhages. The scan on the left is taken after about 1 week. The scan on the right is a month later. The right-sided subdural is larger and the left appears to have resolved; however, close inspection shows that it is still present but isodense. © Anthony Pereira.

Subarachnoid haemorrhage

Introduction

Subarachnoid haemorrhage (SAH) is where bleeding occurs into the subarachnoid space. It most often presents with sudden onset headache and meningism but can cause focal symptoms, i.e. present as a stroke. This occurs when:

- There is a focal haematoma; this is most common for MCA aneurysms
- Secondary vasospasm results in focal ischaemia.

Owing to a high risk of early rebleeding SAH is a medical and neurosurgical emergency and patients should be admitted, and the diagnosis made either with CT scan and/or lumbar puncture.

It has a variety of causes:

- Berry aneurysms cause 70%
- Arteriovenous malformations cause 10%
- Hypertension causes 10%
- Five per cent are idiopathic.

The incidence of SAH is about 10 per 100 000 compared to intracerebral haemorrhage which is just below 30 per 100 000.

It is proportionally commoner in younger stroke patients.

Site of haemorrhage

- Most haemorrhage is from aneurysms which arise intracranially
- A small proportion occur in the spine
- Bleeding is into the subarachnoid space which normally contains CSF
- Therefore, there is no impediment to circulation of this blood.

Risk factors

- Hypertension
- Excess alcohol consumption
- Smoking
- Connective tissue disease predisposing to berry aneurysms.

Further reading

Nilsson OG, Lindgren A, Stahl N, Brandt L, Säveland H (2000) Incidence of intracerebral and subarachnoid haemorrhage in southern Sweden. *Journal of Neurology Neurosurgery and Psychiatry* **69**, 601–7.

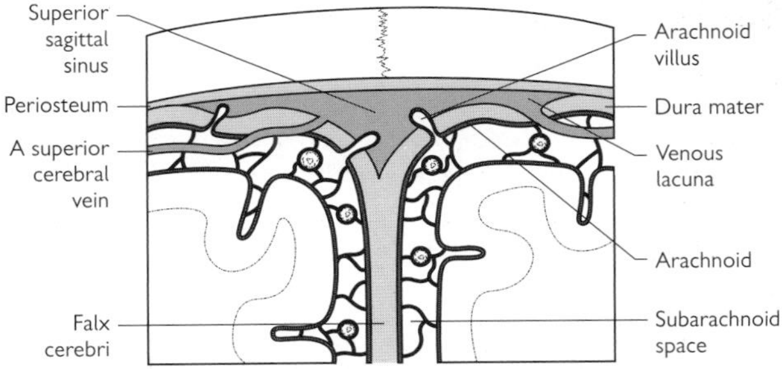

Fig. 13.4 The diagram shows the anatomy of the subarachnoid space. It is a 'potential' space lying between the arachnoid mater and the pia mater. The space is very narrow but blood vessels traverse it.

Berry (saccular) aneurysms

Aneurysms are found in 2% of asymptomatic individuals at post mortem. They are:

- Thin-walled
- Saccular
- They most commonly occur at arterial bifurcations.

Common sites of aneurysms are:

- Posterior communicating artery (30%)
- Anterior communicating artery (25%)
- Middle cerebral artery (25%)
- Fifteen per cent are multiple.

Most are asymptomatic. They cause symptoms either when they rupture or occasionally if they increase in size. A ruptured aneurysm is a common cause of sudden death, particularly in the young.

Rupture rates depend on size and position of the aneurysm. The cumulative 5-year rupture rates for aneurysms in the anterior and posterior circulation are shown below.

Anterior circulation: internal carotid artery, anterior communicating or anterior cerebral artery, middle cerebral artery:

- <7 mm 0%
- 7–12 mm 2.6%
- 13–24 mm 14.5%
- >25 mm 40%

Posterior circulation: posterior cerebral and posterior communicating:

- <7 mm 2.5%
- 7–12 mm 14.5%
- 13–24 mm 18.4%
- >25 mm 50%

Further reading

Wiebers DO, Whisnant JP, Huston J *et al.* (2003) Unruptured intracranial aneurysms: natural history, clinical outcome, and risks of surgical and endovascular treatment. *Lancet* **362**, 103–10.

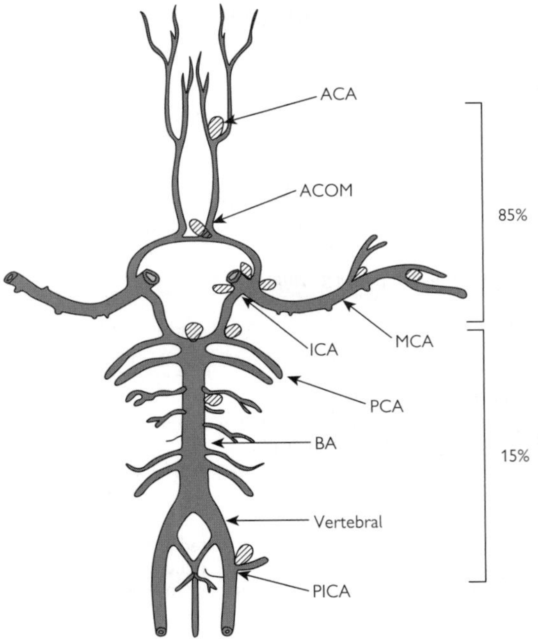

Fig. 13.5 Common sites of berry aneurysms. Adapted from McCormick WF in Rosenberg *et al* (eds). ACA, anterior cerebral artery; ACOM, anterior communicating artery; BA, berry aneurysm; ICA, internal carotid artery; MCA, middle cerebral artery; PCA, posterior cerebral artery; PICA, posterior interior cerebral artery.

Clinical features of SAH

Symptoms

Headache

- The classic presentation is with a very sudden onset (thunderclap) severe headache
- It is often occipital but any new very sudden onset headache should be considered as a potential SAH
- Some patients with a SAH may have had a warning or so-called 'sentinel' headache in the preceding days owing to a minor leak of blood.

Other frequent accompanying symptoms

- Nausea
- Vomiting
- Photophobia
- Neck stiffness.

Conscious level

- This may be reduced and is associated with worse prognosis
- SAH can present with sudden death
- A short period of loss of consciousness may occur at onset.

Signs

- Meningism: marked neck stiffness
  - Kernig's sign—straight leg raising is limited and induces pain
  - Brudzinsky's sign—flexion of the neck induces bending of the legs
  - Interestingly, although flexion of the neck may be impossible, lateral rotation of the neck is unaffected
- Bilateral VI cranial nerve palsy from raised ICP
- Focal neurological signs—these are often not present but may occur depending on the site of bleeding, the presence of focal haematoma and secondary to complication such as vasospasm
- Fundoscopy may show subhyaloid haemorrhage.

Differential diagnoses

- Migraine
- Coital cephalgia
- Meningitis
- Thunderclap headache without SAH
  - This presentation usually occurs without meningism or focal neurology
  - CT imaging and CSF examination are normal
  - It is associated with good outcome and low incidence of subsequent SAH.

Grading of SAH

There are several grading systems used to describe the severity of SAH. Two are given on 📖 p. 383: the Hunt and Hess grading and the World Federation of Neurological Surgeons grading system. Grading is a useful method to describe the severity of SAH and provides some indication of the likely outcome, which is worse with a higher grade.

Hunt and Hess grades

Grade I—asymptomatic, or minimal headache and slight nuchal rigidity
Grade II—moderate to severe headache, nuchal rigidity, only cranial nerve palsy
Grade III—drowsiness, confusion or mild focal deficit
Grade IV—stupor, moderate to severe hemiparesis, possibly early decerebrate rigidity, and vegetative disturbances
Grade V—deep coma, decerebrate rigidity, moribund appearance.

World Federation of Neurological Surgeons

Grade	GCS score	Motor deficit
I	15	Absent
II	14–13	Absent
III	14–13	Present
IV	12–7	Present or absent
V	6–3	Present or absent

Investigation of SAH

Computed tomography

- Diagnosis can often be confirmed by an early CT
- This has become the first line diagnostic test of choice and it often enables one to avoid lumbar puncture
- Sensitivity is 90% if performed within the first 24 hours
- Sensitivity is reduced to 50% by 72 hours as blood is reabsorbed
- CT may also identify the source of haemorrhage
  - Anterior communicating artery aneurysm bleed produces blood at the front of the interhemispheric fissure
  - Middle cerebral artery aneurysm produces blood in the Sylvian fissure
  - Internal carotid artery bleeding produces blood in the suprasellar cistern on one side
  - Posterior communicating artery aneurysm produces blood in the suprasellar and prepontine cisterns
  - Basilar artery aneurysm produces blood in the basal cisterns.

Lumbar puncture

- Indicated if diagnosis is in doubt, i.e. if CT has given equivocal results, lumbar puncture is indicated
- Opening pressure may be raised
- Uniform blood-staining of CSF is seen. If it has been a traumatic or 'bloody' tap, the number of red cells will decline as time goes on. This can be seen if three serial samples are taken and the depth of blood staining visualized when they are held up to light
- The ratio of white cells to red cells will be 1:500, the same as in peripheral blood. A higher proportion of white cells may indicate a different diagnosis
- Xanthochromia (a yellow tinge to the fluid) appears as CSF blood haemolyses. It remains present reliably for about 2 weeks
- Spectrophotometry of CSF for bilirubin quantitation to check for xanthochromia is the recommended method of analysis and should be done on the final bottle of CSF collected.

Cerebral angiography

- This is essential in all cases in which intervention might be possible to determine whether there is an underlying aneurysm and identify its site and size
- CT angiography is good at identifying aneurysms, and technology is continuing to improve but may miss smaller aneurysms
- MR angiography can identify larger aneurysms but may miss those 3–5 mm in diameter or less
- The gold standard is intra-arterial digital subtraction angiography which is necessary if CTA/MRA are negative.

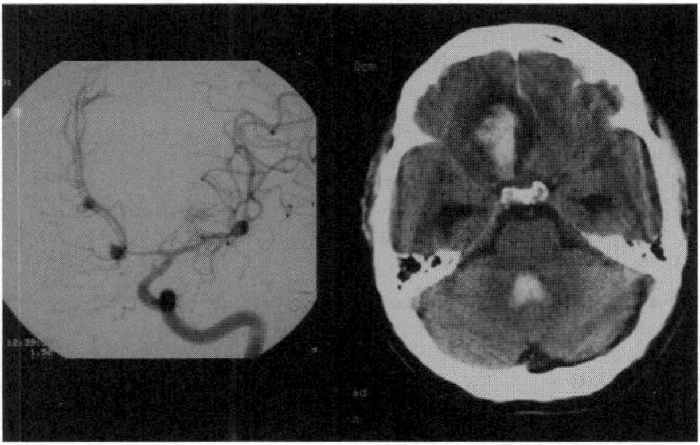

Fig. 13.6 A left anterior communicating artery aneurysm which caused intracerebral haemorrhage which can be seen both in the right frontal region. Blood is also visible on CT in the fourth ventricle. The aneurysm is visible on the angiogram. © Hugh Markus.

Complications of SAH

The major complications follow.

Rebleeding

- Risk of rebleed is 4% at 24 hours, 25% at 2 weeks and 60% at 6 months if no measures are taken to prevent it
- The mean time for rebleeding is about 10 days
- Rebleeding is associated with an 80% mortality or poor outcome
- This high risk is why early identification and treatment of aneurysms to prevent rebleeding is required.

Delayed ischaemic neurological deficit

- Vasospasm resulting from blood in the CSF may produce a secondary ischaemic neurological deficit
- It is most common after about 2 days and lasts up to 2 weeks
- Treatment is by maintaining cerebral perfusion with adequate hydration
- Calcium channel blockers (nimodipine) may also be useful.

Hydrocephalus

- Results from impaired CSF reabsorption through arachnoid villi owing to blockage by blood in the CSF
- Ten per cent of patients will require CSF diversion or shunting.

Seizures

- Ten per cent of patients may suffer seizures
- The risk is higher the more severe the neurological deficit
- Seizures may occur during the acute episode but can also occur months or more after the SAH.

Cardiac abnormalities

- ST elevation on the ECG is often seen and may mimic changes seen in acute myocardial infarction.

Syndrome of inappropriate ADH secretion (SIADH)

- ADH is secreted, causing salt wasting in the kidney
- The plasma sodium concentration drops as does the osmolality
- It is common and electrolytes should be monitored carefully
- It is diagnosed by sending a simultaneous blood and urine sample to calculate the respective osmolalities
- Inappropriately dilute urine in the face of dilute serum makes the diagnosis
- Treatment is fluid restriction
- SIADH normally abates spontaneously.

Management of SAH: medical

The patient should be admitted to hospital and transferred to a neuroscience centre.

General measures

- Maintain airway, breathing, circulation
- Intubate and ventilate if necessary
- Oxygen if needed
- Serum glucose—use sliding scale infusion of insulin if necessary
- Treat fever
- Consider antiemetics for nausea or vomiting
- Treat seizures
- Watch for, and treat, SIADH with fluid restriction
- Elevate the head of the bed 30° to facilitate intracranial venous drainage
- Maintain euvolaemia (central venous pressure, 5–8 mmHg).

Treatment of raised intracranial pressure

- This is a common complication
- ICP monitoring may be necessary
- Intubation with hyperventilation can reduce ICP via reducing carbon dioxide concentrations (induces vasconstriction)
- Osmotic agents such as mannitol can reduce ICP by as much as 50% within 30 minutes. Effect peaks at about 90 minutes, and lasts 4 hours
- Loop diuretics such as furosemide
- Steroids probably do not work.

Cerebral vasospasm

- Nimodipine (dose 60 mg given every 4 hours) is usually given prophylactically. This was associated with a reduction of one poor outcome for every eight patients treated with oral nimodipine. It may improve outcome by reducing vasospasm and/or have a neuroprotective effect
- If cerebral vasospasm is present, maintain hypervolaemia (CVP 8–12 mmHg, or pulmonary capillary wedge pressure (PCWP) 12–16 mmHg)
- Percutaneous transluminal angioplasty has been used to treat vasospasm but has not been proven to be beneficial in controlled trials
- Transcranial Doppler ultrasound can be performed on a regular basis to monitor for the development of vasospasm (seen as increases in velocity in basal intracerebral vessels).

Further reading

Dorhout Mees SM, Rinkel GJ, Feigin VL *et al.* (2007) Calcium antagonists for aneurysmal subarachnoid haemorrhage. *Cochrane Database of Systematic Reviews* **18**, CD000277.

Suarez JI, Tarr RW, Selman WR (2006) Aneurysmal subarachnoid hemorrhage. *New England Journal of Medicine* **354**, 387–96.

Management of SAH: surgical and endovascular

- The early risk of recurrent bleeding can be reduced by surgical clipping of the aneurysm
- Therefore it is essential to identify any underlying aneurysm on angiography (see 📖 Investigation of SAH, p. 384)
- More recently, endovascular treatment of aneurysms, with embolization with platinum coils, has become available
- The ISAT(International Subarachnoid Aneurysm Trial) showed that endovascular treatment could produce better outcome than surgery
- Of 1063 patients allocated to endovascular treatment, 23(5%) were dead or dependent at 1 year, compared to 30(9%) of 1055 patients allocated to neurosurgery. The early survival advantage was maintained for up to 7 years.

Timing of intervention

- The optimal time for coiling has not been studied but, given the high early rebleed risk, the general feeling is that the earlier the better
- Some evidence suggests if surgery is performed it is better to do this within 3 days owing to the high early rebleeding risk. There is an increased risk of complications after this time due to vasospasm which is maximal at 5–7 days. Some authorities wait until 10 days if surgery cannot be performed within the first 3 days. However, patients may die as a result of rebleed during this period.

Indication for surgery versus endovascular treatment

In certain circumstances one or other approach is considered preferable.

Indications for surgery in patients with SAH

- For patients with milder syndromes who are suitable for either surgical or endovascular treatment, endovascular treatment is now the treatment of choice unless there is a delay in performing it
- For Hunt and Hess/WFNS grades 4–5 (i.e. severe), the outcome is poor with or without surgical intervention
- Large and giant aneurysm
- Wide-necked aneurysms
- Vessels emanating from the aneurysm dome
- Mass effect or haematoma associated with the aneurysm
- Recurrent aneurysm after coil embolization clotting. This appears to be a safer procedure and is more appealing and acceptable to patients. However, there is a 5% failure rate and, if not completely obliterated, the aneurysm may reform.

Indications for endovascular treatment

- For patients with milder syndromes who are suitable for either surgical or endovascular treatment, endovascular treatment is preferable
- Patients with poor clinical grade
- Patients who are medically unstable
- Where aneurysm location carries a high surgical risk, e.g. basilar
- Small-necked aneurysms in the posterior fossa
- Patients with early vasospasm
- Patients with multiple aneurysms in different arterial territories if surgical risk is high.

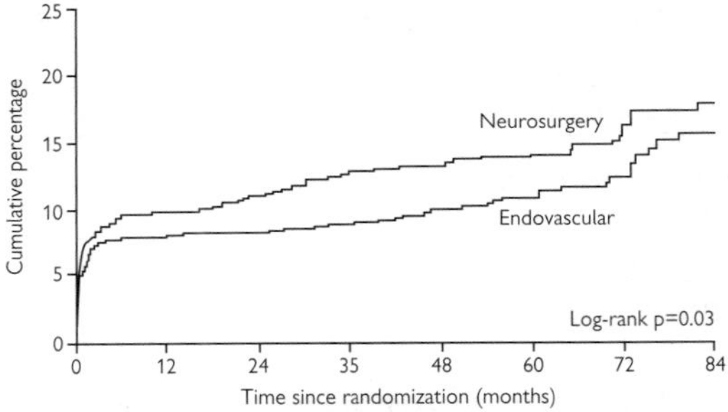

Annual number at risk (deaths)

Endovascular	1073 (85)	974 (3)	887 (5)	717 (8)	541 (4)	373 (5)	215 (6)	103
Neurosurgery	1070 (105)	944 (10)	842 (16)	663 (3)	503 (3)	340 (7)	192 (3)	98

Fig. 13.7 Survival curves for patients treated with neurosurgery and endovascular treatment in the ISAT trial. It can be seen that patients treated with endovascular therapy had a better survival, with the curves separating early. Reproduced from Molyneux AM, Kerr RSC, Yu L-M *et al.* (2005) For the International Subarachnoid Aneurysm Trial (ISAT) of neurosurgical clipping versus endovascular coiling in 2143 patients with ruptured intracranial aneurysms: a randomized comparison of effects on survival, dependency, seizures, rebleeding, subgroups, and aneurysm occlusion. Aneurysm Trial (ISAT) Collaborative Group. *Lancet* **366**, 809–17, with permisssion of Elsevier.

Asymptomatic aneurysms

These can be found:

- Incidentally on neuroimaging performed for another cause
- In patients who have another symptomatic aneurysm
- When family members are screened.

Risk of rupture of asymptomatic intracranial aneurysm

The best data is from the prospective studies ISUIA study cohort of 1692 patients with a mean follow up of 4.1 years.

Risk of haemorrhage over the next 5 years for posterior aneurysms (posterior communicating/posterior circulation)

Size of aneurysm	No SAH (%)	History of SAH (%)
<7 mm	2.5	3.4
7–12 mm	14.5	14.5
13–24 mm	18.4	18.4
>24 mm	50	50

Risk of haemorrhage over the next 5 years for anterior aneurysms (ACA/MCA/ICA)

Size of aneurysm	No SAH (%)	History of SAH (%)
<7 mm	0	1.5
7–12 mm	2.5	2.5
13–24 mm	14.5	14.5
>24 mm	40	40

Screening for intracranial aneurysms

There is an increased risk of aneurysms in family members where one member has already been diagnosed with a berry aneurysm. If they have more than one first-degree relative, their risk is much higher but is still only 10%.

When considering whether to screen one has to consider:

- The risk to the patient of intra-arterial angiography to detect an aneurysm
- Both MRA and CTA can miss small aneurysms (<5 mm for MRA, <2–3 mm for CT)
- Not all aneurysms will rupture
- Aneurysms found will probably require treatment with associated risks
- Some aneurysms found will be untreatable.

Screening should be considered in:

- Individuals with two or more first-degree relatives with aneurysms/ SAH
- Patients with autosomal dominant polycystic kidney disease
- Aneurysms are very rare in childhood and therefore screening is usually started in adult life
- The benefit of screening is reduced in older patients in whom the lifetime risk of aneurysm rupture is less—therefore screening is recommended up to the age of 60–70 years.

In our practice:

- We tend not to advise treatment for aneurysms found to be <7 mm in diameter. However, we normally repeat imaging at yearly intervals for a couple of years to determine whether the aneurysm is enlarging
- In older patients the benefit of treatment is less, especially if there are additional comorbidities that limit life expectancy
- For aneurysms >7 mm we consider treatment if it is technically possible with low risk
- The risk of treating asymptomatic aneurysms depends on many factors, including the aneurysm itself and the patient but as ball park figures:
  - Neurosurgical clipping has a mortality of 2–3% and causes permanent morbidity in another 11%
  - Endovascular treatment has a mortality of 0.5–1% and causes permanent morbidity in another 7%.

Further reading

Risk of rupture of asymptomatic intracranial aneurysm

Wiebers DO, Whisnant JP, Huston J *et al.* (2003) Unruptured intracranial aneurysms: natural history, clinical outcome, and risks of surgical and endovascular treatment. *Lancet* **362**, 103–10.

Screening for intracranial aneurysms

Warlow C *et al.* (2008) Specific interventions to prevent intracranial haemorrhage. In: *Stroke: Practical Management*, 3rd edition, Chapter 15. Oxford, Blackwell.

Intracerebral haemorrhage

- Between 10 and 15% of stroke is due to intracerebral haemorrhage (ICH)
- ICH occurs where blood leaks into the brain parenchyma, resulting in a focal haematoma. Secondary leakage of blood into the subarachnoid space may also occur
- Blood leaks into the brain at arterial pressure and may continue for a prolonged period. Early haematoma growth occurs in 18–38% of patients scanned within 3 hours of ICH
- Mortality is higher after cerebral haemorrhage than after ischaemic stroke.

A list of causes of ICH is shown on 📖 p. 393. This is a bit simplistic as different causes and risk factors interact. For example, in a patient with cerebral small-vessel and leukoaraiosis who bleeds on warfarin therapy and who is also hypertensive, all three factors are contributing. Nevertheless, the classification forms a useful list to work through when assessing a patient with ICH.

Detailed descriptions of specific causes are given later in the chapter along with any specific treatments required for that cause.

Causes of intracerebral haemorrhage

Cerebral haemorrhage may be caused by:

- Abnormal cerebral vessels
- Abnormalities in blood.

These interact with risk factors which increase the risk of bleeding in the presence of many underlying causes.

Abnormal blood vessels

- Cerebral small-vessel disease
  - Hypertension with lipohyalinosis and microaneurysms
- Amyloid angiopathy
- Vascular malformations
  - Arteriovenous malformations
  - Saccular aneurysms
  - Cavernous haemangiomas (cavernomas)
- Cerebral tumours
- Cerebral venous thrombosis
- Moyamoya disease and syndrome
- Septic and mycotic aneurysms
- Cerebral vasculitis.

Abnormalities in the blood

- Systemic bleeding tendency
  - Haemophilia
  - Leukaemia
  - Thrombocytopenia
- Drug therapy
  - Anticoagulants
  - Antiplatelet agents
  - Thrombolytic agents.

Other causes

- Haemorrhagic transformation of a cerebral infarct
- Illicit drugs
  - Amphetamines
  - Cocaine
- Hyperperfusion syndrome post carotid endarterectomy
- Trauma.

Major risk factors for intracerebral haemorrhage

- Hypertension
- Age
- Alcohol excess
- Leukoaraiosis on brain imaging

Clinical features and investigation of ICH

Clinical features

Like ischaemic stroke, ICH presents with the sudden onset of a focal neurological deficit. Prior to the wide availability of brain CT, scales were developed to try to separate ischaemia from cerebral haemorrhage on clinical grounds. Although some features may suggest haemorrhage (e.g. headache at onset or very early symptoms/sign progression), it is impossible to distinguish cerebral haemorrhage from ischaemic stroke reliably on clinical grounds. ICH presents like any other form of stroke with sudden onset neurological deficit.

Therefore the important message is that:
- *It is impossible clinically to differentiate ICH from ischaemic stroke. Therefore urgent brain imaging is essential in all cases of stroke.*

Nevertheless, there are certain clinical features which suggest ICH:
- If blood leaks into the subarachnoid space a severe headache, which may come on very suddenly, can occur. Other features of meningism may also be present (vomiting, neck stiffness)
- Headache is also more common in ICH, even in the absence of subarachnoid blood. However, it can also occur with cerebral infarcts and may be absent in ICH
- Progression early after onset is more common with ICH, but can occur in infarcts as well
- Seizures are more common with ICH, but can also occur with infarcts.

The focal symptoms and signs accompanying ICH depend on the location of the haematoma and are indistinguishable from those caused by infarction.

Investigation of ICH

General tests

These will only rarely identify specific causes of haemorrhage but should be performed. They may include:
- An urgent INR in anyone suspected of being on warfarin
- Blood tests for FBC (particularly platelets)
- Coagulation system screen when indicated
- Testing for illicit drugs should be performed if this is suspected.

However, the key to identifying ICH and determining the underlying causes is brain imaging, described overleaf.

Brain imaging in ICH

CT is most widely used but MRI also has good sensitivity and adds some additional pieces of information.

CT

- Blood appears as high signal
- CT has a high sensitivity for fresh blood
- Usually the hyperdense appearance lasts a few weeks but for small haemorrhages it can be shorter
- Once the blood has been resorbed (over a few weeks) it is impossible to tell whether an old stroke was an infarct or a haemorrhage
- In contrast, MRI can differentiate old haematomas from old infarcts.

MRI

- MRI has a similar sensitivity in diagnosing haemorrhage to CT, as long as the appropriate sequences are done
- Interpreting the scan can be more difficult than for CT
- The time course of symptoms needs to be known when reviewing the scan:
  - Within minutes blood is low density on T1 imaging and bright on T2
  - This remains between hours and a few days
  - Between days and weeks it becomes high signal on T1 and low on T2
  - After weeks it becomes high signal on T1 and high on T2 with a dark rim
- Gradient echo (T2*) sequences should be performed as these are most sensitive to both recent and old haemorrhage
- Gradient echo is very sensitive to haemosiderin from breakdown of blood products which appears as areas of signal loss (black) and this persists for years after haemorrhage. This allows:
  - Detection of old haemorrhage at other sites
  - Determination of whether an old stroke is due to haemorrhage or infarctions (also infarcts which have undergone haemorrhagic infarction will show haemosiderin)
  - Detection of microbleeds.

Other clues from imaging

- Imaging reveals the location of infarction which can give useful clues as to the cause, particularly whether it is lobar or subcortical
- Clues to the cause may be seen, including:
  - Abnormal vessels on an AVM
  - Evidence of cerebral venous thrombosis (filling defects and venous sinus thrombus)
  - Congestion of pial vessels suggesting a dural fistula.

Patterns of haemorrhage

Imaging allows division of haemorrhage into different types according to brain regions affected. This is useful in determing the underlying causes, as different causes tend to have different locations.

- Lobar (cortical) haemorrhage
- Subcortical haemorrhage.

Scans should also be classified as to whether secondary haemorrhage into the subarachnoid space/intraventricular system has occurred.

In some cases multiple ICH are be seen. More common causes of these include:

- Cerebral amyloid angiopathy (MRI may show many old haemorrhages)
- Certain metastatic tumours
  - Melanoma
  - Bronchogenic carcinoma
  - Renal carcinoma
  - Choriocarcinoma
- Cerebral venous thrombosis
- Haematological disorders (including diffuse intravascular coagulation and leukaemia)
- Cerebral vasculitis
- Thrombolytic and other anticoagulant therapy
- Head injury.

Investigation of underlying cause

- Once the patient has recovered from ICH it is important to look for the underlying cause
- Often in the acute phase there is too much blood around and it is impossible to identify an underlying lesion unless a large lesion such as a tumour is present
- Occasionally acute investigation is performed if a lesion with a high early recurrent bleeding risk is suspected, e.g. cerebral aneurysm with a small ICH
- Therefore usually one should wait until the blood has been resorbed; this normally takes 6–8 weeks but may take as long as 3 months
- Imaging is then performed with CT with contrast, or MRI
- MRI is more likely to detect underlying causes than CT, and if gradient echo is included, may give information on other old bleeds; this is particularly helpful in diagnosing amyloid angiopathy
- MRA and CTA may also show underlying vascular malformations
- In a proportion of cases it is necessary to progress to intra-arterial angiography to look for an underlying lesion. Practice varies as to how many patients undergo this. The yield is highest for cortical haemorrhages, in younger individuals (<50 years) and if the patient is not hypertensive.

Treatment of ICH

This includes:

- General supportive measures
- Reversal of any clotting abnormality
- Specific therapies to reduce haematoma size
- Treatment of complications
- Treatment of the underlying cause.

General management

- Admission to a specialized stroke unit is beneficial, as for ischaemic stroke
- General supportive measures (e.g. attention to swallowing and avoidance of aspiration) are as important as for ischaemic stroke
- Optimal management of hypertension is uncertain. Blood pressure rises acutely in ICH. Reducing it might reduce further haemorrhage risk but could reduce perfusion to compromised tissue. Some recent evidence suggests acute treatment is probably safe and may reduce haematoma expansion.

Reversal of any clotting abnormality

- Drugs that can cause bleeding should be stopped, e.g. aspirin and clopidogrel and non-steroidal anti-inflammatory agents
- Clotting and platelet count should be checked
- In warfarin-related ICH, warfarin should be reversed immediately. The best method for doing this is to use a prothrombin complex concentrate which contains coagulation factors II, VII, IX, and X. This provides all the clotting factors that have been removed by warfarin's vitamin K inhibitory action. It acts more quickly than fresh frozen plasma which is a less good alternative. Vitamin K (10–20 mg intravenously at not more than 5 mg/min) is often also given but occasionally patients need to be re-warfarinized after a period of stability and vitamin K may sometimes make this difficult. Vitamin K takes hours to work and since haematomas continue to increase in size up to 24 hours after onset, it is not indicated as reversal treatment monotherapy.

Medical treatment to reduce haematoma size

- Recent imaging studies have shown haematoma size expands in the first hours after ICH; this raises the possibility that it may be possible to give drugs which slow down haematoma expansion
- A phase II trial showed activated recombinant factor VII (NovoSeven) reduced haematoma expansion, and suggested better outcome
- However, a phase III trial showed no clinical benefit despite a reduction in haematoma size. This was because any benefit was outweighed by thrombotic side effects (myocardial ischaemia and other thrombotic events)
- Instilling a low dose thrombolytic agent into the ventricles to break down the clot is currently under evaluation in cases with intra-ventricular blood.

Neurosurgery

- The first surgical clinical trial was done at Atkinson Morley Hospital in Wimbledon by Wylie McKissock. It showed that patients with suspected ICH who underwent neurosurgery did worse than those who were treated conservatively
- The landmark large randomized, multicentre STICH trial was published in 2005. In 1003 patients, it compared surgical evacuation (craniotomy in 75%) scheduled within 24 hours with medical therapy. It was confined to supratentorial haemorrhage. The trial included four times as many patients as all the previous surgical trials in ICH combined
- No difference in outcome was found between the two treatment approaches. A 'favourable outome' was seen in 26% of those randomized to surgery and 24% of those randomized to medical therapy (OR 0.89, 95% CI 0.66–1.19)
- Subgroup analysis suggested that there might be a possible benefit for patients with cortical haematomas, while surgery for subcortical haemorrhage was not beneficial. A futher STICH trial is comparing surgery with medical therapy for cortical ICH only
- Currently, therefore, neurosurgery is not warranted for patients with supratentorial ICH
- The exception to the rule is patients with posterior fossa haemorrhage, i.e. cerebellar haemorrhage
- This can be life-threatening because the posterior fossa space is taken up by haematoma and brainstem compression occurs, causing coning and death
- Patients may make remarkable recoveries from cerebellar lesions and early neurosurgery should be contemplated
- The cut-off haematoma size derived from trials is about 4 cm but patients with any substantial cerebellar haematoma should be notified to the local neurosurgical unit and patients with larger haematoma (above 4 cm) should be transferred in anticipation of urgent neurosurgical intervention.

Treatment of complications

- Raised ICP is common in ICH. There is no good evidence how to manage it
- Hyperventilation has been used to reduce ICP but will reduce cerebral blood flow. There is no trial evidence to support this approach
- Osmotic agents such as mannitol and glycerol are also used but there is no good trial evidence supporting their use.

One should be vigilant for hydrocephalus which is common after ICH with secondary intraventricular haemorrhage. This may need shunting.

Further reading

Medical treatment to reduce haematoma size

Aguilar MI *et al.* (2007) Treatment of warfarin-associated intracerebral hemorrhage: literature review and expert opinion. *Mayo Clinic Proceeddings* **82**, 82–92.

Treatment of complications

Mendelow DM, Gregson BA, Fernandes HM *et al.* (2005) Early surgery versus initial conservative treatment in patients with spontaneous supratentorial intracerebral haematomas in the International Surgical Trial in Intracerebral Haemorrhage (STICH): a randomised trial. *Lancet* **365**, 387–97.

Prognosis of ICH

- This is much worse than that for ischaemic stroke
- Population-based studies report a 1-month mortality rate of about 40% compared with 10–20% for ischaemic stroke. After this the risk falls to 8% per annum (similar to that for ischaemic stroke)
- Factors associated with worse prognosis include:
    - Increasing age
    - Early reduction in the level of consciousness
    - Larger haematoma volume
    - Intraventricular extension of ICH
    - Anticoagulant therapy
    - Secondary hydrocephalus.

Cerebral small-vessel disease, lipohyalinosis, and microaneurysms

- Hypertension is the major risk factor for ICH
- The risk increases as blood pressure increases, both within the normal and elevated range
- Treatment reduces cerebral haemorrhage risk
- Haemorrhage is usually subcortical in the white matter, deep grey matter nuclei or brainstem
- A number of pathological changes may relate to the haemorrhage:
    - Lipohyalinosis and other degenerative changes seen in small perforating arteries. Segmental changes of fibrinoid necrosis and local vessel wall thickening can be seen. This is assumed to lead to vessel fragility and rupture
    - Charcot–Bouchard aneurysms. First described in 1869 these are tiny out-pouchings on the small perforating blood vessels in the basal ganglia and pons and cerebellum which are much more common in hypertensive patients. However, the role of these, and how common they are, has been debated
- Small-vessel disease is associated with leukoaraiosis which is a risk factor for haemorrhage
- Asymptomatic microbleeds seen on gradient echo MRI are common in patients with cerebral haemorrhage, as they are also in patients with small-vessel disease. They are more common in patients with lacunar infarcts and with increasing degrees of leukoaraiosis.

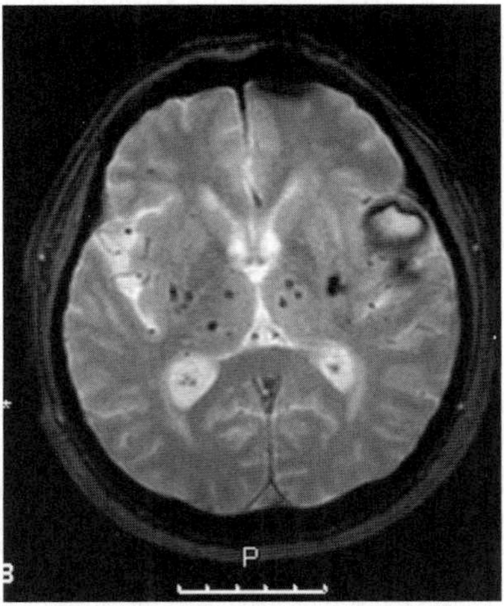

Fig. 13.8 Gradient echo MRI showing multiple microbleeds (appearing as black spots) and a more recent left frontal cortical haemorrhage. © Anthony Pereira.

Cerebral amyloid angiopathy

Pathology

- Cerebral amyloid angiopathy (CAA) is characterized pathologically by deposition of amyloid in small and medium sized arteries of the cortex and leptomeninges
- Classical birefringent amyloid material is seen on histology in the media and adventitia and this stains positive for Congo red
- The amyloid seen in CAA is closely related to the amyloid seen in Alzheimer's disease but is quite different from that in systemic amyloidosis
- It is restricted to the vessels of the leptomeninges and grey matter and usually stops abruptly when a perforating vessel reaches the junction of cortex and subcortex. This explains why haemorrhages in CAA are almost always lobar with the site of rupture usually at the grey–white matter junction
- CAA makes the vessels fragile and more likely to rupture.

Epidemiology

- Amyloid angiopathy becomes increasingly common with age and may occur in over half of unselected post mortems in those aged over 90 years
- It is therefore an important cause of ICH in the elderly
- Most cases are sporadic, although there are a few familial forms but these are very rare:
    - Dutch familial amyloid: autosomal dominant, mutations are in the beta-amyloid precursor protein and therefore the abnormal protein is a beta protein similar to that seen in sporadic CAA and Alzheimer's disease
    - Icelandic amyloid: autosomal dominant, the abnormal protein is antigenically different, being the cystatin C protein.

Clinical features

Amyloid angiopathy can present with:

- Intracerebral haemorrhage—usually lobar
- Cognitive impairment

Brain imaging appearances can be:

- ICH—this is usually lobar or in the grey–white matter boundary
- On gradient echo MRI old larger haemorrhages and/or microbleeds are seen, particularly in the cortex and at the grey–white matter boundary
- White matter hyperintensities/leukoaraiosis.

Diagnosis

- This is suggested by multiple cortical haemorrhages, particularly in an elderly person
- The presence of multiple microbleeds in the typical location in a patient with cortical haemorrhage strongly supports the diagnosis
- Definitive diagnosis requires brain biopsy—the amyloid can be diagnosed with biopsy as a characteristic apple green birefringence under polarized light. It also stains positive with Congo red. However, this is rarely done in most units as it does not alter treatment

- The Boston criteria have been developed to help with *in vivo* diagnosis, and validated against pathological diagnosis, and have reasonable sensitivity and specificity.

Boston criteria for diagnosis of CAA

- Definite: post-mortem evidence of CAA
- Probable: clinically likely with some pathological evidence (e.g. from biopsy) or clinically likely with MRI evidence in a patient older than 60 years
- Possible: MRI evidence of a lobar (or multiple lobar) haemorrhage without a primary cause in a patient over 60 years.

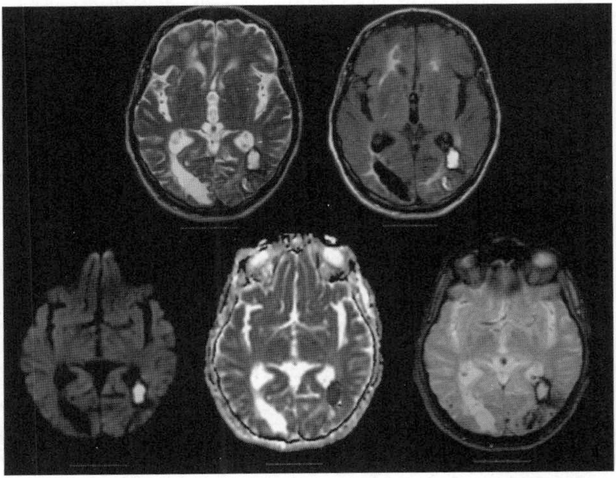

Fig. 13.9 MRI scans from a patient with amyloid angiopathy. Sequences are from left top row: T2, FLAIR; bottom row: DWI, ADC, and gradient echo. An acute haemorrhage is present in the left parietal lobe. The gradient echo GRE is very sensitive to the paramagnetic effect of blood and shows multiple little haemorrhages mainly in the left hemisphere as well as some dots in the right. © Anthony Pereira.

Further reading

Knudsen KA, Rosand J, Karluk D, Greenburg SM (2001) Clinical diagnosis of cerebral amyloid angiopathy: validation of the Boston criteria. *Neurology* **56**, 537–9.

Arteriovenous malformations

- Arteriovenous malformations (AVMs) are caused by an abnormal communication between arteries and veins
- One or more feeding arteries supplies blood directly into a draining vein, without a capillary network between the two. The vein is therefore exposed to high (arterial) blood pressure
- The cause of rupture may be because high pressure blood is continually pumped into the venous system. Associated aneurysms may also be found on the feeding vessel in about 20% of AVMs and these can rupture
- Most are probably congenital malformations but some can be acquired, e.g. dural fistulas occurring after trauma
- About 1% of intracranial haemorrhage is associated with an AVM
- These are more usually lobar rather than subcortical haemorrhages, although can be subcortical depending on the site of the AVM
- Sometimes AVMs may be multiple, and rarely are caused by an underlying systemic disorder such as hereditary haemorrhagic telangiectasia
- AVMs are associated with epilepsy, independent of ICH.

Dural AVMs or fistulas

- These are a specific type of AVM. In a dural AVM the arteries are derived from the dural and meningeal branches of the external carotid artery, and drainage is most commonly into the dural sinuses, most often the transverse and sigmoid
- They can occur secondary to blockage of drainage of a venous sinus after cerebral venous thrombosis or can be due to other causes such as neoplasia. They also occur secondary to trauma
- They can also cause pulsatile tinnitus if the fistula is near the temporal bone
- They are an important cause of ICH particularly in the young as they require specific treatment but are rare. Treatment can be surgical or endovascular. Fistulas are anatomically heterogenous so treatment needs to be tailored to the individual case.

Diagnosis of AVMs

- The tangled vessels may be seen on routine brain CT (particularly with contrast) or MRI (flow voids in the vessels)
- They can often be well seen on CTA or MRA
- Small AVMs and dural fistulas may require an intra-arterial angiogram to diagnose, and this will also be necessary for larger AVMs to plan treatment
- It may be impossible to visualize an AVM following cerebral haemorrhage owing to it being obscured by a haematoma; therefore further imaging is often delayed for 2–3 months.

Prognosis

- The risk of rebleeding in AVMs is about 2–3% per annum
- This increases to as high as 7% if there is an associated aneurysm on a feeding vessel
- The risk appears to be higher in the first few months after a bleed.

Treatment of AVMs

- There are the following treatment options:
  - Do nothing—conservative
  - Surgical excision
  - Stereotactic radiotherapy (radiosurgery)
  - Endovascular embolization
  - Very large AVMs may not be amenable for surgery
- There are no randomized trials looking at which AVMs need treating and which is the best approach. The following is a possible guideline until evidence is available:
  - Superficial or large aneurysms may be amenable to neurosurgery
  - Small AVMs in eloquent sites or smaller than 3 cm in diameter may be treated by radiosurgery. Larger lesions are not suitable as too much normal tissue has to be included in the radiation field. Radiation leads to obliteration of vessels but this takes some time and therefore the reduction is bleeding risk is delayed
  - Endovascular treatment aims to occlude the feeding vessels by the use of embolic agents such as coils or Onyx liquid polymer. This is often used to reduce the size of the AVM to make it suitable for surgery or radiosurgery.

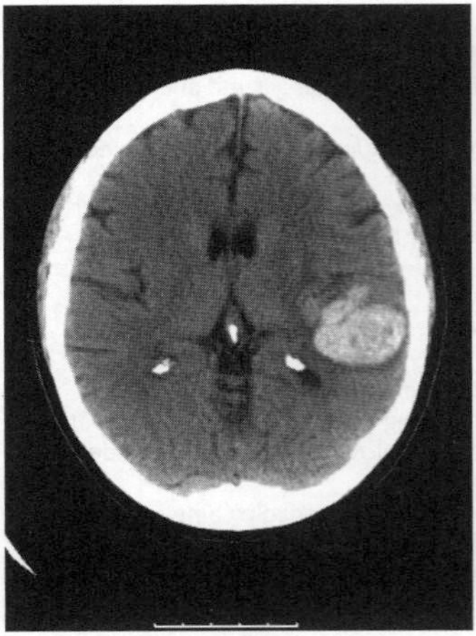

(a)

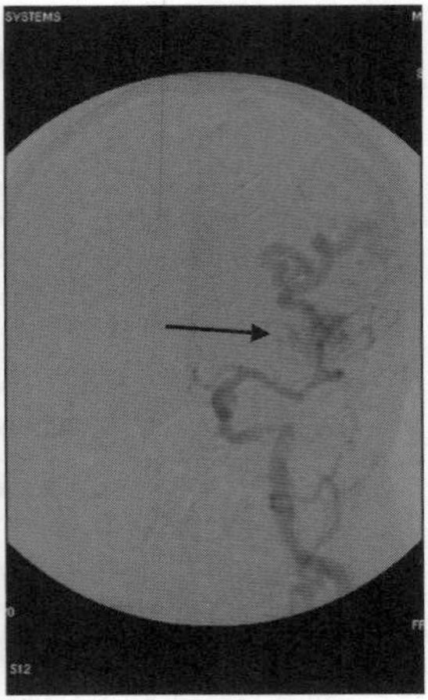

(c)

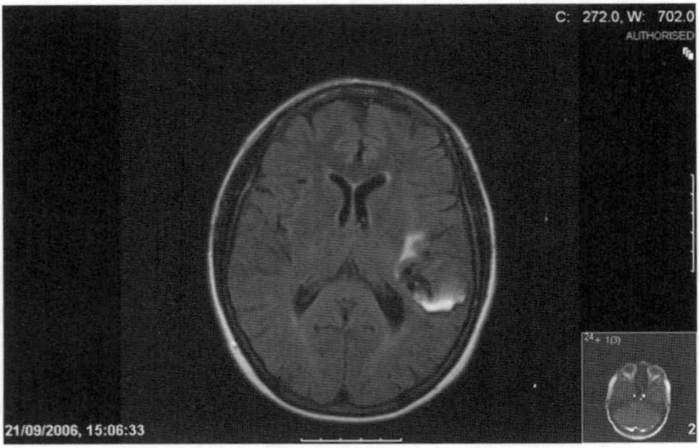

(b)

Fig. 13.10 An AVM presenting with an ICH. This patient presented to the acute stroke unit. **(a)** The initial CT showed a left-sided cortical haemorrhage; **(b)** MR in the subacute stage showed a resolving haemorrhage as well as flow voids owing to dilated vessels; **(c)** an intra-arterial angiogram shows an AVM (arrowed). © Hugh Markus.

Cavernous malformations

- Cerebral cavernous malformations are small (mm to a few cm) thin-walled vascular malformations, lined by endothelium without muscular or elastic layers and with no intervening brain tissues. They may be single, multiple, and are sometimes calcified
- Usually sporadic and of unknown aetiology
- Present asymptomatically in 0.5% of post mortems and MRIs
- Rare familial variants exist. CCM1 and CCM2 are caused by mutations in the *Krit1* and *MGC4607* genes, respectively. The underlying genes of other familial cases are not yet known. These familial forms are associated with multiple cavernomas
- Occur in hemispheric white matter or cortex in one-half, posterior fossa (most commonly the brainstem) in one-third, and basal ganglia or thalamus in one-sixth
- They can be associated with ICH, but more commonly blood leaks out, slowly causing a ring of haemosiderin deposition.

Imaging

Easily diagnosed on MRI:

- On T2-MRI: mixed signal intensity core, with surrounding rim of decreased signal intensity corresponding to haemosiderin
- The surrounding haemosiderin is better seen on gradient echo MRI which is the most sensitive technique for their detection. Gradient echo MRI may show multiple cavernomas
- Imaging studies have shown they may grow, or regress, and may occur *de novo* in familial cases
- No abnormalities are seen on angiography.

Clinical features

- Cerebral haemorrhage—these are usually small and, depending on the site, may not cause much in the way of symptoms
- Local compressive symptoms—these occur for some brainstem cavernomas which compress the surrounding tightly packed brainstem nuclei and tracts. Chronic leakage and gradual expansion can occur
- Epileptic seizures
- Asymptomatic— the most common clinical picture is an incidental finding on brain imaging.

Usually no treatment is required. The risk of recurrent haemorrhage is low; estimates vary between 0.25 and 6%. Occasionally surgical exicison is performed, particularly if compressive symptoms are occurring, although excision of brainstem cavernomas can have high surgical risk. Stereotactic 'gamma knife' radiation has also been used, although there is no controlled trial data to support its use. Brainstem cavernoma lesions may normally be watched but sometimes these bleed very slowly, causing brainstem compression. Treatment is very hazardous and may cause permanent deficit from damage to the brainstem.

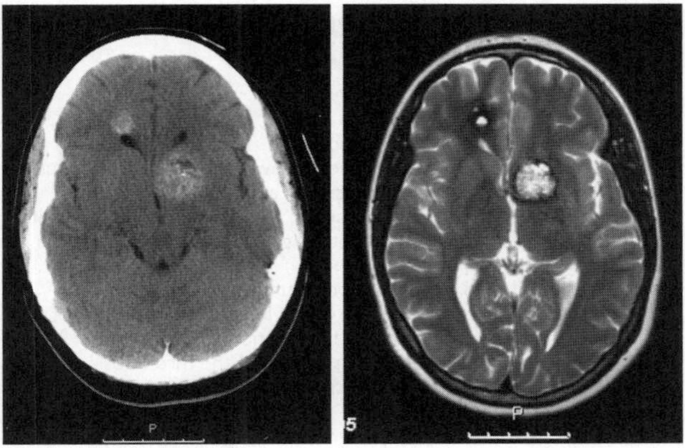

Fig. 13.11 A left thalamic cavernoma can be seen on CT on the left and on T2-weighted MRI on the right. On MRI a typical dark ring can be seen corresponding to haemosiderin deposition caused by bleeding. A second right frontal lesion can also be seen. © Hugh Markus.

Other vascular abnormalities causing ICH

Cerebral venous thrombosis

- This is an important cause of haemorrhage and is often diagnosed late
- As haemorrhage occurs from the veins (low pressure), it is often not as devastating as in an arterial haemorrhage and its onset is slower
- Often the ICH is preceded by ischaemic symptoms with focal deficits, seizures or encephalopathy without imaging evidence of haemorrhage which may occur hours or days later
- Occasionally ICH can be the first presentation
- It can be more difficult to diagnose and, if left untreated, may progress
- The diagnosis can be suspected by the location and pattern of haemorrhage which will depend on the site of the thrombosis:
  - Superior sagittal sinus thrombosis, in the parasagittal region, often bilateral
  - Transverse sinus tends to cause haemorrhage in the temporal lobes
  - Cerebral convexity with leakage from a cortical vein
  - Straight sinus causing bilateral thalamic oedema
- More details on this topic are are given in 📖 Chapter 12.

Moyamoya disease and syndrome

- This is a rare condition affecting children and young adults. Stenosis or occlusion occurs in childhood in the basal intracerebral arteries. This is followed by new vessel formation to try to bypass the obstruction. These new vessels are fragile and can leak
- The syndrome can be primary (of unknown cause but more common in individuals from the Far East) or secondary to other causes of basal cerebral artery occlusion (e.g. sickle cell disease)
- More details are given on 📖 p. 338.

Vasculitis

- CNS vasculitis, either primary or as part of a systemic vasculitis, can occasionally cause haemorrhage
- It can cause the combination of separate infarcts and haemorrhage, and is also a cause of multiple haemorrhages.

Septic arteritis and mycotic aneurysms

- Infective endocarditis is complicated by ICH in 5% of cases
- This can occur due to:
  - Acute pyogenic necrosis of the arterial wall caused by virulent organisms such as *Staphylococcus aureus*
  - Mycotic aneurysms which can rupture; this may occur later, including during therapy and with less virulent organisms.

Haemostatic factors causing ICH

Anticoagulation treatment

- Treatment with warfarin increases the risk of ICH 8–10-fold
- In patients with previous stroke, the risk of ICH is approximately 1% per annum
- The risk increases with the intensity of coagulation (INR)
- The risk of haemorrhage is related to the degree of anticoagulation
- It is markedly increased in the presence of leukoaraiosis, particularly if the INR is higher, as shown in data from the SPIRIT trial
- ICH is usually subcortical, reflecting the distribution of cerebral small-vessel disease. It can also be lobar, especially in the elderly, perhaps because of the increasing prevalence of underlying cerebral amyloid angiopathy in this age group
- ICH in patients on anticoagulants are on average larger than those in patients not on anticoagulants.

Antiplatelet agents

- The absolute risk of haemorrhage from aspirin is low: about 1 per 1000 extra ICH per 3–5 years of treatment on aspirin
- A meta-analysis of all available data until 1997 from randomized trials of antiplatelet agents (mostly aspirin) for all indications showed a 22% relative increase in the risk of ICH, but this was outweighed by a 30% relative reduction in ischaemic stroke
- The MATCH study demonstrated that the combination of aspirin and clopidogrel was associated with a small but statistically increased risk of ICH compared with clopidogrel alone
- The PROFESS trial showed that the combination of dipyridamole and aspirin was associated with a slightly higher bleeding risk than clopidogrel alone.

Thrombolytic agents

- Haemorrhage can be associated with thrombolysis for stroke or myocardial infarction
- When thrombolysis is given for acute ischaemic stroke, the haemorrhagic transformation usually occurs at the site of the infarct.
- For other thrombolysis, most commonly myocardial infarction, haemorrhage may occur at any site in the brain.

Systemic bleeding tendency

- Disorders such as haemophilia are rare causes of ICH. ICH may be provoked by minor trauma
- ICH is a well recognized complication of acute myeloid leukaemia, occurring in about 20% of cases. It is rare in lymphatic leukaemia
- Disseminated intravascular coagulation can be complicated by ICH which may be multiple
- Thrombocytopenia can be complicated by ICH, but this will usually only occur if the platelet count is $\leq 20 \times 10^9$/L.

Haemorrhagic transformation of a cerebral infarct

- Haemorrhagic transformation is a common complication of cerebral infarction. It occurs because of blood–brain barrier disruption secondary to the ischaemia
- It is most common a few days after the infarct
- It is usually minor but can sometimes causes massive haemorrhage with space-occupying effects and secondary oedema
- Risk factors include thrombolysis and hypertension
- Symptomatic parenchymal haemorrhage occurs in about 0.6% of stroke not treated with thrombolysis
- Thrombolysis with tPA for myocardial infarction is associated with an approximately 0.5% risk of ICH
- Thrombolysis with tPA for stroke is associated with an approximately 3–6% risk of symptomatic haemorrhage depending on the definition used
- The degree of haemorrhagic transformation can be defined according to the NINDS and ECASS definitions, which are particularly used in clinical trials.

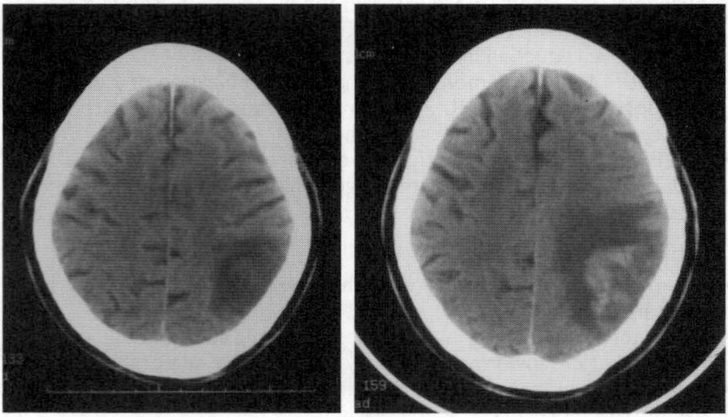

(a) (b)

Fig. 13.12 Haemorrhagic transformation on CT. This patient presented with right homonymous hemianopia and dysphasia. **(a)** A scan on day 1 shows a left parietal infarct; **(b)** on day 15 she deteriorated with worsening dysphasia. A repeat scan showed haemorrhage within the infarct. © Hugh Markus.

Further reading

Trouillas T, von Kummer R (2006) Classification and pathogenesis of cerebral hemorrhages after thrombolysis in ischemic stroke. *Stroke* **37**, 556–61.

Imaging scales for haemorrhagic transformation

NINDS definitions

HI: Acute infarction with punctate or variable hypodensity or hyperdensity, with an indistinct border within the vascular territory

PH: Typically homogeneous, hyperdense lesion with a sharp border with or without oedema or mass effect

ECASS (1 and 2) definitions

HI: Petechial infarction without space-occupying effect
HI1: small petechiae
HI2: more confluent petechiae

PH: Haemorrhage (coagulum) with mass effect
PH1: <30% of the infarcted area with mild space-occupying effect
PH2: >30% of the infarcted area with significant space-occupying effect

Other specific causes of ICH

Cerebral tumours

- Bleeding into cerebral tumours may account for up to 5% of ICH
- Often the diagnosis is easy if the patient has a known cerebral tumour, or an extracranial malignancy
- Some secondary (metastatic) tumours have a particular tendency to bleed:
  - Malignant melanoma
  - Choriocarcinoma
  - Renal cell carcinoma
  - Breast and lung metastases have a lower tendency to bleed individually but as they are very common they are relatively frequent causes of ICH-related tumours
- Primary tumours tend not to bleed, but glioblastoma multiforme is the exception and can bleed
- Clues to an underlying tumour on imaging include:
  - A disproportionate amount of oedema or mass effect
  - Nodular enhancement of surrounding tissue with IV contrast
  - Irregular patchy appearance of haematoma with low density area in the centre on CT suggesting necrotic tissue
  - Multiple haemorrhages
- Therefore the underlying tumour can often be suspected on the original brain imaging. However, it cannot be excluded and therefore repeat imaging (CT or preferably MRI) is required for all ICH cases when the haematoma has resolved (usually at about 3 months).

Illicit drugs

There are two classes of drugs that cause intracerebral haemorrhage.

Amphetamines

- These cause haemorrhage from minutes to a few hours after administration
- Contributing factors include:
  - A hypertensive surge
  - Fibrinoid necrosis in small and medium sized vessels—seen angiogaphically as 'beading' (areas of narrowing and dilatation and occlusion)
- Underlying vascular abnormalities (e.g. aneurysm, AVM) are often found, suggesting that amphetamines increase the risk of bleeding from these.

Cocaine

- Cocaine haemorrhages occur soon after ingestion
- They are more common with crack cocaine
- Most common in the white matter and may be multiple
- As for amphetamines, an underlying vascular malformation is often present. Haemodynamic factors may be important. Otherwise at post mortem blood vessels are usually normal
- For more details on stroke caused by illicit drugs see 📖 Chapter 11.

Hyperperfusion syndrome

- This is rare but a well recognized complication of carotid endarterectomy, and carotid stenting, affecting <1% of cases
- The haemorrhage usually occurs within a week of the operation, with haemorrhages and oedema in the carotid artery territory distal to the endarterectomy
- It can also cause seizures
- It is more likely to occur in hypertensive individuals with haemodynamic compromise to the cerebral circulation and a poor collateral supply
- There is some evidence that careful control of blood pressure postoperatively, avoiding hypertension and fluctuations, can reduce the risk of this syndrome.

Recovery and rehabilitation

Introduction

Life is never the same after stroke. The processes that go into picking up the pieces and returning to a pre-stroke life and lifestyle are outlined in this chapter.

Rehabilitation is an active, participatory process to minimize the neurological impairment resulting from stroke translating into disability and handicap.

Rehabilitation interventions are designed to:

- Reduce impairment (*restorative*)
- Help people adapt to impairment (*compensatory*).

Rehabilitation requires a multiprofessional team of healthcare workers.

For those of conventional working age, *vocational rehabilitation* may be appropriate. Returning to employment or an alternative meaningful occupation is always a major challenge after stroke. Returning to work is not only fundamental to psychosocial wellbeing for many but has significant financial implications. Vocational rehabilitation is designed specifically to maximize potential for a successful return to work. It frequently involves a collaboration between health and social services (including the Job Centre) and independent and voluntary organizations.

The 5 'R's of rehabilitation

- Realization of potential—to help the patient improve so their recovery plateaus close to their best anticipated function
- Re-enablement—to maximize functional independence
- Resettlement—to provide safe and confident transfer of care
- Role fulfilment—to re-establish personal status and autonomy
- Readjustment—to adapt to and accept new lifestyle after stroke.

Further reading

Introduction

Young J, Forster A (2007) Review of stroke rehabilitation. *BMJ* **334**, 86–90.

The 5 'R's of rehabilitation

Kalra L, Ratan R (2007) Recent advances in stroke rehabilitation 2006. *Stroke* **38**, 235–7.

Basic science of stroke recovery

After stroke, early recovery of function is thought to be due to reperfusion of hypoxic brain or reduction in vasogenic oedema associated with ischaemic brain tissue. All subsequent recovery is thought to be related to the brain's ability to compensate and remodel after injury, termed 'neuronal plasticity'. Dead brain tissue does not regenerate or re-grow but the remaining brain is not 'hard wired'.

Mechanisms underlying neuronal plasticity may include:

- Change in balance of excitation and inhibition: 'unmasking' of connections and neuronal pathways
- Strengthening or weakening of existing synapses: long-term potentiation or depression of key pathways
- Change in neuronal membrane excitability
- Anatomical changes such as sprouting new axons/synaptic connections.

The way in which these mechanisms are implemented is thought to influence functional outcome. The ability to utilize or recruit adjacent areas of undamaged cortex is thought to be associated with good outcome, using contralateral pathways and cortical 'maps' is less good and using deep short connections leads to the least good outcome.

A key aspect of neuronal plasticity with important implications for rehabilitation is that the modifications in neuronal networks are use-dependent. Animal experimental studies and clinical trials in humans using functional imaging have shown that forced use and functional training contribute to improved function. On the other hand, techniques that promote non-use may inhibit recovery.

Further reading

Hallet M (2001) Plasticity of the human motor cortex and recovery from stroke. *Brain Research Review* **36**, 169–74.

Natural history of stroke recovery

The rate of recovery differs between stroke severity and is fastest early on.

It is influenced by site, size of lesion, age, concomitant brain disease, and other systemic physical and psychological comorbidities.

The greatest rate of recovery is within the first 3–4 months after stroke and it is within this window that therapy intervention is thought to have the biggest impact. Functional change often continues beyond this stage, so each patient should be taken as an individual case when considering the spectrum of outcome after stroke.

It is currently accepted that:

- Approximately 35% (one in three) of survivors with leg paralysis do not regain useful function and about 25% of all stroke survivors are unable to walk independently
- Six months after stroke, 65% (two of three) of those with upper limb weakness cannot use their affected hand in normal functional tasks.

While acute treatment is targeted at reducing the extent of brain injury from stroke, rehabilitation has much to do to improve these statistics.

Good prognostic features:

- Absence of coma
- Early motor recovery, especially thumb and foot
- Continence.

Poor prognostic features:

- Coma
- Older age
- Incontinence
- Marked communication deficits
- Cognitive impairment
- Spatial neglect
- No leg movement at 2 weeks
- Flaccid upper limb with no selective finger movement at 4 weeks.

Trials have shown that coordinated stroke unit care saves lives and improves outcome, but the evidence base for the efficacy of specific components of stroke rehabilitation is scant with respect to randomized, controlled trial data.

Trial design is difficult as stroke is so heterogeneous in terms of subtype and natural history, where physical deficits recover spontaneously and variably over time. For example, a weak arm may be part of a large hemispheric cortical infarct, a small subcortical lacune or a brainstem lesion affecting the corticospinal pathway; all of these recover differently.

As well as stroke type, the rate of recovery is dependent on comorbidity which influences neuronal plasticity.

Furthermore, many interventions are difficult to 'control', e.g. what is placebo physiotherapy?

As a result, most evidence on therapy intervention comes from case-controlled series. In the UK Royal College of Physicians Concise Guide for Stroke, the evidence base for the majority of rehabilitation and therapy is Grade 'D', based on expert committee reports, opinion, and/or experience of respected authorities.

The stroke team

- Members of the multiprofessional stroke team and their roles are listed here
- All are involved in goalsetting and discharge planning
- A functional and cohesive multidisciplinary/professional team (MDT) is essential for comprehensive and successful stroke care.

Nursing

Nursing staff have a pivotal role in inpatient stroke rehabilitation as they are the only members of the multiprofessional team who are with the patient 24 hours a day. Rehabilitation should be a 24/7 process with all members of staff working together with the patient to achieve agreed goals and promote recovery.

Nursing staff have important roles in many areas of stroke care, including:

- Practising transfers
- Supervising mobility
- Promoting continence
- Being vigilant for signs of breakdown in skin integrity
- Identifying disturbance of mood
- Supervising patients' nutritional intake and monitoring their weight
- Liaising with carers and families outside office hours and managing their expectation of recovery as well as facilitating transfer of care back to the community.

Medical team

The diagnosis of stroke is made by doctors, as is the management of secondary prevention, early complications, and recovery.

In the acute stages of stroke, different specialties will contribute to care, including the stroke physician/neurologist/radiologist/cardiologist, and vascular surgeon.

Later on, medical input is from the primary care physician/family doctor with the help of hospital- or community-based specialists.

Physiotherapy

This is 'physical', often 'hands-on' therapy, which predominantly aids motor recovery (mobility and upper limb function).

With all therapies, but especially physiotherapy, there is a 30% or more placebo component.

Also, it is difficult to separate spontaneous recovery from the effects of therapy.

Physiotherapists use different approaches:

- Bobath—here the ethos is to maintain symmetry and correct adverse compensations such as 'pushing' with the good side. 'Hands-on' approach
- Carr and Shepherd—this approach uses a motor re-learning programme. Patients are given repeated functional movement pattern exercises, e.g. bending and stretching the arm. This improves strength and specific functional movements but not all the movements used in normal life. It is less 'hands-on', making it difficult in patients with cognitive or low arousal states to participate

- Neurofacilitation—here abnormal muscle tone is inhibited through weightbearing, sustained stretch and more normal movement promoted by trying to recruit paretic muscle activity through functional strength training in 'conventional' physiotherapy.

Traditionally, the Bobath approach has influenced UK physiotherapy practice more than any other. In practice, most physiotherapists use a combination based on their experience and the individual needs of the patient of:
- 'Conventional' physiotherapy approaches (usually a combination of those listed above)
- Assistive devices, e.g. treadmill retraining
- Novel approaches, e.g. constraint therapy, 'robot training', mirror imagery
- Functional electrical stimulation (FES)
- Use of orthoses.

Potential promoters of plasticity by physical therapy include:
- Repetition
- Functional goal-directed activity
- Attention during learning
- Electrical stimulation
- Immobilization.

Occupational therapy

Occupational therapists (OT) work closely with physiotherapists but particularly are involved in:
- Seating
- Functional assessment of personal care, including transfers (e.g. bed-to-chair), washing, dressing, using the toilet, working in the kitchen, and other high level assessments such as fitness to drive and vocational assessment
- Training motor and sensory function (e.g. 'errorless learning', a technique particularly helpful in managing dyspraxia)
- Provision of splints, static or dynamic for the affected upper limb
- Training compensatory skills
- Training cognitive function
- Advice and instruction over assisted devices, from adaptive cutlery to the appropriate use of rails, wheelchairs, and hoists
- Education of primary caregiver and family. The pre-discharge home visit is part of this as well as advising over assisted devices and adaptations.

Speech and language therapy (SALT)

This therapist has four major roles in the assessment and treatment of stroke patients:
- Swallow (dysphagia) assessment in complex cases or in those patients who fail an initial bedside swallow
- Assessment and treatment of patients with speech/communication disorders, including:
  - Dysarthria
  - Dysphasia
  - Cognitive communication disorder.

They also serve as facilitators and advocates for those with communication problems in a wide range of issues.

Dietician

Dieticians help assess nutritional status and prescribe regimens of enteral nutrition for those who cannot swallow. They also help in establishing PEG feeding in patients who have longer term feeding problems.

- It is estimated that between 8 and 18% of acute stroke patients are malnourished on admission
- Nutritional status can be judged by anthropometric factors, including body mass index, skinfold thickness, and biochemical markers such as serum albumin
- Stroke patients are at high risk of worsening malnutrition
- The number of malnourished patients increases significantly during the first week after stroke
- Stroke size, location, and severity have no effect on resting energy expenditure, but infection will increase energy requirements
- Dysphagia will also result in decreased intake, as will functional deficits such as weakness, sensory, and visual disturbance
- Texture modified diets often have a relatively low nutritional content and low patient tolerability
- In the FOOD trial, early tube feeding was associated with a non-specificant reduction in risk of death of 5.8% (95% CI –0.8 to 12.5, P=0.09)
- Stroke patients are at risk of metabolic and multiorgan crisis called 're-feeding syndrome' if they are given enteral feed:
    - After 10 days or more of no nutritional intake
    - Are depleted in potassium, phosphate, magnesium pre-feeding
    - Have unintentional weight loss of >15% usual body weight in the previous 3–6 months.

In managing patients at risk of re-feeding syndrome, enteral feeding usually starts at a low rate—10 ml/hour, increasing up to 120 ml/hour as tolerated. The calorie delivery would typically start at 10 kcal/kg/day, increasing slowly to meet full requirements by the end of the first week. Thiamine 200–300 mg is given daily for the first 10 days and daily measures of potassium, magnesium, and phosphate to guide oral/enteral or intravenous supplements are required. After a week of enteral feeding, the risk of metabolic crisis is rare and feeding can be increased as normal.

Clinical psychology

Neuropsychologists help with:

- *Diagnosis*—detecting the presence and nature of cognitive impairment, discriminating psychiatric and neurological symptoms, and diagnosing mood disorder
- *Management and goal planning*—neuropsychological assessment provides a detailed analysis of an individual's current cognitive function and outlines areas of strengths and weakness, providing a descriptive basis for rehabilitation goal planning. Clinical psychology can also help provide insight and techniques to help with psychological adjustment issues after stroke for both patient and carers or family members

- *Monitoring change/evaluation*—the individual's performance on the neuropsychological tests provides baseline data against which their degree of recovery can be measured. It can also be an important form of feedback for families and carers.

Domains of cognitive testing include:
- Overall intellectual ability
- Attention and concentration
- Speed of processing information
- Memory and learning
- Language and communication
- Visuospatial and spatial–constructional skills
- 'Executive functions', including complex abstract reasoning, planning, organization and flexibility of thinking.

Social work

- The social work team works alongside multidisciplinary colleagues to assist patients and carers in adjusting to and managing the impact of stroke
- The emphasis is on working in partnership with a client and their social network to promote independence and provide care in the community
- This involves assessment of individual need, care planning, implementing a care plan, monitoring, and review
- There is also a separate assessment of the needs of the carer
- Social workers assess the psychosocial impact of stroke and issues around welfare and benefits
- Patients may have a 'continuing care assessment', after which social services will instigate an appropriate care package and, if necessary, help facilitate day centre, respite or long-term care, applications for re-housing, and access to voluntary based resources
- More recently in England and Wales, the social work team has a role in organizing an independent advocate for those patients who lack the ability to make competent decisions with regard to treatment and discharge planning and who have no appropriate next of kin.

Further reading

Dennis MS, Lewis SC, Warlow C (2005) FOOD Trial Collaboration. Routine oral nutritional supplementation for stroke patients in hospital (FOOD): a multicentre randomised controlled trial. *Lancet* **365**, 755–63.

Steultjens E, Dekker J, Bouter L *et al.* (2003) Occupational therapy for stroke patients. A systematic review. *Stroke* **34**, 676–87.

Woldag H, Hummelsheim H (2002) Evidence-based physiotherapeutic concepts for improving arm and hand function in stroke patients. A review. *Journal of Neurology* **249**, 518–28.

UK Royal College of Physicians Stroke Guidelines. http://www.rcplondon.ac.uk/pubs/books/stroke/stroke_guidelines_2ed.pdf

Common problems after stroke

Seating

Mobilization and seating is a cornerstone of early stroke care aimed to:

- *Maximize*
  - Function
  - Comfort
- *Minimize*
  - Development of deformities
  - Development of tissue trauma
- *Improve*
  - Self-esteem
  - Eating, swallowing, digestive function
  - Visual, cognitive, and perceptual ability
  - Cardiovascular efficiency
  - Functional symmetry and balance
- *Decrease*
  - Risk of chest infection
  - Effects of abnormal reflexes and muscle tone.

The timing of seating a stroke patient needs to be assessed on an individual basis. Effective seating should:

- Control alignment
- Provide an appropriate and stable base
- Relieve stress on loaded structures.

Four types of seating commonly used outside of a standard hospital armchair include:

1. *Standard wheelchairs*—used for mobility, transfers, patients with poor exercise tolerance, outdoor use.
2. *Standard wheelchairs with adaptations*—used for patients with:
   - Good head and trunk control
   - Poor pelvic stability
   - One-sided weakness—hemiplegia, pusher syndrome
   - Perceptual problems in addition to hemiplegia.
3. *Recliner wheelchairs*—used for patients with:
   - Perceptual problems in addition to hemiplegia
   - Good head control
   - Moderate trunk control
   - Poor pelvic stability.
4. *Tilt in space wheelchairs*—used for patients with:
   - Poor head and trunk control
   - Compromised haemodynamic status
   - Overactivity in non-hemiplegic side
   - Dense hemiplegia
   - Decreased alertness and arousal.

Weakness

Predictors of motor recovery

- Early, selective movement across joints is a good prognostic marker
- Early thumb movement is a good indicator of future useful hand function.

Patterns of recovery

- In MCA territory stroke, leg weakness recovers before arm because the cortical area controlling leg function is in the vascular territory of the anterior cerebral artery
- Subcortical strokes affecting the arm may recover distal function early; this is attributed to preserved hand cortex
- Cortical infarcts typically recover better proximally; late selective finger movement is associated with poor dexterity
- Striatocapsular infarcts may show cortical signs which recover rapidly but hemiparesis which is longer term. They usually result from embolic proximal trunk MCA occlusions which rapidly re-canalize. Transient widespread MCA hypoperfusion occurs but there is only permanent infarction in the striatal region supplied by the perforating arteries which have no collateral supply. This pattern is often seen following thrombolysis.

References

Diserens K, Michel P, Bogousslavsky J (2006) Early mobilisation after stroke: review of the literature. *Cerebrovascular Diseases* **22**, 183–90.

Mulley G (1993) Nursing elderly patients out of bed. *BMJ* **307**, 80–1.

Communication

Communication problems are common after stroke—up to 70% of stroke patients have altered speech at time of presentation and persistent problems are a major adverse factor in rehabilitation.

The major types of speech and language disorder after stroke are listed below. They frequently coexist, and correct interpretation of brain imaging can help guide treatment and predict recovery. Dysarthria is a disorder of speech and articulation; aphasia/dysphasia is a disorder of language. They are often confused if adequate examination is not performed (see 📖 Speech and language, p. 120).

- *Dysarthria* or slurred speech is common after stroke
- *Anarthria* is severe dysarthria where no intelligible sound is made
- *Dysphasia/aphasia* is a disorder of language comprehension and/or production
- *Dysphonia* is marked reduction in voice with preserved language and articulation (e.g. due to vocal cord palsy).

Dysarthria

- Occurs owing to motor weakness of muscles involved in speech or brain areas involved in control of articulation (e.g. cerebellum)
- Exacerbated by non-stroke factors, e.g. dry mouth, ill-fitting dentures
- Treatment includes facial muscle exercise and education around breaking sentences and words into discrete intelligible blocks
- Give dysarthric patients time to articulate and never pretend to understand when you haven't—this leads to frustration for the patient. Alternative lines of communication may be available—writing, gesture, or using assisted devices such as a sign-writer.

Aphasia/dysphasia

The terms aphasia and dysphasia are used interchangeably, which can cause confusion. Aphasia really means loss of speech owing to a disorder of language rather than articulation, and dysphasia is a disorder without complete loss. However, in some countries aphasia is the preferred terminology for primary disorder of language.

Aphasia can comprise:

- Poor understanding of language (*receptive* component)
- Poor verbalization of language—reduced verbal fluency, paraphrasic syntax, grammatical, and naming/nominal errors (*expressive* component).

Whilst aphasia is nearly always made up of these two components, it is not unusual for one component to dominate. Global aphasia is where there is no apparent understanding or language output. Usually, it is a mixture of receptive and expressive language problems, characterized by poor verbal fluency, naming or nominal difficulties, paraphrasic, syntax and semantic errors with speech.

Features of aphasia

- Aphasia is caused by dominant hemisphere stroke (usually left hemisphere but remember to determine handedness) and can be isolated as part of a branch MCA cortical stroke or more often associated with hemiparesis if the stroke is extensive. It can also be part of a subcortical stroke, e.g. thalamic aphasia
- Between 20% and 40% or one in three of all acute stroke patients present with primary language disturbance or aphasia
- Approximately 80% of aphasic patients have persistent language problems at 1 year
- Aphasia is associated with post-stroke depression
- The relationship between stroke type, location, and aphasia recovery is complex and needs to be considered on an individual basis. Young age and good early comprehension are positive prognostic indicators
- The ability to reorganize language within the dominant hemisphere (especially left temporal area) seems to be associated with better recovery
- May be associated with inability to read (dyslexia) and write (dysgraphia).

Aphasia treatment

- Patients with predominant receptive problems are far more challenging to treat
- There is little RCT data but some suggestion that SALT may improve outcome. Interventions include melodic intervention therapy (MIT), lexical semantic therapy, and other focused techniques to develop verbal output and understanding. Computer programmes are sometimes helpful
- The minimum effective SALT intervention is thought to be 2 hours a week, with improved outcome demonstrated if the intensity is increased to 9 hours a week. SALT is most effective when delivered in the acute period of recovery (first 3 months), but apparent benefits have been shown after more than 1 year
- It is possible that biological treatment that increases brain acetylcholine levels may help conventional SALT treatment. Piracetam may help experimentally but there is no demonstrable long-term effect proven to date.

Cognitive communication disorder (CCD)

This is poorly understood and under-recognized. CCD may be more prominent in right hemisphere stroke.

There are no typical features of aphasia but:

- Altered non-verbal communication, e.g. monotone voice, flat facial expression, reduced eye contact
- Verbose and tangential output with poor self-monitoring
- Reduced awareness of the listener
- Associated with other signs of cognitive impairment such as altered attention, affect, and neglect.

Low mood and post-stroke depression

Depression is extremely common after stroke, and the diagnosis is frequently missed. Treatment can have a dramatic effect on recovery and quality of life.

- Up to 70% of stroke patients experience low mood after stroke and 25–30% show significant post-stroke depression (PSD)
- The later the symptoms present after stroke onset, the worse depression is likely to be
- Early emotionalism may be considered a 'normal/expected' accompaniment to stroke and usually resolves spontaneously
- Depression is not predicted by the stroke subtype or lesion site but is particularly common in aphasic patients
- Previous history of major depression is associated with developing PSD
- The cognitive effects of stroke may mimic PSD, making the diagnosis difficult
- There are many different assessment tools and scales, including GDS, HAMDS, PHQ9 (see 📖 Useful stroke scales, pp. 535–552)
- VASES can be helpful to assess mood in some aphasic patients
- Patients with PSD have worse functional outcome, slower recovery, and increased mortality, so timely detection and intervention is important
- Differential diagnosis includes intercurrent illness, drugs, adjustment.

The DSM-IV Major Depressive Episode definition includes duration, pervasiveness, and five of the following, including at least one of the first two.

- *Depressed mood*
- *Diminished pleasure/interest*
- Weight disturbance
- Sleep disturbance
- Psychomotor changes
- Fatigue
- Worthlessness/guilt
- Diminished concentration/indecisiveness
- Thoughts of death.

Treatment of PSD

- Prompt identification and treatment improves outcome. Explain it is a very common complication of stroke and responds to treatment. Warn stroke patients it may occur and what to watch out for. This reduces the stigma often attached to the diagnosis
- *Non-pharmacological*: counselling. Often underused and helpful
- *Pharmacological:* little RCT evidence but:
  - Symptoms need to be present continually for at least 2 weeks to be significant and warrant drug treatment
  - Most classes of antidepressants seem safe post-stroke
  - Anticholinergic side effects should be avoided (dry mouth, constipation, confusion, and worsening cognitive impairment)
  - SSRIs: citalopram and fluoxetine are commonly used (some supportive trial data)

- If there is no improvement after 6 weeks with SSRI, consider venlafaxine. Minimum treatment period should be 6 months
- If possible use in conjunction with psychological therapy/counselling.

Emotional lability

- This describes excessive crying and/or laughing, to trivial or no obvious stimuli, in the absence of depression
- Also called involuntary emotional expression disorder (IEED), pseudobulbar affect, or emotional incontinence
- Most common after bilateral anterior frontal cortical lesions, or subcortical disease leading to white matter tract disruption and bilateral frontal cortical disconnection
- Can be extremely distressing for both patient and family/carers
- Crying alone can be mistaken for depression although it can coexist with depression
- There is some evidence that emotional lability can be helped with SSRIs and it is often worth a therapeutic trial for a couple of months but stop if no benefit is seen. Cochrane review concluded that there was evidence that antidepressants helped but no particular drug or drug class was superior
- Advice to patients on how to manage with this disabling symptom is available on: http://www.stroke.org/site/PageServer?pagename=IEED

Further reading

Bennett HE, Thomas SA, Austen R, Morris AM, Lincoln NB (2006) Validation of screening measures for assessing mood in stroke patients. *British Journal of Clinical Psychology* **45**, 367–76.

Carson AJ, MacHale S, Allen K *et al.* (2000) Depression after stroke and lesion location: a systematic review. *Lancet* **356**, 122–6.

Hackett ML, Yapa C, Parag V, Anderson CS (2005) Frequency of depression after stroke. A systematic review of observational studies. *Stroke* **36**, 1330–40.

House AO, Hackett ML, Anderson CS, Horrocks JA (2004) Pharmaceutical interventions for emotionalism after stroke. *Cochrane Database of Systematic Reviews*, Issue 2. Art. No.: CD003690. DOI: 10.1002/14651858.CD003690.pub2.

Unsafe swallowing (dysphagia)

Forty per cent of acute stroke patients have altered swallow or dysphagia—20% will go on to have significant prolonged swallowing difficulties.

- A bedside swallow test is mandatory in all acute stroke patients (see Fig. 14.1)
- Patients with severe facial weakness are at particularly high risk of unsafe swallow and lung aspiration
- Oropharyngeal weakness, poor coordination, and other comorbidity such as poor dentition worsen swallowing problems
- Dysphagia will result in decreased oral intake, a problem magnified by functional deficits such as weakness, sensory and visual disturbance
- Patients with large cortical strokes predictably deteriorate clinically over the ensuing 4–7 days owing to worsening brain oedema. These patients become drowsy and may no longer be alert enough to swallow safely. Therefore, swallowing should be screened repeatedly even if the initial screen was successful.

For patients with an unsafe swallow, most stroke units instigate early enteral nutrition using nasogastric (NG) feeding within the first 24–48 hours.

Early feeding in the FOOD trial showed a (non-significant) trend towards improved functional outcome and reduced mortality. The same trial showed no evidence to suggest routine percutaneous endoscopic gastrostomy (PEG) feeding was better than NG feeding. In the first 3–4 weeks, NG feeding should be the preferred route unless there are strong practical reasons for PEG.

Where patients repeatedly pull out the NG tube, placement with a 'nasal bridle' is an alternative. Such tubes have a bridle 'tape' which is looped behind the nasal septum and secured to the feeding tube. If the patient pulls on the tube it will be uncomfortable and deter further pulling but remain *in situ*. With significant force, the bridle will stretch and the NG tube loosen and still come out but without nasal septum injury.

Most units consider PEG insertion at 4–6 weeks if there has been no improvement in swallow and patients are likely to rely on enteral nutrition in the medium term (few patients fail to regain any swallow by 6 months after stroke). Percutaneous endoscopic jejunostomy (PEJ) tubes are rarely indicated after stroke.

Management involves graded reintroduction of oral intake with trials of varied consistencies of diet and fluid supervised by SALT, nursing staff, and dietician. Exercises for facial weakness, tongue base movement, laryngeal elevation, and sensory stimulation with ice may also help.

Flow chart for nutritional management of acute stroke patients.

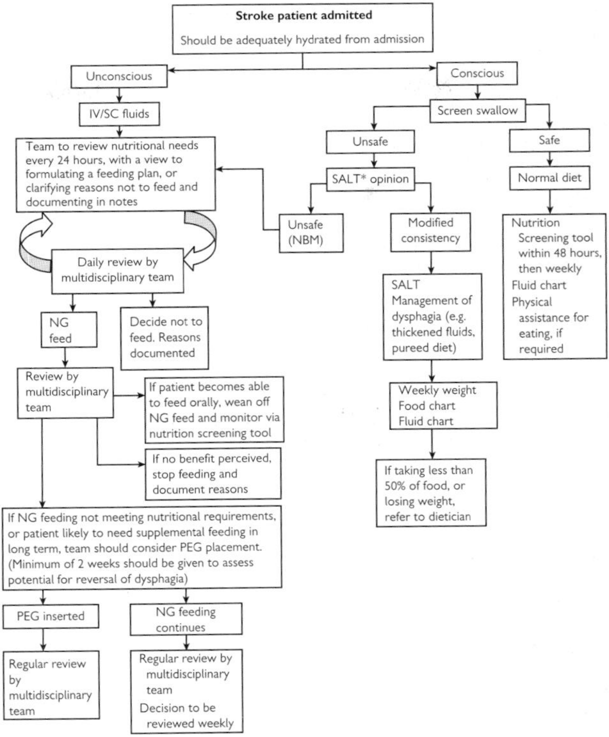

Fig. 14.1 Algorithm of swallowing assessment from St George's acute stroke unit (with thanks to Helen Mann for permission).

Indications for videofluoroscopy to assess swallowing

A videofluoroscopy swallow study (also known as a dysphagia barium swallow) is a dynamic X-ray taken while swallowing a bolus containing X-ray contrast. Usually, videofluoroscopy will only be carried out after a bedside evaluation of swallowing to give an objective view of the pharyngeal stage of swallowing. It was considered the gold standard for dysphagia assessment but there is variability in the interpretation of the procedure.

In terms of management, it allows:

- Visualization of structure and function of the oral, pharyngeal, and upper oesophageal stages of the swallow
- Specific recommendations for food/fluid consistencies and non-oral feeding
- Trialling of therapy.

Indications for videofluoroscopy include:

- Unclear signs on bedside evaluation
- Silent aspiration suspected or seen on previous videofluoroscopy
- To establish a baseline of swallowing function with progressive disorders (this may be relevant in patients with previous stroke and pre-existing swallow problems or patients with extensive subcortical cerebrovascular disease)
- Known or suspected dysphagia of structural origin
- To try therapeutic manoeuvres, e.g. supraglottic swallow, Mendelssohn's manoeuvre.

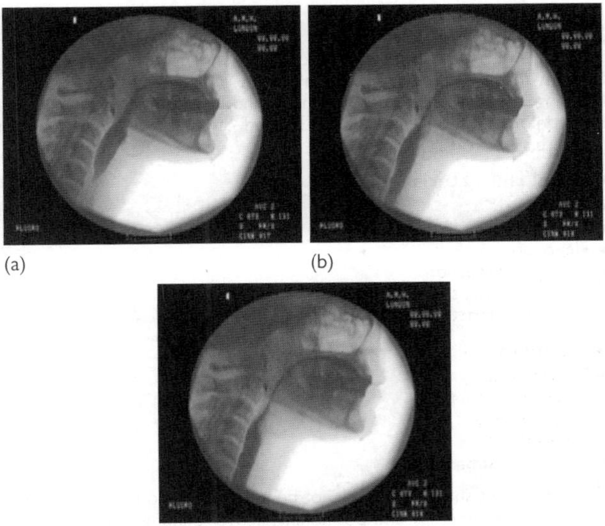

(a) (b) (c)

Fig. 14.2 Videofluoroscopy showing passage of liquid bolus without aspiration. © Geoff Cloud

References

Dennis MS, Lewis SC, Warlow C (2005) FOOD Trial Collaboration. Effect of timing and method of enteral tube feeding for dysphagic stroke patients (FOOD): a multicentre randomised controlled trial. *Lancet* **365**, 764–72.

Smithard DG, O'Neill PA, England RE *et al.* (1997) The natural history of dysphagia following a stroke. *Dysphagia* **12**, 188–93.

Spasticity

Symptoms relating to spasticity are present in up to 60% of strokes. Spasticity is excessive, inappropriate, and involuntary muscle activity resulting in stiffness, loss of movement, and pain. At worst it produces fixed deformity known as contracture and can lead to development of pressure sores.

Clinical characteristics

- High tone
- Hyperreflexia
- Flexor spasms
- Clasp knife reaction
- Extensor spasms
- Associated reactions.

Treatments

- Physiotherapy
- Drug treatments
  - Systemic
  - Local
- Surgical treatments (rarely).

Drug treatment should generally not be used in isolation but in combination with physiotherapy and positioning, active splinting, and positioning. Drugs are either systemic or targeted/focal.

Systemic treatment of spasticity: drugs

Baclofen

- Structurally related to GABA
- GABA agonist, acts presynaptically on $GABA_B$ with inhibitory effect
- Starting dose 5 mg bd increasing gradually up to a maximum of 100 mg in divided doses
- Side effects include drowsiness, hallucinations, confusion, and generalized weakness
- Abrupt withdrawal causes seizures.

Tizanidine

- Alpha-2-adrenergic receptor agonist
- Inhibitory effect on spinal interneurons
- Some anti-nocioceptive action on spasticity-related pain
- Less muscle weakness than baclofen (and diazepam)
- Side effects: drowsiness
- Main trials in multiple sclerosis patients.

Dantrolene

- Acts directly on contractile apparatus of muscles
- Inhibits release of intramuscular calcium
- Can cause irreversible liver damage
- No CNS action and therefore can be used in combination with other centrally acting agents
- Useful if baclofen causes excessive drowsiness

- More useful in spinal causes of spasticity
- Start at 25 mg od and increase slowly to maximum dose of 400 mg daily. Stop if no benefit demonstrable within 6 weeks
- Side effects: nausea, vomiting, and muscle weakness.

Diazepam

- Increases GABA-mediated inhibition by increasing affinity of the receptors
- More helpful in spinal causes
- May cause CNS depression and drowsiness, respiratory depression, paradoxical anxiety, and hallucinations
- Risk of addiction
- Start at low dose 2 mg bd and increase to maximum of typically 60 mg in divided doses.

Clonidine

- Central alpha-2-agonist (like tizanidine) and antihypertensive
- Mechanism of action not understood
- Helpful in reducing flexor spasms.

Other drugs used predominately in spasticity of traumatic spinal origin but on occasion trialled on stroke patients include gabapentin, vagabatrin, tetrazepam, orphenadrine and cannabinoids.

Focal treatment of spasticity: botulinum toxin

Introduction

- Since 1817 when Justinus Kerner first described foodborne botulism, the Gram-negative anaerobic bacterium *Clostridium botulinum* has been known to produce a potent neurotoxin resulting in muscle paralysis by blockade of neuromuscular transmission
- When injected directly into a muscle, it causes chemical denervation of peripheral cholinergic nerve endings and local paralysis, an effect which has been shown to have therapeutic use for treating dystonia and spasticity
- Nerve sprouting and muscle reinnervation lead to functional recovery and reversal of effect within 2–4 months.

Subtypes

- There are seven immunologically distinct serotypes of botulinum toxin labelled A–G
- Only A is in routine clinical use currently and is produced commercially in purified form as either Dysport© (Ipsen) or Botox© (Allergan)
- A vial of Dysport contains 500 units and a vial of Botox 100 units. Botox is considered 3–4 times more potent than Dysport
- A commercial preparation of botulinum toxin B (NeuroBloc©) has recently been licensed.

Advantages over other spasticity treatments

- Unlike systemic antispasticity drugs, which are non-selective and commonly associated with generalized weakness and functional loss, botulinum toxin is targeted therapy
- Unlike chemical neurolysis with alcohol or phenol, botulinum toxin injection does not cause skin sensory loss or dysaesthesia.

Disadvantages over other spasticity treatments

- Expensive.

Indications in post-stroke spasticity

- In randomized studies, botulinum toxin injection in the post-stroke spastic upper and lower limb has been shown to reduce spasticity and improve function
- Best results are gained with concomitant physical therapy, which may involve the use of splints/orthoses
- The decision to inject a muscle with botulinum toxin after stroke should always be made together with a neurophysiotherapist and ideally be attached to the aim of achieving a functional goal, e.g. being able to put a spastic arm through a garment sleeve. It should rarely be considered in the first 3 months after stroke. Injection may also give some short-term relief from pain associated with chronic post-stroke spasticity and reduce carer burden
- Treatment should be individualized and reviewed as part of a rehabilitation programme
- It is contraindicated in myasthenia gravis, Lambert–Eaton syndrome and other neuromuscular disorders, pregnancy, and with the use of aminoglycoside antibiotics.

Administration

- Both should be reconstituted in a small (2 ml) volume of saline (reconstituting in water makes for a painful injection)
- The motor endplate zone of the muscle to be injected should be identified using conventional EMG surface anatomy landmarks. Where this is difficult, EMG guidance should be used. A needle appropriate to the size of the muscle to be injected (size 10–12 G) should be used
- The suggested dose for injections of muscles commonly treated after stroke is outlined in Fig. 14.4. Spasticity reduction and muscle weakness are dose-dependent
- The peak effect usually occurs 4 weeks after injection. Physiotherapy review is recommended within 7–14 days after injection
- Treatments may be safely repeated at intervals of 12 weeks but a total dose of 1500 units Dysport or equivalent should not be exceeded in any one treatment.

Side effects

- The most common local side effect is weakness, which is usually mild and transient. Pain at injection site and local irritation are reported in less than 5% of cases
- More systemic flu-like symptoms, anaphylaxis, and excessive fatigue are rare
- Occasionally, antibody formation can occur which makes repeated injection ineffective. Higher and more frequent doses increase the chance of immunoresistance and non-responsiveness
- Ref: http://www.rcplondon.ac.uk/pubs/books/botox/

Surgical treatments for spasticity

Surgical treatment is rarely used. It may be a last resort to enable proper seating, fitting of orthoses or enable appropriate hygiene. Examples include adductor tenotomies or obturator neurectomies.

Muscle	Action	Injection point	Dose
Gracilis (inferior pubic ramus to posterior aspect of medial tibial condyle)	Adducts thigh and flexes knee. Medially rotates flexed leg	Posterior medial edge of thigh—several points of injection down medial thigh	80–120 u (B) 300–400 u (D)
Semi membranosus/tendinosus (ischial tuberosity to posterior medial aspect of medial tibial condyle)	Flexes knee. Medially rotates flexed leg and extends hip	Medial muscles in posterior thigh—multiple injection sites	100–150 u (B) 400–600 u (D)
Biceps femoris (ischial tuberosity to head of fibula)	Flexes knee, rotates leg externally, and extends hip	Lateral muscle in posterior thigh—multiple injection sites	100–150 u (B) 400–600 u (D)
Biceps brachii (short—coracoid process, long—supraglenoid tubercle of scapula, both inserting into bicipital aponeurosis)	Supination and elbow flexion	Anterior aspect of upper arm—inject both heads	75–100 u (B) 300–400 u (D)
Brachialis (front of distal half humerus to coracoid process of ulna)	Flexes elbow	Lower anterior humerus medial and lateral of biceps tendon	50 u (B) 200 u (D)
Brachioradialis (left supracondylar ridge of humerus to lateral surface of distal radius)	Flexes elbow	Radial side upper forearm	50 u (B) 200 u (D)
Flexor digitorum profundus (proximal two-thirds ulna to terminal phalanges of fingers)	Flexes all fingers	Upper third forearm—deep muscle above lateral border of ulna	30–40 u (B) 120–160 u (D)
Flexor digitorum superficialis (humeral head from medial epicondyle and coracoid process, radial head from upper half of anterior border of radius inserting in to middle phalanges of medial four digits)	PIP and MCP joint flexor	Middle of forearm half way down to either side of palmaris tendon	25–30 u (B) 100–120 u (D)
Flexor carpi ulnaris (humeral head from medial humeral epicondyle, ulna head from olecranon and upper two-thirds of its posterior border into pisiform bone in wrist)	Flexes and adducts hand and wrist	Upper forearm medial aspect of flexor surface below bicipital aponeurosis, medial to flexor carpi radialis (observe action of wrist flexion)	30–40 u (B) 120–160 u (D)
Flexor carpi radialis (medial humeral epicondyle to base of second metacarpal)	Flexes wrist and elbow	Upper forearm just below bicipital aponeurosis and medial to pronator teres	30–40 u (B) 120–160 u (D)

B=Botox® D=Dysport®

Fig. 14.3 Botox administration table.

Hemiplegic shoulder pain

- The shoulder is a shallow 'ball and socket' type joint with a relatively small surface area of articulation which makes for a wide range of movement but poor joint stability
- The 'rotator cuff' comprises muscles around the joint which acts as a lever for elevation during abduction
- Weakness of the rotator cuff can cause subluxation of the humeral head, impingement and inflammation in the joint and tendon insertions of the rotator cuff muscles.

Hemiplegic shoulder pain (HSP) is common (9–40% of hemiplegic stroke) and typically occurs 2–3 months after stroke onset. It may be classified into four groups:

- Joint pain caused by misaligned joint producing sharp pain on movement (active or passive). This is a frequent complication of a flaccid arm
- Overactive or spastic muscle pain—deep pulling pain on movement. Can be associated with adhesive capsulitis
- Diffuse pain from altered sensation from stroke—constant ache around shoulder
- Reflex sympathetic dystrophy pain—diffusely involving the whole limb and shoulder together. May be associated with vasomotor changes (sweating and altered coloration), trophic changes, and oedema.

HSP is associated with motor loss, sensory loss, and low mood. Shoulder X-rays are of little use in management.

Prevention and treatment

- HSP can be prevented by attention to handling and position, especially in those with flaccid arms early in stroke recovery. Slings or supports may be useful in reducing subluxation and tension in the shoulder capsule. Wearing a support device may promote immobility and possible contracture formation. Such devices, therefore, need to be worn as part of a regimen in conjunction with active therapy treatment. Pillows to support the shoulder and maintain alignment whilst seated are standard. Elevation of the arm supported on a pillow may also prevent dependent oedema. Positions that avoid patterns of spasticity are key. The Bexhill arm rest on wheelchairs is commonly used to facilitate this
- Functional electrical stimulation (FES) has shown some success in maintaining tone and reducing atrophy of rotator cuff muscle groups, so reducing the incidence of subluxation acutely. The effects tend to be short-lived, however, and benefits disappear on discontinuation of treatment
- Local steroid joint injection may help adhesive capsulitis
- Transcutaneous electrical nerve stimulation (TENS) may relieve pain to enable passive movement around the joint and improve functional range for purposes of dressing and hygiene
- Drug therapy may require only simple analgesics or specific anti-spasticity medication such as baclofen.

Further reading

Bender L, McKenna K (2001) Hemiplegic shoulder pain: defining the problem and its management. *Disability Rehabilitation* **23**, 698–705.

Turner-Stokes L, Jackson D (2002) Shoulder pain after stroke: a review of the evidence base to inform the development of an integrated care pathway. *Clinical Rehabilitation* **16**, 276–98.

Central post-stroke pain syndrome

Central post-stroke pain syndrome (CPSP) is pain of central neurogenic origin. It is unusual after stroke but when it occurs it can be extremely distressing.

- It occurs in approximately 4–8% of patients with stroke
- At least half have moderate to severe pain
- More common in older stroke patients (those over 80 years) and is, therefore, likely to be under-reported
- CPSP syndrome typically develops between 4 and 8 weeks after stroke but can develop over a year after stroke
- Classically associated with thalamic lesions—previously known as 'thalamic pain'. It is now appreciated that it can also occur with extrathalamic strokes and only around 60% cases have thalamic involvement
- The mechanism of CPSP is poorly understood. Strokes involving either the thalamic nucleii (particularly ventrocaudal and ventroposterior inferior nuclei) or the spinothalamic cortical pathway may cause alterations in thalamocortical processing and altered sensory perception.

CPSP syndrome has several distinct characteristic forms:

- Muscle pain—typically cramping
- Dysaesthesia—unpleasant, delayed onset after stimulus—burning
- Hyperaesthesia—heightened response to trivial stimuli
- Allodynia—present in up to 60% of CPSP patients, this is the interpretation of non-painful stimuli such as thermal or light touch as being painful or the location of the pain in an area remote from that being stimulated
- Shooting pain—intermittent and localized usually
- Circulatory pain—pins and needles, insect bites, walking on broken glass
- Peristaltic/visceral pain—fullness of bladder, dysuria with urinary urge, abdominal bloating.

Treatment

- Low dose tricyclic antidepressant drugs, amitriptyline 10–25 mg od (remember these are not antidepressant doses, however)
- Antiepileptic drugs—lamotrigine (doses of at least 200 mg/day required) has more evidence than carbamazepine. Gabapentin/pregabalin may be the best of this class
- A recent meta-analysis concluded evidence only for amitriptyline and lamotrigine, but there is emerging evidence for gabapentin
- IV drugs such as lidocaine, propofol, and ketamine have shown efficacy for short-term control of CPSP, but their application and potential side effects make them unsuitable for long-term treatment
- Opiates can help in acute exacerbations but are not recommended for chronic pain management
- Non-pharmacological—there is experimental work with deep brain stimulation for the most refractory and debilitated cases.

Further reading

Frese A, Husstedt IW, Ringelstein EB, Evers S (2006) Pharmacologic treatment of central post-stroke pain. *Clinical Journal of Pain* **22**, 252–60.
Nicholson BD (2004) Evaluation and treatment of central pain syndromes. *Neurology* **62**(Suppl.), S30–6.

Post-stroke epilepsy

- Seizures can occur at the time of stroke or in the recovery phase. The implication and treatment of the two are quite different
- More common with cortical, versus subcortical, strokes
- Cerebrovascular disease (which may be previously asymptomatic) is the most common cause of late-onset epilepsy. A first fit in a person aged over 65 years is likely to be due to underlying cerebrovascular disease and such patients are at increased risk of developing stroke
- Remember, a diagnosis of epilepsy should only be made if there are repeated unprovoked seizures. A single seizure is not epilepsy
- Seizures are more common if there is pre-existing dementia and there is some evidence that post-stroke seizures may increase the risk of subsequent dementia.

Seizures during the acute phase

- The reported frequency of seizures during the first days of stroke ranges from 2% to 23% depending on study designs. The true risk is probably at the lower end of the range
- Likely to be partial with or without secondary generalization. Status epilepticus is rare
- Haemorrhagic stroke is associated with seizure activity more than ischaemic stroke
- There is some controversy as to whether they are more common with cardioembolic stroke.

Late seizures after stroke

- Late seizures have been reported in between 3% and 67% of strokes in different series. The true incidence is again probably at the lower end
- Most seizures occur within the first year of stroke
- It is unusual to develop seizures more than 2 years after stroke onset
- Perhaps half will have recurrent seizures (epilepsy).

Treatment of seizures

Seizures at stroke onset

- A seizure at stroke presentation does not generally warrant regular antiepileptic drug medication
- Nor does it merit IV benzodiazepine therapy at the time of seizure to terminate it. It usually self-terminates and this can lead to unnecessary respiratory depression. This is only required for continuing seizures (status epilepticus)
- For those who present with prolonged and generalized seizures, usually in the context of large and haemorraghic infarcts or primary intracerebral bleeding, anticonvulsants should be started.

Seizures occurring after the acute stroke presentation

- For seizures not associated with the immediate stroke presentation, it needs to be ascertained whether they were 'provoked', e.g. due to intercurrent metabolic disturbance, severe infection, or change in medication which may lower seizure threshold or new stroke episode

- For unprovoked seizures, an individual risk:benefit assessment needs to be carried out—risk of further potentially harmful seizures against risk of side effects and drug interactions caused by antiepileptic drugs
- Bear in mind that even small, shortlived partial seizures can cause considerable anxiety and morbidity in older people living alone and having suffered the consequences of a previous stroke.

Choice of anticonvulsants

- There is no good quality trial data evaluating anticonvulsant in post-stroke epilepsy. Therefore there is no evidence that one antiepileptic drug is superior in this setting and the choice of agent will be influenced by age, concomitant medication, and comorbidity
- It has been suggested that phenytoin is not the most appropriate choice in stroke patients because of potential harmful impact on functional recovery and bone health
- Common first-line choices include sodium valproate, carbamazepine, and lamotrigine. Levetiracetam also seems to be safe and useful in refractory cases
- There are no data on whether prophylactic anticonvulsants can prevent seizure onset.

Lifestyle and seizures

- It is important to warn of lifestyle risks, e.g. danger of drowning in bath water
- Warn of risk of driving and inform of local regulations. These differ in different countries. For example, in the UK driving is forbidden until free of seizures for 1 year (although occasionally an exception may be made for provoked seizures).

Further reading

Camilo O, Goldstein LB (2004) Seizures and epilepsy after ischemic stroke. *Stroke* **35**, 1769–75.

Kammersgaard LP, Olsen TS (2005) Poststroke epilepsy in the Copenhagen stroke study: incidence and predictors. *Journal of Stroke and Cerebrovascular Disease* **14**, 210–14.

Ryvlin P, Montavont A, Nighoghossian N (2006) Optimizing therapy of seizures in stroke patients. *Neurology* **67**(Suppl. 4), S3–S9.

Neglect and inattention

- Defined as a disorder of 'attention' and often described in behavioural terms
- Normal attention is reliant on intact sensory registration, and neglect can occur in any sensory modality (tactile, auditory, visual)
- Visual and spatial inattention are the most frequently recognized after stroke
- Right-sided brain lesions typically result in the most severe neglect
- Left-sided stroke with right-sided inattention is probably less common and is poorly understood—principally as it often coexists with marked language disorder in patients with left hemispheric stroke. It also appears to resolve rapidly in many cases.

Neglect behaviours

- *Extinction*—simultaneous stimuli to left and right result in failure to recognize the stimulus on the neglected side
- *Allesthesia*—mislocation of stimulus
- *Anosognosia*—lack of awareness of the problem
- Decreased spontaneous movement of side demonstrating neglect:
    - *Hypokinesia*—delayed movements
    - *Hypometria*—decreased amplitude of the movement
    - *Akinesia*—no movement.

The implications for patients with inattention in daily living can be numerous. Examples of these may include: reading, writing, drawing, walking, driving, socializing, and with activities of personal care. Patients with neglect have poor or slow recovery because of loss of awareness, and tend to have difficulty relearning to dress, walk, and care for themselves. Lack of awareness can undermine participation in the rehabilitation process.

Treatment

- Sitting or addressing patients from the neglected side, scanning, and auditory feedback are thought to be ineffective
- Environmental modifications
- Prisms
- A half field patch (for patients with no hemianopia)
- Cognitive strategies
- Limb activation treatment (grading position, trunk rotation, other adaptive approaches).

Dyspraxia and abnormal perception

Praxis is the ability to use the limbs and body in skilled tasks in order to function. It has three stages—ideation, motor planning, and execution.

Dyspraxia is a disorder of the execution of learned movement which cannot be accounted for by weakness, incoordination, sensory loss, incomprehension or inattention to command.

It can be categorized clinically into:

1. *Ideational*
- Incorrect object use (e.g. using a toothbrush to comb hair)
- Incorrect order of elements of activity
- Sections of the sequence omitted
- Two or more elements of an activity blended
- Overshooting of action
- After interruption unable to continue an action
- Perseveration.

2. *Ideomotor*
- Spatial orientation errors
- Initiation and timing mistakes
- Poor distal differentiation
- View body part as object
- Verbalization instead of action
- Gestural enhancement
- Fragmentary responses.

The type of deficit can be related to location of stroke. Ideational dyspraxia tends to be caused by lesions in the left posterior parietal, occipital, and temporal lobes. Ideomotor is seen more in left frontal lobe strokes. Dyspraxia is also seen in right hemisphere stroke but equivalent lesions on the right do not necessarily produce dyspraxic symptoms.

Treatment is based on principles of 'errorless learning' and needs to be structured, goal-based, and functional.

Further reading

Jackson T (1999) Dyspraxia: guidelines for intervention. *British Journal of Occupational Therapy* **62**, 321–6.

McClain M, Foundas A (2004) Apraxia. *Neurology and Neuroscience Reports* **4**, 471–6.

Stone SP, Wilson B, Wroot A *et al.* (1991) The assessment of visuo-spatial neglect after acute stroke. *Journal of Neurology Neurosurgery and Psychiatry* **54**, 345–50.

Stone SP, Halligan PW, Greenwood RJ (1993) The incidence of neglect phenomena and related disorders in patients with an acute right or left hemisphere stroke. *Age Ageing* **22**, 46–52.

Hemianopia (visual field loss)

This is common in stroke. Patients are often unaware of homonymous hemianopia.

Examination for and determination of the site of lesion causing hemianopia is described on 📖 p. 132. Usually accurate assessment can be obtained on bedside examination, but full visual field testing may be necessary, particularly for partial defects and where assessment for driving or other vocational activities is required.

Hemianopia causes problems such as being unaware of things on one side, bumping into things on one side (especially when walking through doorways), and reading difficulty.

Bilateral occipital lobe stroke can cause 'cortical blindness'. Up to 10% of such patients deny their visual difficulties (Anton's syndrome).

- *Orthoptists* specialize in eye movement disorders
- *Ophthalmologists* specialize in medical disorders of the eye
- *Optometrists or opticians* generally practise in High Street locations and deal with disorders of vision correctable with spectacles.

Management

- Functional assessment and counselling (especially with respect to driving)
- Head posture and movement
- Lighting
- Mirrors
- Prisms
- Stimulation—computer-based training (visual restitution training; VRT) for an hour a day for 6 months can improve visual field typically by 5°. VRT is still not widely available and awaits further validation.

Pressure sores

These are a disaster on a stroke unit and are always avoidable with appropriate assessment and management. However, a number of patients present to acute stroke services after a 'long lie' on the floor as a consequence of the acute stroke, and every stroke unit will see pressure sores. They are traditionally graded from 1 to 4 (see Fig. 14.4).

The Waterlow score (Fig. 14.5) can be used to triage those most at risk and stratify the need for low air flow ripple mattress, soft mattress or normal mattress with regular turning.

Common sites are bony prominences such as heels, sacrum, pelvic prominences, and over kyphotic spines. They can be caused by ill-fitting TED stockings or even periods as short as 30 minutes immobilized on a hard surface in X-ray.

Vigilance is required as, once established, they are a considerable cause of morbidity (principally through pain) and are associated with poor stroke recovery. Treatment often takes months and may even require surgical intervention.

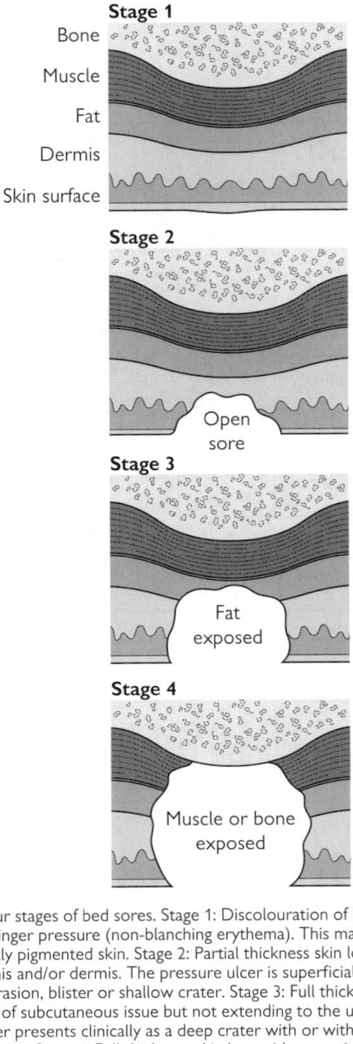

Fig. 14.4 The four stages of bed sores. Stage 1: Discolouration of intact skin not affected by light finger pressure (non-blanching erythema). This may be difficult to identify in darkly pigmented skin. Stage 2: Partial thickness skin loss or damage involving epidermis and/or dermis. The pressure ulcer is superficial and presents clinically as an abrasion, blister or shallow crater. Stage 3: Full thickness skin loss involving damage of subcutaneous issue but not extending to the underlying fascia. The pressure ulcer presents clinically as a deep crater with or without undermining of the adjacent tissue. Stage 4: Full thickness skin loss with extensive destruction and necrosis extending to underlying tissue.

WATERLOW PRESSURE ULCER PREVENTION/TREATMENT POLICY

RING SCORES IN TABLE, ADD TOTAL. MORE THAN 1 SCORE/CATEGORY CAN BE USED

BUILD/WEIGHT FOR HEIGHT	◆	SKIN TYPE VISUAL RISK AREAS	◆	SEX AGE	◆
AVERAGE BMI = 20–24.9	0	HEALTHY	0	MALE	1
ABOVE AVERAGE BMI = 25–29.9	1	TISSUE PAPER	1	FEMALE	2
OBESE BMI > 30	2	DRY	1	14–49	1
BELOW AVERAGE BMI < 20	3	OEDEMATOUS	1	50–64	2
BMI=Wt(Kg)/Ht $(m)^2$		CLAMMY, PYREXIA	1	65–74	3
		DISCOLOURED GRADE 1	2	75–80	4
		BROKEN/SPOTS GRADE 2-4	3	81+	5

MALNUTRITION SCREENING TOOL (MST)
(Nutrition Vol.15, No.6 1999 – Australia)

A – HAS PATIENT LOST WEIGHT RECENTLY?	B – WEIGHTLOSS SCORE
YES – GO TO B	0.5–5kg = 1
NO – GO TO C	5–10kg = 2
UNSURE – GO TO C AND SCORE 2	10–15kg = 3
	>15kg = 4
	Unsure = 2

C – PATIENT EATING POORLY OR LACK OF APPETITE 'NO' = 0; 'YES' SCORE = 1	NUTRITION SCORE If > 2, refer for nutrition assessment/intervention	

CONTINENCE	◆	MOBILITY	◆
COMPLETE/ CATHETERIZED	0	FULLY	0
URINE INCONT.	1	RESTLESS/FIDGETY	1
FAECAL INCONT.	2	APATHETIC	2
URINARY + FAECAL INCONTINENCE	3	RESTRICTED	1
		BEDBOUND e.g.TRACTION	4
		CHAIRBOUND e.g.WHEELCHAIR	5

SCORE
10+ AT RISK
15+ HIGH RISK
20+ VERY HIGH RISK

SPECIAL RISKS

TISSUE MALNUTRITION	◆	NEUROLOGICAL DEFICIT	◆
TERMINAL CACHEXIA	8	DIABETES, MS, CVA	4–6
MULTIPLE ORGAN FAILURE	8	MOTOR/SENSORY	4–6
SINGLE ORGAN FAILURE (RESP., RENAL, CARDIAC)	5	PARAPLEGIA (MAX OF 6)	4–6
PERIPHERAL VASCULAR DISEASE	5	**MAJOR SURGERY or TRAUMA**	
ANAEMIA (Hb < 8)	2	ORTHOPAEDIC/SPINAL	5
SMOKING	1	ON TABLE > 2 HR#	5
		ON TABLE > 6 HR#	8

MEDICATION – CYTOTOXICS, LONG-TERM/HIGH-DOSE STEROIDS, ANTI-INFLAMMATORY MAX OF 4

Scores can be discounted after 48 hours, provided patient is recovering normally

©J Waterlow 1985 Revised 2005*
Obtainable from the Nook, Stoke Road, Henlade TAUNTON TA3 5LX
* The 2005 revision incorporates the research undertaken by Queensland Health.
www.judy-waterlow.co.uk

Fig. 14.5 The Waterlow pressure score scale. © J. Waterlow 1985, revised 2005.

Urinary incontinence

- Occurs in 40–60% of patients admitted to hospital following stroke
- Pre-stroke incontinence prevalence is 2.5–17%
- Twenty-five per cent of stroke patients have urinary incontinence at discharge and 15% are still incontinent at 1 year
- Incontinence is associated with any stroke lesion except for occipital lobe. Anteromedial region (ACA territory) and frontal lobe are frequently associated with urinary incontinence. The micturition centre is located in the pons
- Strokes with cortical and subcortical involvement (i.e. large volume strokes) are five times more likely to be associated with incontinence than lacunar infarcts, suggesting that size of the stroke may be more important than location. The extent of cortical damage is likely to affect levels of arousal and awareness which are more likely to lead to incontinent state.

Prognostic significance

- Urinary incontinence is a key indicator of mortality after stroke. Of stroke patients with urinary incontinence, 52% are dead at 6 months compared with 7% of continent stroke survivors. Urinary incontinence 30 days after stroke is associated with almost four times the 1-year mortality compared with continent stroke survivors and two times increased mortality within 5 years
- Early urinary incontinence after stroke is a strong predictor of severe/moderate disability at 3 months: in one study the OR was 5.4 (95% CI 3.3–9.0). It is associated with poor functional outcome, immobility, and increased likelihood for discharge to institutionalized care home
- May also predict recovery of limb strength and activities of daily living
- The presence of continence is a better predictor of recovery at 4 weeks than almost any other predictive scoring
- Urinary incontinence after stroke is also associated with falls
    - Incontinence is associated with 2.3 times (1.3–4.1) relative risk of falls
    - Twenty per cent of falls occurred during visits to the toilet or bathroom
    - Other factors: cognitive impairment, heart disease, previous fall.

Causes

Mechanisms of urinary incontinence after stroke are unclear. Few studies have performed urodynamic examinations in stroke patients. Simple bladder scanning is of benefit in establishing the cause of incontinence if urodynamic studies are not practicable.

No specific type of incontinence is associated with stroke—a number of different types can occur:

- Detrusor hyperreflexia is the commonest lesion, in 50–82%. This is thought to be caused by disruption of neuromicturition pathways causing urge incontinence
- Acontractile bladder in 17–25%. This may be caused by concurrent neuropathy or medication use, resulting in overflow type incontinence

- Outflow tract obstruction (excluding faecal impaction which may cause this)
- Incontinence owing to stroke-related cognitive and language deficits, with normal bladder function is common. A new subtype of post-stroke incontinence, 'impaired awareness urge incontinence' (AI-UI) has been described. This group of patients, often with parietal lobe damage, have little urge to urinate and frequently no sense of full bladder or leakage and, as such, tend to fail to recognize and report their incontinence. Bladder training is usually unsuccessful in such cases.

Management of urinary incontinence

- Exclude exacerbating/precipitating features, particularly urinary tract infections, drugs (e.g. diuretics), faecal impaction
- Comprehensive assessment is paramount. Portable bladder scanners can give useful estimates of post-voiding residual volume (PVR) at the bedside. A PVR of greater than 50 cm^3 may indicate the need for further urodynamic studies
- Importance of lower urinary tract symptoms, rather than 'incontinence'
- Mobility
- Dexterity
- Environment
- Scheduled voiding/bladder retraining
- Drugs (anticholinergics are the mainstay)
- Botulinum toxin intravesical injection (for detrusor instability)
- Pads and continence aids (female urinal, penile pouch, convenes)
- Catheterization as a last resort
- Approaches used include behavioural interventions, such as timed voiding and pelvic floor muscle training, professional input interventions (e.g. structured assessment and management by continence nurse advisors), and drug therapy (e.g. meclofenoxate, oxybutinin or oestrogen)
- Cochrane review concluded that good quality trial data is not available, but there is suggestive evidence that professional input through structured assessment and management of care and specialist continence nursing may reduce urinary incontinence and related symptoms after stroke.

Further reading

Patel M, Coshill C, Rudd AG, Wolfe CD (2001) Natural history and effects on 2 year outcomes of urinary incontinence after stroke. *Stroke* **32**, 122–7.

Pettersen R, Stien R, Wyller TB (2007) Post-stroke urinary incontinence with impaired awareness of the need to void: clinical and urodynamic features. *The British Journal of Urology Int* **99**, 1073–7.

Thomas LH, Cross S, Barrett J *et al.* (2005) Treatment of urinary incontinence after stroke in adults. *Cochrane Database of Systematic Reviews*, Issue 3. Art. No.: CD004462. DOI: 10.1002/14651858.CD004462.pub

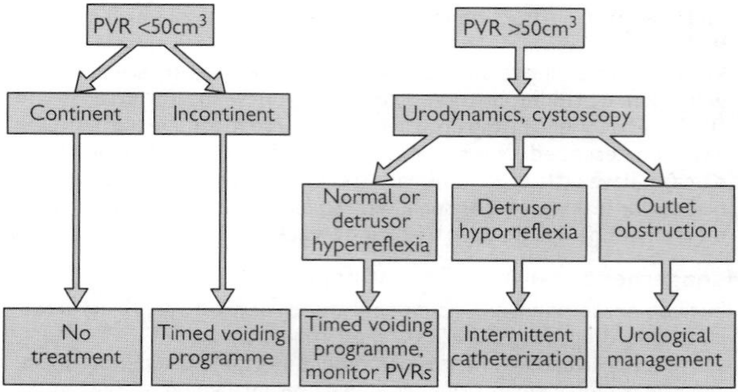

Fig. 14.6 Management of post-stroke urinary incontinence. First exclude infection and other exacerbating factors. PVR, post-voiding residual volume.

Bowel management

Bowel incontinence

New-onset faecal incontinence after stroke is sadly very common: 56% acutely, 30% (7–10 days) and 11% (3 months). Older patients, women, and those with severe strokes are most at risk. The impact of faecal incontinence is always devastating:

- Social taboo
- Poor self-image
- Depression
- Tissue viability
- Carer stress
- Reduced rehabilitation participation.

Comprehensive assessment requires:

- Bowel history
- Medication review
- Diet/fluid intake
- Mobility
- Current bowel movement status
- Abdominal exam
- Rectal exam (by trained person).

Incontinence is more likely when stool is loose, commonly caused by:

- Drugs—proton pump inhibitors, antibiotics, laxatives, NSAIDS, antihypertensives, and potassium supplements
- Artificial feeding (NG/PEG)
- Infection (*Clostridium difficile*).

Functional bowel incontinence may be caused by impairments in mobility, dexterity, communication and vision, and be improved with:

- Communication aids (call bell/picture cards)
- Regular toileting programme (in line with normal bowel habits)
- Simple bold signage.

Bowel urgency

- Bladder training has been found to be useful with urgency or frequency of micturition, and similar training may help bowel incontinence
- Patients distressed by faecal incontinence may become hypervigilant and hypersensitive, and any bowel sensation may be interpreted as urgency. This may then result in anxiety or panic if a toilet is not readily available. A vicious circle can then develop as anxiety is a known bowel stimulant
- A progressive programme of urge resistance is recommended
- Smoking cessation may be useful in patients with urgency.

Management of ongoing bowel incontinence

- Skin care (repeated wiping can spread digestive enzymes and bacteria contained within the stool and cause local skin irritation)
- Difficult to find any product that reliably disguises bowel leakage and smell
- Pads
- Faecal collectors
- Anal plugs.

Bowel programmes, e.g. daily codeine phosphate with twice-weekly enemas resulted in 75% of nursing home patients achieving bowel continence.

Use of loperamide 2 mg up to three times per day according to symptoms can be a last resort.

Constipation

Constipation is a common problem in older people and is particularly common after stroke. Constipation is present in up to 60% of stroke patients in rehabilitation wards.

The cost of prescribed laxatives to the NHS is £48 million (and a further over-the-counter cost estimated at £27 million).

Constipation can be defined by Rome II criteria by two or more of the following:

- Fewer than three bowel movements per week
- Hard stool or sense of incomplete emptying in 25% of bowel movements
- Excessive straining in 25% of bowel movements
- Necessity of digital manipulation to facilitate evacuation.

Objective recording of bowel opening is key. The Bristol Stool chart can be helpful.

Studies show that 65% of older people reporting constipation had their bowels open at least once a day, and 25% of people have no symptoms of constipation but feel that a regular stool is necessary. One man's constipation is another man's diarrhoea!

Poor evidence base underlies treatment of constipation after stroke.

Predisposing factors to acquired constipation are:

- Drugs
- Tricyclic antidepressants
- Opiates
- Anticonvulsants
- Drugs for Parkinson's disease
- Beta blockers, diuretics
- Anticholinergic drugs
- Diet/dehydration
- Immobility
- Constipation can be behaviourally induced by deliberately ignoring the urge to defecate. This is not common in acute debilitating stroke where toileting independence has been lost.

Constipation can result in faecal impaction with overflow incontinence.

Faecal impaction may result in urinary retention as impaction may impinge on bladder neck emptying (as well as cause external compression of deep pelvic veins).

Constipation invariably causes abdominal discomfort and distension, and commonly increases confusion.

Treatment of constipation

- Keep a bedside stool chart (e.g. Bristol Stool chart)
- Review current medication
- Consider metabolic disorder (hypothyroidism, hypokalaemia, hypercalcaemia)
- Review diet, fluid intake
- Bulk forming agents
- Movicol
- Glycerine suppositories may be used to soften stool
- If no result after 2 days consider use of an enema
- If problems remain, consider adding in senna for 1 week (overuse or misuse of senna can cause water, sodium, and potassium depletion)
- Education (what constitutes normal bowel habit, correction of misperceptions, misuse of laxatives)
- Individuals should have the opportunity to attempt defecation within half an hour of breakfast. Comfort and privacy are required
- Positioning correctly to facilitate bowel opening—it is far easier sitting forward than lying back.

Further reading

Harari D, Coshall C, Rudd AG, Wolfe CD (2003) New-onset fecal incontinence after stroke: prevalence, natural history, risk factors, and impact. *Stroke* **34**, 144–50.

Lewis SJ, Heaton KW (1997) Stool form scale as a useful guide to intestinal transit time. *Scandinavian Journal of Gastroenterology* **32**, 920–4.

Potter J, Wagg A (2005) Management of bowel problems in older people: an update. *Clinical Medicine* **5**, 289–95.

Driving after stroke

In the UK, all patients with group 1 licence (car, moped or motorcycle) who experience a stroke episode (including TIA or amaurosis fugax)* should not drive for 1 month. If they have neurological deficit at 1 month that may impair driving ability, they are obliged to inform the Driver Vehicle Licensing Authority (DVLA) and need a medical assessment of their fitness to drive before attempting to drive again. Seizure associated with stroke onset (provoked seizure) is not considered epilepsy, but seizures more than 24 hours from stroke onset also require DVLA notification.

Holders of LGV or PCV licences should notify the DVLA of any stroke episode and should not drive such vehicles until after further medical enquiry.

All patients should inform their insurers of their change in health circumstances.

Persistent limb disability following a stroke may not prevent a patient holding a driving licence again. Adaptations to a vehicle and/or restriction to automatic types of vehicle may help to overcome driving difficulties even with quite complex disabilities.

The law requires adaptations or restriction to certain types of vehicles to be noted on the licence. Therefore, the DVLA should be notified if adaptations are necessary.

In the UK, a series of charity funded mobility centres offer assessment of driving ability and potential for driving adapted vehicles, e.g. http://www.qefd.org/mobilitycentre/

Flying after stroke

- There is no absolute medical bar on flying after a stroke and no central UK guidance
- Each airline has its own rules about whom it allows on its planes
- British Airways suggests that, providing symptoms are stable or improving, air travel is possible 3 days after stroke but wish to be notified in advance if a stroke episode has occurred within the last 10 days
- The oxygen pressure during flight is lower than that at sea level, so there is a theoretical risk of harm to someone who has suffered a recent stroke
- Most advise not flying for a fortnight after the stroke unless it is imperative. After that, there is no medical reason why an otherwise fit stroke patient shouldn't fly
- Patients with physical disability should notify the airline that they will need extra help at the airport or on the plane. They should also inform their insurers.

*If there are multiple TIAs and no underlying reversible cause, then 3 months should be taken off driving (assuming no further events).

Measuring outcome and progress

Goal planning

This is a central ethos in neurorehabilitation, particularly in recovery from complex neurological deficits associated with stroke. After a period of multidisciplinary assessment, the patient, their carer and family are engaged in a process of setting relevant goals over an agreed time period. Long-term goals are then broken down into 'stepping stone' goals that are reviewed and reassessed at regular intervals. For example, a long-term goal may be to achieve independent transfers from bed to chair at 3 months. In this case, these would be the interim 'stepping stone' goals: obtaining independent sitting balance, then assisted sliding board transfers, then assisted pivot transfers, and then independent standing transfers. Goals need to be specific for individual patients and measurable.

Remember SMART goals:

- **S**pecific
- **M**easurable
- **A**chievable
- **R**elevant
- **T**ime-limited.

Goals achieved is a valid and individualized outcome measure.

Goal attainment scaling tool

The goal attainment scaling (GAS) tool was developed for 'goal-driven management mentoring' in the 1960s and has been used in industry, relationship counselling, and recently neurorehabilitation.

GAS is able to judge progress against goals set jointly between the MDT and the patient, as part of a case management process. To do this, the expected outcome needs to be defined when identifying goals. The MDT and patient need to agree what would constitute 'more than expected' or 'less than expected' outcomes. A time for review of achievement of the goal is set when completing the form.

The expected outcome is defined as the result that could reasonably be expected to be achieved within a given time; it is scored as '0'. These outcomes are tailored to each individual. GAS involves identifying descriptors, preferably behavioural, to provide evidence that the goal has been achieved.

The first step is identifying high priority goal areas. Write the first in the box labelled 'Goal 1' and add others as appropriate for the patient's needs and period of neurorehabilitation.

The next step is to identify possible outcomes in each chosen goal area. Outcomes should be specific and, where possible, expressed as a behavioural statement or something that is observable. Examples of a completed form are shown in the Table.

Start with the most likely outcome. This is what you would reasonably expect to occur within the time agreed and indicates success. This is recorded as 0. Then describe what would be considered a higher or better outcome (+1) and an even higher or better outcome (+2). Then do the same for lower levels of success (–1) and (–2). An example is below.

At the end of the agreed time frame the level of achievement is reviewed. If the team and patient are setting realistic goals for the timeframe available you would expect most outcomes to be the 0 result.

Advantages of GAS

- Cheap
- Goals can be completely individualized
- Goals can be changed or abandoned if circumstances change.

Disadvantages of GAS

- Bias (make goals overly easy to attain, problems with multiple 'raters')
- Assumption that outcomes can be determined in advance (crystal ball gazing)
- Staff will need training in using the approach
- There is an additional time commitment involved in developing the outcome levels, though this is less of an impact if such discussion is part of the practice approach
- Expected outcomes need to be set at a realistic level for the client's needs and circumstances, and the time period set for review, or results will be distorted
- Research has shown that a maximum of five goals is likely to be manageable at any one time and that most people would be working on two goals in any one period of time.

GAS FORM

Level of expected outcome	Goal 1: Decision-making	Goal 2: Self-esteem	Goal 3: Isolation
Review date:			
Much more than expected (+2)	Makes plans, follows through, modifies if needed, and reaches goal	Expresses realistic positive feelings about self	Actively participates in group or social activities
More than expected (+1)	Makes plans, follows through without assistance unless plan needs changing	Expresses more positive than negative feelings about self	Attends activities, sometimes initiates contact with others
Most likely outcome (0)	Makes plans and follows through with assistance/ reminders	Expresses equally both positive and negative feelings about self	Leaves house and attends community centre. Responds if approached
Less than expected outcome (−1)	Makes plans but does not take any action to follow through	Expresses more negative than positive feelings about self	Leaves house occasionally, no social contact
Much less than expected (−2)	Can consider alternatives but doesn't decide on a plan	Expresses only negative feelings about self	Spends most of time in house except for formal appointments

When measuring goal attainment, the box which matches the outcome achieved is marked and the scores for each goal are added. This total is the GAS and again is an individualized outcome measure. Taken from Kiresuk TJ, Sherman RE (1967) Goal attainment scaling: a general method for evaluating comprehensive community mental health programs. *Community Mental Health Journal* **4**, 443–53, with kind permission of Springer Science and Business Media.

Discharge planning

Discharge planning is an active process that 'aims to reduce hospital length of stay and unplanned readmission to hospital and improve the coordination of services following discharge from hospital thereby bridging the gap between hospital and place of discharge'.

Frequently suggested advantages to discharge planning include:

- Reduced readmission rates
- Shortened length of stay
- Preventing unsafe discharges
- Improved patient/carer satisfaction.

However, the evidence for this is not robust.

Discharge planning should start at the earliest possible opportunity by ensuring a full history is taken at the time of stroke presentation, including the patient's previous level of functioning and social circumstance. Preparing for discharge includes the entire multidisciplinary stroke team and is a focus of MDT meetings. Where appropriate, a provisional expected date of discharge should be set at the earliest opportunity.

Throughout the recovery and rehabilitation process the patient should remain central to the process but carers and family need to be engaged particularly with discharge planning. A survey by Carers UK found that 43% of carers felt they had inadequate support when the person returned home. This should not be ignored given that voluntary carers provide a huge amount of support which would otherwise need to be provided by health service. For example, in England alone carers provide in the region of £2 billion stroke care per year.

Admission to hospital is a vulnerable time for patients. As a result of stroke, patients frequently experience a loss of functional ability, and require either a temporary increase in support or rehabilitation or more prolonged support. For most patients the ideal situation is to return to their premorbid state so that they can function as they previously had done. Less than 50% do.

Stroke patients with irreversible loss of function may require additional support at home. This can be achieved by increased care services (via social services), aids or home modifications (via occupational therapy), community nursing or via the patient's informal care network. Ultimately, a small proportion of patients who are no longer able to manage at home will require long-term placement into a residential home (providing 24-hour care) or a nursing home (if specific nursing needs are evident). Finding a suitable placement for patients is something that should be started only after discussion with the patient, relatives, and the rest of the MDT.

To bridge the transition to home, and reduce length of stay in more expensive specialized hospitals, intermediate care has become popular in some countries. 'Packages' of multidisciplinary care lasting a few weeks can be tailored to meet specific needs of stroke patients who no longer need acute hospital stay. These may be delivered in community hospitals, or at home with support from early supported discharge teams.

On discharge into the community, the quality of transfer of care relies on multidisciplinary and multiagency handover and communication. A good example of an immediate discharge document has been developed by the Royal College of Physicians http://www.rcplondon.ac.uk/pubs/books/stroketoc/

Causes of increase risk of 'failed' discharge/early readmission include:

- Great age
- History of repeated unplanned admissions
- Social isolation/living alone
- In receipt of care package prior to stroke
- Lack of informal care network
- Admitted patient being a carer
- Marked loss of physical or mental function
- Issues of neglect or abuse.

Role of carers and voluntary sector

- The presence of an immediate support network is an important factor in not only discharge planning but also adjustment to life after stroke
- Carer burden is well documented in stroke
- Voluntary sector organizations can provide financial, emotional, and practical help for both stroke patients and carers
- Post-stroke groups can help with regaining confidence after stroke. These are often facilitated by former users or patients and can improve measures of anxiety and depression and 'self-efficacy'.

Further reading

Shepperd S, Parkes J, McClaren J, Phillips C (2004) Discharge planning from hospital to home. *Cochrane Database of Systematic Reviews* (1):CD000313.

Chapter 15

Vascular dementia

Vascular dementia: concepts

Various definitions of dementia exist but all require a decline in intellectual function involving several separate cognitive domains. Cognition is the process by which internal or external stimuli are transformed into purposeful thought or action. Cognition relies upon a number of higher cerebral functions or domains, including attention, speed of processing, visual special skills, language, and, importantly (but not exclusively), memory.

A wide variety of vascular pathologies can cause dementia.

Dementia resulting from vascular disease must be distinguished from:

- Confusion—an acute and reversible disturbance of cognitive function
- Focal disturbances affecting single cognitive domains, e.g. amnesia or aphasia.

The field of vascular dementia is challenging for the following reasons:

- It is a syndrome not a specific disease and can be caused by multiple pathologies
- The cognitive features of vascular disease affecting different parts of the brain differ markedly (e.g. the cognitive profile of dementia caused by multiple cortical infarcts is quite different from that caused by diffuse subcortical disease)
- Many different definitions of vascular dementia have been used
- Most of the definitions are designed for Alzheimer's type 'cortical dementias' and describe the features of vascular dementia, particularly subcortical vascular dementia, less well
- Vascular pathology and Alzheimer's pathology frequently coexist. Some studies suggest mixed dementia is more common than pure vascular dementia
- Assessing dementia can be difficult in patients with stroke, particularly those with communication problems.

Classification of vascular dementia

It is most useful to classify vascular dementia according to the site of vascular damage as this determines the cognitive profile. A classification is shown on 📖 p. 475.

Frequently more than one subtype can coexist, and vascular disease may coexist with a wide variety of other dementias, not only Alzheimer's disease but also Lewy body dementia and other dementias.

Strategic infarcts

- Single infarcts in specific sites may result in cognitive impairment which may meet the criteria for 'dementia'. Whether they meet the criteria for dementia depends largely on the definition of dementia used (see 📖 Definitions of vascular dementia, p. 476).They cause 'dementia' by resulting in discrete 'disconnections' within complex neuronal pathways concerned with cognitive processes
- Usually other signs of stroke make the diagnosis clear
- Diagnosis of the lesion is often more useful than making a diagnosis of dementia
- The following lesions may produce specific cognitive disturbances:
  - Frontal lesions (anterior cerebral artery)—apathy and emotional blunting (usually when bilateral)
  - Medial temporal lobe lesions—severe amnesia (especially when bilateral)
  - Thalamic infarcts—disturbances of attention, memory, language, and abstract thinking
  - Caudate head infarcts—apathy, disinhibition, and affective symptoms.

Multiple cortical infarcts

Here the pattern of cognitive impairment depends upon the site of the lesion. Whether patients with such lesions develop dementia depends upon the infarct size, the total infarct volume, and age of the patient.

Small-vessel (subcortical) dementia

This occurs because of multiple subcortical lacunar infarcts usually accompanied by more diffuse ischaemic changes (leukoaraiosis) (see 📖 p. 228). Patients may or may not have clinical evidence of lacunar stroke. A typical cognitive profile occurs with predominant impairment of executive function, attention, and speed of information processing. In contrast, memory and visuospatial cognition is relatively preserved.

Hypoperfusion dementia

This is a rare cause of dementia and the clinical picture will depend upon the mechanism. For example, patients with subcortical vascular disease and impaired autoregulation in the white matter may deteriorate markedly following a period of hypoperfusion which worsens white matter ischaemia. In contrast, patients with large extracranial vessel occlusion (carotid and vertebral) may suffer watershed infarction following hypoperfusion involving both cortical and subcortical watershed regions.

Dementia caused by cerebral haemorrhage

This encompasses both subcortical and cortical pathologies. Cerebral haemorrhage is a frequent feature of subcortical vascular disease coexisting with small-vessel disease. The other major pathology producing dementia and cerebral haemorrhage is amyloid angiopathy.

Subtypes of vascular dementia

Multiple large cortical infarcts
Small-vessel dementia (subcortical dementia)
Strategic infarct dementia
Hypoperfusion dementia
Dementia secondary to cerebral haemorrhage
Mixed dementia (vascular disease with Alzheimer's disease)

Definitions of vascular dementia

The term vascular dementia has been, and is still, widely used both clinically and in research studies. However, there are problems inherent in the use of the term dementia. Multiple definitions exist and some of these, such as the Diagnostic and Statistical Manual (DSM-IV) and International Classification of Disease (ICD-10), require the presence of memory impairment as an absolute requirement, and, in addition, the presence of one or more (for DSM-IV) or two or more (ICD-10) other cognitive domains to be affected. This approach has been criticized because memory impairment, which is commonly (though not universally) seen early in the course of Alzheimer's disease, is much less often seen in patients with cerebrovascular disease. It is a particular problem for subcortical dementia, which presents predominantly with executive dysfunction rather than memory impairment. As many definitions of vascular dementia are so influenced by Alzheimer's disease, there is a circularity in the argument; if the criterion requires memory impairment, then it is likely that a number of patients fulfilling such criteria for vascular dementia may also have concurrent Alzheimer type pathology.

In view of these difficulties, it has been suggested that a definition of vascular dementia should not absolutely require the presence of memory impairment. Furthermore, because there is a continuum of cognitive impairment associated with vascular disease, some authorities suggest a broader term of 'vascular cognitive impairment' rather than dementia.

The definition used has a marked effect on the prevalence of vascular dementia, as shown in Table 15.1 (Erkinjuntti *et al.*, 1997).

Table 15.1 Effect of using different definitions of vascular dementia on the prevalence of the disease

Criteria	Prevalence (%)
ICD-9	5.0
ICD-10	3.1
CAMDEX	4.9
DSM-III	29.1
DSM-IV	13.7
Clinical consensus	20.9

Data from Erkinjuntti *et al.*, 1997.

Reference

Erkinjuntti T *et al.* (1997) The effect of different diagnostic criteria on the prevalence of dementia. *New England Journal of Medicine* **337**, 1667–74.

Further reading

O'Brien JT (2006) Vascular cognitive impairment. *American Journal of Geriatric Psychiatry* **14**, 724–33.

Epidemiology

- Vascular dementia is the second most common cause of dementia after Alzheimer's disease
- Historically, prevalence rates have been higher in Asian compared with western countries, although recent studies have shown a shift from vascular to Alzheimer's disease in these countries, perhaps reflecting longevity
- Rates increase exponentially with age
- Men are more affected than women, but sex differences narrow at older age groups
- Stroke is a major risk factor
- Dementia is seen in up to 20–30% of subjects 3 months after stroke. However, this figure depends greatly on the definition of dementia used
- Risk factors for developing dementia after stroke include advanced age, previous stroke, lacunar infarction, diabetes mellitus, and left hemisphere stroke
- One epidemiological study from Sweden found that the lifetime risk of developing vascular dementia was 30% in men and 25% in women, very similar to that for developing Alzheimer's type dementia. Estimates from other populations have differed markedly owing to both differing definitions and differing populations.

Small-vessel disease dementia (subcortical vascular dementia)

Subcortical vascular dementia results from ischaemia in the deep white matter and deep grey matter nuclei secondary to diffuse disease of the small perforating blood vessels supplying these regions.

Recent data has shown it is an important cause of vascular dementia, and in treatment trials it accounted for more than half of cases of vascular dementia.

The true burden is likely to be underestimated because the major cognitive features are executive dysfunction and impairment of information processing speed. These deficits are not well identified by the screening tools often used (such as the MMSE), which were designed to detect impairments due to 'cortical' dementias such as Alzheimer's.

Causes

- Sporadic small-vessel disease (90% hypertensive)
- Monogenic forms of small-vessel disease (CADASIL and others)
- Small-vessel vasculitis
- Other rare causes.

The vast majority of cases are caused by hypertensive small-vessel disease. In only approximately 10% of sporadic small-vessel disease is hypertension not present. Diabetes and elevated serum homocysteine have also been identified as risk factors for small-vessel disease.

Radiological features

A combination of lacunar infarction (often multiple) and leukoaraiosis is usually seen. Leukoaraiosis is seen as periventricular and deep white matter low signal on CT or much better seen as high signal on T2-weighted or FLAIR MRI. Other common features include diffuse cerebral atrophy and multiple microbleeds on gradient echo MRI.

Mechanism of dementia

Disruption of cortical–subcortical and cortical–cortical white matter tracts, with an ensuing 'disconnection' syndrome, is believed to play a central role. This could occur due to both lacunar infarcts and leukoaraiosis (which have been shown to disrupt white matter tracts using diffusion tensor imaging).

Diffuse atrophy may also contribute to cognitive impairment, although whether this is secondary to white matter tract disruption remains to be determined.

Clinical features

Some or all of the following may be present. Clinical lacunar stroke is not essential for the diagnosis, although neuroimaging evidence of small-vessel disease is.

- Lacunar stroke (see 📖 p. 78)
- Subcortical cognitive impairment
- Parkinsonian features
- Gait apraxia

- Depression
- Emotional lability.

Cognitive profile

There is a characteristic cognitive profile with major deficits seen in:

- Attention
- Speed of information processing
- Executive function.

Such functions, predominantly served by frontostriatal–thalamic circuits, which are most disrupted by subcortical vascular change, are not well detected on current screening and assessment instruments for dementia. For example, there can be significant cognitive deficit despite an MMSE which is normal or slightly impaired.

Other bedside tests are more useful to screen for this deficit, including:

- Verbal fluency
- Trail making or maze tests
- Clock drawing
- Reverse digit span.

Other clinical features

- Bradyphrenia, a slowing of mental agility, may be a marked feature in subcortical dementia. The patient may be slow to remember a list of items but eventually respond correctly, in contrast to patients with cortical dementia who tend to remember immediately or not at all
- Confusional episodes may occur, particularly in the latter stages. Marked deterioration can occur in response to systemic disorders (e.g. infection or following a seizure)
- Gait apraxia with poor gait ignition ('stuttering standing start'), wide base and small steps (*march a petit pas*). Occasionally, patients present with an extrapyramidal, seemingly Parkinsonian, syndrome, but this is non-DOPA responsive and there is a lack of tremor
- In advanced cases, other features include pseudobulbar palsy, emotional lability, extensor plantar responses and urinary incontinence
- Chronic hypertension is usually present, but it is important to note that in the later stages of the disease, blood pressure measurements may decline to the normal range. Therefore taking a premorbid history of hypertension is important
- Depression is common. Recent evidence suggests many white matter diseases disrupting subcortical–cortical circuits predispose to depression.

Overlap with Alzheimer's disease

Increasing evidence has shown that Alzheimer's and vascular pathology can coexist in many patients. This has important implications clinically and for research studies.

- In the prospective clinicopathological Nuns study in the US, in which cognitive testing was performed in life and then compared with pathology at post mortem, a lesser degree of Alzheimer's (tangle) pathology was needed to produce the same degree of cognitive impairment during life if one or more infarcts was present
- In most autopsy studies on selected older people, mixed Alzheimer and vascular pathology was the most common cause of cognitive impairment. Many studies have shown it is at least as common, if not more common, than 'pure' vascular dementia
- Several risk factors for vascular disease have also been shown to be risk factors for Alzheimer's, including hypertension, smoking, diabetes, ischaemic heart disease, and, in some studies, cholesterol and homocysteine
- Commonly used definitions of dementia have been designed for Alzheimer's or cortical type dementias and these are not sensitive to subcortical dementias. The requirement of memory impairment may lead to overrepresentation of Alzheimer pathology in patients with dementia
- White matter hyperintensities and leukoaraiosis on MRI can be seen in up to 50% of Alzheimer's patients.

How do vascular and Alzheimer's pathologies interact?

This is uncertain but a number of mechanisms have been suggested.

It has been suggested the two pathologies are independent but frequently coexist. If any pathology damages 'brain reserve' this is likely to exacerbate the damage caused by a second pathology.

- Two independent co-occurring pathologies
- Vascular changes reduce the elimination of amyloid through the perivascular (lymphatic) system
- Vascular changes (hypoxia, hypoperfusion) increase formation of Alzheimer's disease pathology (beta-amyloid and phosphorylated-tau)
- Amyloid angiopathy contributes to and/or accelerates vascular damage.

More recent data has suggested that vascular changes may actually stimulate or exacerbate the formation of Alzheimer type pathology. For example, by contributing to vessel wall thickening and reducing the efficiency of the perivascular drainage system, this could lead to reduced elimination of amyloid. Secondary to this, increased accumulation of amyloid and a greater likelihood of plaque formation could occur.

Vascular pathology can also lead to hypoxia and hypoperfusion, and in animal models both have been clearly demonstrated to increase Alzheimer pathology. Ischaemia has also been shown to accelerate hyperphosphorylation of tau, a crucial step in tangle formation, and increase the cleavage of amyloid precursor protein, which would lead to increased plaque accumulation.

Further reading

O'Brien JT (2006) Vascular cognitive impairment. *American Journal of Geriatric Psychiatry* **14**, 724–33.

Snowdon DA, Greiner LH, Mortimer JA *et al.* (1997) Brain infarction and the clinical expression of Alzheimer disease. The Nun Study. *JAMA* **277**, 813–17.

Investigation of the vascular dementia patient

History

- Details of cognitive decline
  - Time scale
  - Relationship to stroke
- Social setting
  - Effect on patient and carer.

Examination

- Full neurological examination
- Check for gait apraxia.

Cognitive assessment

- MMSE (but remember, may be insensitive to subcortical cognitive deficit)
- Simple tests of higher cortical function, e.g. parietal function
- Assessment of executive function, e.g. trail making test.

Investigations

- CT
- MRI
  - Better than CT, particularly for small-vessel disease
  - Gradient echo will show old microbleeds—these occur in small-vessel disease and amyloid angiopathy
- Bloods
  - Routine stroke screen
  - Rare tests (e.g. CADASIL genetic analysis) when indicated.

Apart from vascular causes, one should also screen for common or reversible causes of dementia:

- Full blood count (anaemia)
- ESR/CRP (vasculitis)
- Renal function—renal failure can cause cognitive impairment
- Liver function—hepatic encephalopathy, when chronic, may masquerade as dementia
- Thyroid function is very common in the elderly
- B12
- Antinuclear antibodies and ANCA—ANA for lupus and ANCA for vasculitis
- Anticardiolipin antibodies
- VDRL (venereal disease research laboratory) test
- In young people with vascular disease, don't forget HIV.

Management

One should follow this plan:

- History, examination, and investigation as above
- Classification of type of dementia
- Treat rare/reversible causes
- Look for intercurrent depression and treat
- Secondary prevention
  - Antithrombotic therapy
  - Identify and treat vascular risk factors
- Identify and treat complications
- Provide family and social support.

Therapy of dementia

This can be divided into:
- Prevention and treatment of risk factors
- Symptomatic treatments
- Treatment of complications, including depression
- General supportive care of patient and carers.

Prevention and treatment of risk factors

Few studies have specifically investigated treatment of risk factors in preventing cognitive decline as opposed to stroke. Nevertheless, it seems sensible to treat risk factors as one would for stroke. These include:
- Hypertension
- Diabetes mellitus
- Raised cholesterol
- Smoking.

Treating hypertension is particularly important in prevention of small-vessel disease and was shown to reduce progression of MRI white matter hyperintensities which represent early cerebral small-vessel disease.

In patients with advanced subcortical dementia it has been suggested that excessive blood pressure lowering may reduce cognitive function. This is a controversial area. This should not be used as an excuse for failing to treat blood pressure aggressively in the vast majority of patients.

Antiplatelet therapy

There is little data specifically assessing antiplatelet therapy in preventing dementia. Nevertheless, most authorities recommend antiplatelet treatment with aspirin ± dipyridamole. Warfarin is contraindicated except for specific reasons (e.g. cardioembolic source). Leukoaraiosis is associated with an increased risk of cerebral haemorrhage in anticoagulated patients as shown in the SPIRIT trial. Some data suggest aspirin plus clopidogrel may increase risk of haemorrhage in these patients.

Homocysteine

A number of studies have shown that homocysteine is particularly raised in small-vessel disease with leukoaraiosis. Whether treating this reduces cognitive decline remains to be determined.

Symptomatic pharmacological treatments

Symptomatic treatments for vascular dementia have been explored:
- Cholinesterase inhibitors
  - Donepezil
  - Galantamine
- Memantine—an NMDA antagonist.

Trials in vascular and mixed dementia have suggested modest benefits in some outcomes but no major benefit.

Interpretation of the data is difficult because:
- Many patients may have coexistent Alzheimer's disease which could account for the benefit seen

- The outcome scores are more suited to assessing cognitive deficits in cortical or Alzheimer's-type dementia rather than subcortical vascular dementia (which comprised the majority of patients in some studies)
- To determine whether the cholinesterase inhibitor donepezil is effective in pure vascular cognitive impairment, a randomized double-blind study was performed in CADASIL. This autosomal dominant form of small-vessel disease causes a similar cognitive impairment to that seen in sporadic small-vessel disease. However, it occurs at an earlier age when coexistent Alzheimer pathology is very rare. No effect was found on a traditional trial endpoint, the VADASCog, but a significant (but small) improvement occurred in executive function. This has two implications:
  - Cholinesterase inhibitors do result in improvement in some cognitive features in subcortical dementia although the effect is small and of questionable clinical benefit
  - Treatment effects will be detected best using tests targeted to the deficits seen in this group of patients, i.e. executive dysfunction and speed of information processing.

Currently most bodies (e.g. NICE in the UK) do not recommend the widespread use of cholinesterase inhibitors or memantine for vascular dementia, and suggest more data from well designed clinical trials is required.

Treatment of complications

If there is a sudden or unexpected deterioration in cognitive state, a thorough assessment should be made of treatable comorbid states or complications, including:

- Intercurrent infection
- Medication side effects
- Cardiovascular compromise leading to hypoperfusion
- Seizures and post-ictal worsening
- Depression.

Non-pharmacological therapy

This is an important part of dementia care and suggested patterns of care are well described in the UK NICE guidelines for dementia (http://www.nice.org.uk); a modified version of these is presented below.

Dementia is associated with complex needs and, especially in the later stages, high levels of dependency and morbidity. As the condition progresses, people with dementia can present carers and healthcare staff with complex problems, including aggressive behaviour, restlessness and wandering, eating problems, incontinence, delusions and hallucinations, and mobility difficulties that can lead to falls and fractures. The impact of dementia on an individual may be compounded by personal circumstances such as changes in financial status and accommodation, or bereavement.

Wherever possible and appropriate, agencies should work in an integrated way to maximize the benefit for people with dementia and their carers.

Further reading

Prevention and treatment of risk factors

Birns J, Markus HS, Kalra L (2005) Blood pressure reduction for vascular risk – is there a price to be paid? *Stroke* **36**, 1308–13.

Dufouil C, Chalmers J, Coskun O *et al*; PROGRESS MRI Substudy Investigators (2005) Effects of blood pressure lowering on cerebral white matter hyperintensities in patients with stroke: the PROGRESS (Perindopril Protection Against Recurrent Stroke Study) Magnetic Resonance Imaging Substudy. *Circulation* **112**, 1644–50.

Gorter JW (1999) Major bleeding during anticoagulation after cerebral ischemia: patterns and risk factors. Stroke Prevention In Reversible Ischemia Trial (SPIRIT). European Atrial Fibrillation Trial (EAFT) study groups. *Neurology* **53**, 1319–27.

Symptomatic pharmacological treatments

Dichgans M, Markus HS, Salloway S *et al.* (2008) Donepezil in patients with subcortical vascular cognitive impairment: a randomised double-blind trial in CADASIL. *Lancet Neurology* **7**, 310–18.

Kavirajan H, Schneider LS (2007) Efficacy and adverse effects of cholinesterase inhibitors and memantine in vascular dementia: a meta-analysis of randomised controlled trials. *Lancet Neurology* **6**, 782–92.

Promoting independence of people with dementia

Health and social care staff should aim to promote and maintain the independence, including mobility, of people with dementia. Care plans should address activities of daily living (ADLs) that maximize independent activity, enhance function, adapt and develop skills, and minimize the need for support. Important considerations in helping maintain independence include:

- Consistent and stable staffing
- Retaining a familiar environment
- Minimizing relocations
- Flexibility to accommodate fluctuating abilities
- Assessment and care planning advice regarding ADLs, and ADL skill training from an occupational therapist
- Assessment and care planning advice about independent toileting skills; if incontinence occurs, all possible causes should be assessed and relevant treatments tried before concluding that it is permanent
- Environmental modifications to aid independent functioning, including assistive technology, with advice from an occupational therapist and/or clinical psychologist
- Physical exercise, with assessment and advice from a physiotherapist when needed
- Support for people to go at their own pace and participate in activities they enjoy.

Capacity and dementia

People with dementia should have the opportunity to make informed decisions about their care in partnership with their health and social care professionals. If they do not have the capacity to make decisions, health professionals should follow national guidelines; for example, in the UK the Department of Health guidelines *Reference guide to consent for examination or treatment* (2001), *Seeking consent: working with older people* (2001), and *Seeking consent: working with people with learning disabilities* (2001) (all available from www.dh.gov.uk). Since April 2007 healthcare professionals in the UK need to follow the Mental Capacity Act 2005 (summary available from www.dca.gov.uk/menincap/bill-summary.htm). It has five key principles:

- Adults must be assumed to have capacity to make decisions for themselves unless proved otherwise
- Individuals must be given all available support before it is concluded that they cannot make decisions for themselves
- Individuals must retain the right to make what might be seen as eccentric or unwise decisions
- Anything done for, or on behalf of, individuals without capacity must be in their best interests
- Anything done for, or on behalf of, individuals without capacity must be the least restrictive alternative in terms of their rights and basic freedoms.

Good communication between care providers and people with dementia and their families and carers is essential.

Depression in vascular dementia

- Depression is common in vascular dementia. This is due not only to the physical and emotional stress caused by the disease and its diagnosis and effects but also (for small-vessel dementia) because of a direct effect of white matter damage on cortical–subcortical circuits
- Depression complicating dementia can be difficult to detect and is frequently missed
- A high index of suspicion is essential because good treatment responses can be obtained
- Dementia patients with depression do not necessarily present with biological symptoms, but it may result in a global deterioration which may be taken as a progression of their underlying disease instead of depression
- It is difficult to diagnose. Multidisciplinary team assessment and carer opinion is important. Sometimes a carefully monitored trial of therapy is required
- Treatment should consider both pharmacological and non-pharmacological approaches.

Psychological interventions

- Care packages for people with dementia should include assessment and monitoring for depression and/or anxiety
- For people with dementia who have depression and/or anxiety, cognitive behavioural therapy, which may involve the active participation of their carers, may be considered as part of treatment
- A range of tailored interventions, such as reminiscence therapy, music therapy, multisensory stimulation, animal-assisted therapy, and exercise, should be available for people with dementia who have depression and/or anxiety.

Pharmacological treatment

- People with dementia who also have major depressive disorder should be offered antidepressant medication
- Antidepressant drugs with anticholinergic effects should be avoided because they may adversely affect cognition, particularly in patients with coexistent Alzheimer's pathology or a mixed dementia picture.

Vascular mild cognitive impairment

This describes cognitive impairment resulting from cerebrovascular disease which does not meet the criteria for dementia. It is increasingly being used as a concept.

This follows from the use of the term 'mild cognitive impairment' (MCI) to describe patients with a pre-Alzheimer syndrome of mild cognitive impairment, not meeting the criteria for Alzheimer's dementia. Patients with MCI have a high probability of progressing to Alzheimer's disease, although not all do. The hope is that the identification and treatment may delay progression, although this has not yet been supported by clinical trials.

Community studies have shown that vascular mild cognitive impairment is more common than vascular dementia (2.6% versus 1.5% in the Canadian Study of Health and Ageing). In the same study, the prevalence of vascular MCI increased with age (from 1.4% at >65 years to 3.8% in those >85 years).

Vascular MCI may identify a group with high risk of dementia. In one study, 50% of patients progressed to frank dementia in a 5-year period.

The concept is still in its infancy. Whether it is a useful concept is disputed. If more appropriate and sensitive criteria are used (particularly those sensitive to the cognitive features of subcortical dementia), many patients with vascular MCI may in fact have dementia. Because of the difficulties in applying conventional dementia criteria to vascular dementia, some authorities suggest using the term vascular cognitive impairment to include both vascular MCI and vascular dementia.

Further reading

O'Brien JT (2006) Vascular cognitive impairment. *American Journal of Geriatric Psychiatry* **14**, 724–33.

Chapter 16

Organization of stroke services

Introduction

- Stroke has been recognized in medicine for more than 3000 years but only recently has stroke medicine been considered a specialty in its own right
- As a disease of ageing, stroke has been susceptible to age-related prejudice which has hindered development of services and investment in research
- In the context of a worldwide ageing population, stroke care is changing all over the world with the recognition that stroke is now a treatable condition
- Since the landmark work of the Stroke Unit Trialists' Collaboration in the 1990s, stroke units now feature in hospitals worldwide, although large geographical disparities remain. South Africa gained its first stroke unit in a public hospital in 2000. In India (a country with 1.4 million strokes per annum), stroke units exist in the main only in private and a few teaching hospitals. In the UK NHS, the RCP Sentinel stroke audit has shown a steady increase in access to stroke unit care, but still only two-thirds of eligible patients in 2006 went anywhere near a stroke unit
- There is still much to be done and an organizational (evidence-based) framework is the cornerstone of delivering effective stroke care. In England and Wales this has been set out for the first time since the creation of the NHS in The National Stroke Strategy documentation, published in December 2007, available at http://www.dhgov.uk/en/Publicationsandstatistics/publications/publicationspolicyandguidance/dh_081062
- Stroke services should be organized to fit within the structure of the existing healthcare system but require a systematic approach to provide a 'pathway' along which a patient with stroke may 'journey'. Such a pathway should have five components:
  - Effective primary prevention and public awareness of stroke symptoms
  - Direct access to specialist acute stroke services for diagnosis, treatment, and secondary prevention
  - Stroke unit care in hospital
  - Specialist stroke rehabilitation
  - Re-integration into community life after stroke.

The pathway will involve primary and secondary healthcare as well as social care providers and voluntary sector bodies.

For the purpose of this chapter, the stroke pathway will be divided into three phases:

- Pre-hospital care
- Acute hospital care
- Post-hospital care.

Pre-hospital care

- Acute stroke care begins with the timely recognition of the symptoms of stroke and treating stroke as a 'medical emergency'. This involves both public education and education of the wider healthcare community
- With the advent of thrombolytic therapy, the need for an acute stroke 'pathway' and early symptom recognition is paramount
- Rapid transportation to an acute stroke centre (alerting the hospital in advance to the patient's imminent arrival) is a prerequisite to receiving thrombolytic treatment of threatened ischaemic stroke as there is such a narrow therapeutic window—administration has currently to be within 4.5 hours of symptom onset—and requires prior brain imaging
- A key concept when planning pre-hospital care is that *'Time is brain'*
- Simple tools have been developed to help with stroke symptom recognition by paramedics. Pre-hospital stroke recognition instruments were first introduced in the mid 1990s in the USA (Los Angeles Paramedic Stroke Scale [LAPSS] and Cincinnatti Prehospital Stroke Scale [CPSS]) and in the late 1990s in the UK (Face Arm Speech Test [FAST], a modification of the Cincinnatti scale)
- The **F**ace **A**rm **S**peech **T**est was designed to be an integral part of a training package for UK ambulance personnel. As with the CPSS, the FAST consists of three items (facial weakness, arm weakness, and speech disturbance) but avoids the need for the patient to repeat a sentence as a measure of speech. Instead, language fluency and clarity are assessed by the paramedic during conversation with the patient
- The FAST test is being increasingly used as a method for the public to be alerted to the symptoms of stroke.

The FAST test

- *F–FACE:* Ask the person to smile. Does one side of the mouth or face droop?
- *A–ARMS:* Ask the person to raise both arms. Does one arm drift downward or can't be raised?
- *S–Speech:* Ask the person to repeat a sentence. Can they repeat it correctly? Do they slur the words?
- *T–TIME:* If the person exhibits any problems with these call for emergency help.

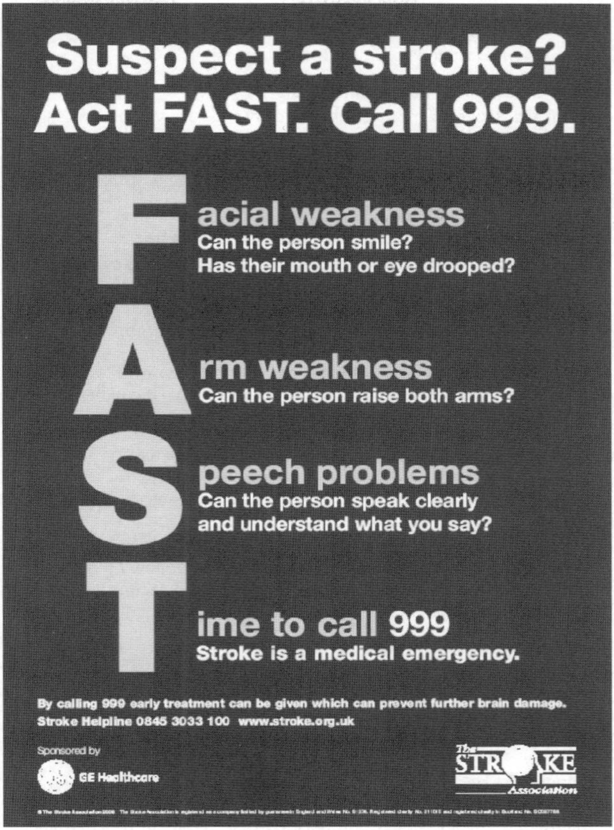

Fig. 16.1 A poster designed to promote public awareness of stroke using the FAST test. © Stroke Association. Reproduced with permission.

Further reading

Nor AM, McAllister C, Louw SJ *et al.* (2004) Agreement between ambulance paramedic- and physician-recorded neurological signs with Face Arm Speech Test (FAST) in acute stroke patients. *Stroke* **35**, 1355–9.

Acute hospital care

This starts with fast and accurate stroke diagnosis.

Initial emergency room diagnosis

In hospital a stroke diagnosis can be speedily and relatively accurately and reliably carried out by non-specialist healthcare professionals using the ROSIER scoring system (Fig. 16.2). The aim of this assessment tool is to enable medical and nursing staff to differentiate patients with stroke from stroke mimics.

Other aspects of acute stroke care organization

- Brain imaging is always required to confirm the diagnosis of stroke
- In all cases, especially in cases potentially suitable for thrombolysis, imaging is an emergency
- A formal thrombolysis protocol (see 📖 p. 242) with appropriate training for staff is essential
- Acute stroke should be managed in an organized acute stroke unit
- If the stroke diagnosis is subarachnoid haemorrhage, the patient is best managed in a centre with neuroradiology and neurosurgical expertise as well as a specialist intensive care unit
- The use of documented protocols for major aspects of management and of proformas for data collection is important
- Audit of processes and outcome is an essential part of a good stroke service
- Transfer of care from acute hospital should involve a comprehensive multidisciplinary discharge summary. Appropriate follow up is needed if there are outstanding matters involving diagnosis, secondary prevention or other issues.

Thrombolysis as a driver for change

Thrombolysis treatment for acute stroke, offering the possibility for the first time of cure for stroke, is the one thing more than any other that has changed how stroke services are being organized. It is this treatment that has predominantly led to stroke now being considered a 'medical emergency'.

Potential barriers to stroke thrombolysis occur in both the pre-hospital and acute hospital care pathway and include:

- Failure of recognition of symptoms of stroke by patient or family and/ or failure to seek urgent help
- Failing to go directly to hospital (i.e. calling the general practitioner/ family doctor rather than an ambulance first)
- Paramedics and emergency department staff triaging stroke as non-urgent or failing to diagnose stroke
- Delays in neuroimaging
- Inefficient process of in-hospital emergency stroke care
- Physicians' uncertainty about administering thrombolysis.

Exclude BM <3.5 mmol/L, treat urgently, and reassess once blood glucose normal		
Has there been loss of consciousness or syncope?	Y (−1)✍	N (0)✍
Has there been seizure activity?	Y (−1)✍	N (0)✍
Is there a *new acute* onset (or on awakening from sleep)?		
I. Asymmetric facial weakness	Y (+1)✍	N (0)✍
II. Asymmetric arm weakness	Y (+1)✍	N (0)✍
III. Asymmetric leg weakness	Y (+1)✍	N (0)✍
IV. Speech disturbance	Y (+1)✍	N (0)✍
V. Visual field effect	Y (+1)✍	N (0)✍
*Total score ____ (−2 to +5) Provisional diagnosis: ✍ Stroke ✍ Non-stroke (specify) ____________		
*Stroke is likely if total scores are >0. Scores of </=0 have a low possibility of stroke but it is not completely excluded		

Fig. 16.2 The ROSIER scale designed to aid in emergency room diagnosis of stroke patients. Reproduced with permission from Nor AM, Davis J, Sen B *et al.* (2005) The Recognition of Stroke in the Emergency Room (ROSIER) scale: development and validation of a stroke recognition instrument. *Lancet Neurology* **4**, 727–34, with permission from Elsevier.

Further reading

Kwan J, Hand P, Sandercock P (2004) A systematic review of barriers to delivery of thrombolysis for acute stroke. *Age Ageing* **33**, 116–21.

Stroke units

The evidence from over 30 trials, in 7000 stroke patients, is that organized care on a specialized stroke unit reduces death, disability, and the number of stroke patients needing discharge into institutionalized long-term care.

- Although the evidence is based on a number of different models of stroke unit care, the best results come from those which are based in a dedicated ward (as opposed to a 'mobile stroke unit' or team).

What is a stroke unit?

There are a number of models of stroke unit—acute, rehabilitation, mixed, all of which have the same core features of:

- Geographically defined area in a hospital
- Evidence-based protocols for treating stroke and its complications
- Ethos of promoting stroke recovery and rehabilitation
- Co-ordinated multidisciplinary care
- Programmes of education in stroke.

Acute stroke units must have:

- Brain imaging
- Rapid assessment protocols for thrombolysis
- Proactive/anticipatory management of common complications of stroke
- Non-invasive physiological monitoring for:
  - HR (arrhythmia)
  - BP
  - RR
  - O_2 saturation
  - Temperature
  - Glucose
- Protocols and guidelines in all areas of acute stroke management.

Why do stroke units succeed?

Although evidence shows that stroke units reduce mortality there is no definite information on what aspects of care result in this improvement. It is likely that many aspects of care result in this improvement, including:

- Interested and motivated staff
- Evidence-based, protocol-driven, management
- Reduction of complications (e.g. DVT, pneumonia)
- More intensive medical intervention
  - Observational studies have shown interventions such as IV fluids in the first 24 hours, insulin therapy, antibiotic therapy, and oxygen are more common in stroke units
- More organized and intensive therapy
  - For example, observational studies have shown that early mobilization is more common on stroke units
- What is clear is that thrombolysis does not account for the difference in the stroke unit trials. Only a small minority of patients received it in the trials.

Staffing a stroke unit

- There is no single correct answer to how many staff are required on a stroke unit although there are some interesting proposals
- Most of the time the issue is limited resources
- Stroke units should have an establishment of medical, nursing, physiotherapy and occupational therapy, speech and language therapy, dietician, and clinical psychology healthcare staff
- In England, the Department of Health suggested a workforce establishment based on consensus views and compared it to a recent actual survey. A survey of recommendations is shown in Table 16.3
- Within the table, the estimated number of whole working-time equivalent members of each profession per 10 beds of stroke unit are shown
- Sources of data include the Stroke Unit Trialists' Collaboration (SUTC), the National Sentinel Stroke Audit, the British Association of Stroke Physicians (BASP), and the University of Central Lancashire data set (UCLan). There are also figures from a survey carried out by the Royal College of Physicians on behalf of the Department of Health (DH). A further source of information comes from the consensus statements produced by professional bodies involved in UK stroke care. Some of these sources have further broken down their analysis into staffing levels for acute (ASU) and rehabilitation (SRU) stroke units
- Staffing in stroke units inevitably varies. In another western European country, Austria, an acute stroke unit of 4–8 beds would typically have:
  - One neurologist
  - One nurse per bed
  - One physiotherapist, one occupational therapist, and one speech and language therapist per four beds.

This is similar to the aspirational levels of staffing proposed by the English Department of Health.

Actual

	No. working time equivalents of each profession per 10 bed ward						
Profession	SUTC*	NSA*	BASP – ASU	BASP – SRU	UCLan – ASU	UCLan – SRU	DH – Survey*
Nurses	7-12	3.3 (2.9-3.7)^	8	10.1	8.5	12.8	10.9 (9.3-13.1)
Occupational therapists	0.6-1.7 (1-1.3)	1 (0.7-1.3)	0.7	0.6	0.3	1.2	1.3 (0.8-1.6)
Physiotherapists	1.2-1.7 (1-2)	1.3 (0.9-1.6)	0.9	0.8	2	3	1.7 (1.2-2.1)
Speech and language therapists	0.25-0.75 (0.2-0.6)	0.3 (0.2-0.6)	0.35	0.25	0.2	0.4	0.4 (0.2-0.6)

*Median (IQR)
^Relates to number of staff on duty at a particular time per 10 bed unit

Aspirational

	No. working time equivalents of each profession per 10 bed ward			
	Consensus statements	UCLan – ASU	UCLan – SRU	DH – Survey
Nurses	12.5	12.00	11.59	12.9
Occupational therapists	1 (ASU) 2 (SRU)	2.56	2.89	3.3
Physiotherapists	3.74 (ASU) 4.67 (RSU)	3.22	3.40	3.7
Speech and language therapists	1	1.89	1.14	1.4
Psychologists		0.92	0.92	

Fig. 16.3 Illustrative Stroke Unit Staffing Grid (English Department of Health). Reproduced from the Department of Health website (2008). http://www.dh.gov.uk/en/Healthcare/NationalServiceFrameworks/Stroke/DH_081389. Reproduced under the terms of the Click-Use Licence.

Further reading

BASP: Cassidy TP *et al.* on behalf of British Association of Stroke Physicians (2006) Specialist stroke services: Consultant workforce requirements. http://www.basp.ac.uk/portals/15/BASP-Consultant-Manpower-Report.pdf

Department of Health and Royal College of Physicians (2007) Survey of Stroke Unit Staffing and Patient Dependency. London, DH.

NSA: Clinical Effectiveness and Evaluation Unit (2007) Royal College of Physicians. National Sentinel Stroke Audit 2006

Stroke Unit Trialists' Collaboration. (2007) Organised inpatient (stroke unit) care for stroke. *Cochrane Database Systematic Reviews* **17(4)**, CD000197.

Stroke Unit Trialists' Collaboration (1997) Collaborative systematic review of the randomised trials of organised inpatient (stroke unit) care after stroke. *BMJ* **314**, 1151–9.

SUTC: Langhorne P, Pollock A, in conjunction with The Stroke Unit Trialists' Collaboration (2002) What are the components of effective stroke unit care? *Age and Ageing* **31**, 365–71.

UCLan: Leathley MJ *et al.* (1997) Pre/post discharge audit of stroke services and care in Liverpool and Sefton: delivery,timelines and targeting. Report to Liverpool Health Authority.

Post-hospital care

Early supported discharge

- For patients with mild to moderate disability after stroke, there is some evidence now that 'early supported discharge' by a specialist multidisciplinary (rehabilitation) team reduces death and disability (as well as length of hospital stay)
- Such models of stroke care have, however, been associated with a suspicion of increased carer burden
- Whilst a promising approach, early supported discharge is likely to be only part of a portfolio of services required in the post-acute stroke care pathway.

Bed-based stroke rehabilitation

- This is likely to be the most appropriate post-acute stroke care for patients with severe and complex neurological disability from stroke
- Coordinated multidisciplinary care with a 'goal planning' approach is usual in a bed-based setting which would have 24-hour nursing supervision and a geographical setting removed from the acute hospital (see 🕮 Chapter 14).

Community stroke services

- Unidisciplinary or multidisplinary community-based rehabilitation services are an important part of post-acute stroke care
- Ideally, patients should move seamlessly into a bespoke programme of community-based neurorehabilitation according to their need, as early intervention is likely to have the greatest impact on functional outcome
- This may be either administered at home or in a community-based rehabilitation centre
- Such a service is also essential for management of ongoing symptoms for those left with chronic long-term neurological conditions as a result of stroke (e.g. wheelchair services, spasticity clinics, and orthotics).

Role of the voluntary sector

- Voluntary sector organizations can help with regaining confidence after stroke and provide valuable social, emotional, as well as practical support, enabling integration back into a community setting.

Further reading

Early supported discharge

Langhorne P, Holmqvist LW (2007) Early supported discharge trialists. Early supported discharge after stroke. *Journal of Rehabilitation Medicine* **39**, 103–8.

Langhorne P, Taylor G, Murray G *et al.* (2005) Early supported discharge services for stroke patients: a meta-analysis of individual patients' data. *Lancet* **365**, 501–6.

Chapter 17

Ethical issues in stroke care

Background and legal framework

When making any clinical decision, a healthcare professional needs to be sure that they are firmly on the 'playing field of medical ethics' which has as its boundaries the four cornerstones of:

- **Autonomy** (what the patient wants/patient choice)
- **Beneficence** (to do good by the patient)
- **Non-malificence** (to do no harm to the patient)
- **Justice/equity** (to be 'fair').

The final consideration is *legality*. Healthcare professionals cannot act outside the law. Considerations of legality differ between countries. For example, physician-assisted suicide is a criminal offence in the UK, but is legal within strictly regulated guidelines in some other countries.

Whilst much of what is outlined in this chapter is directly relevant to those practising in the UK NHS, the principles discussed are generally applicable to all those working with stroke patients.

European Law of Human Rights—The Human Rights Act 1998

This came into force in the UK at the beginning of October 2000.

The articles of the act most relevant to clinical care are:

- Article 2: right to life
- Article 3: prohibition of torture and inhuman and degrading treatment. This was termed as an 'absolute human right'
- Article 5: right to liberty
- Article 8: right to respect for private and family life, home, and correspondence
- Article 10: freedom of expression and right to information
- Article 14: right not to be discriminated against on grounds of, for example, race, sex, etc.

Details of the act can by found at the following web address: http://www.opsi.gov.uk/ACTS/acts1998/ukpga_19980042_en_1.

Confidentiality

It is essential to respect a patient's confidentiality. The following points are taken from guidance issued by the General Medical Council (GMC)—the regulatory body of the medical profession in the UK. They are, however, widely applicable and represent a good standard of practice.

- Patients have a right to expect that a doctor will not disclose any personal information which they learn during the course of their professional duties, unless the patient gives permission
- Disclosure of medical information between medical teams in hospital and between hospital and general practitioner (family doctor) is clearly required for treatment to which a patient has agreed and, as such, the patient's explicit consent is not needed. The same goes in cases of medical emergency
- Disclosure to employers and insurance companies should only be undertaken with the patient's written consent
- The following are circumstances where disclosure without the patient's consent may be appropriate:
  - 'In the patient's medical interests'
  - 'In the best interests of others', i.e. in the public interest.

The GMC guidance can be found in full at the following web address: http://www.gmc-uk.org/guidance/current/library/confidentiality.asp.

Capacity

- The terms competence and capacity are often used interchangeably
  - Competence is a legal concept
  - Capacity is a more pragmatic concept related to a clinical setting where a clinician determines the patient's ability to make an informed decision about his or her healthcare
- The law presumes all adults to have capacity until proven otherwise
- Competence is specific to the task being considered, not global. For example, in the first few days after a stroke, a patient who has capacity to decide whether they prefer tea or coffee may not have capacity to decide on whether they wish to enter a research trial of a novel pharmacological agent
- Owing to the high incidence of communication problems following stroke, capacity decisions are often difficult. The common issues that need assessment of capacity involve: treatment decisions (e.g. insertion of feeding gastrostomy tube); discharge planning (e.g. a patient with high level care needs who refuses help or adaptations but insists on returning home); and finances
- Many patients with aphasia still have capacity provided the assessment is conducted using supported communication techniques, such as 'total communication' which utilizes verbal, written, and gestured communication. In trying to assess capacity in a patient with aphasia, a joint review with a speech and language therapist is helpful. Where there is doubt (either way), provided there is no life-threatening urgency to the decision, it is always better to wait and return at a different time or day to form a final opinion
- On 📖 p. 509 are several examples of guidance showing how the concept of assessing capacity has developed—all of which have a similar theme.

Applebaum and Grisso: Standards for Determining Capacity

New England Journal of Medicine 1988; **319**, 1635–8.

- The ability to maintain and communicate stable choices
- The comprehension of information presented
- The appreciation of the likely consequences
- The ability to manipulate the information rationally.

Case Law (UK)—Legal Capacity and Consent to Treatment: Re C [Adult Refusal of Medical treatment 1994, 1 A11 ER 819]

- An adult has legal capacity to give consent or refuse consent to medical treatment if he or she can:
  - Understand and retain the information relevant to the decision in question
  - Believe that information
  - Weigh that information in the balance to arrive at a choice.

British Medical Association and Law Society—Assessment of mental capacity guidance for doctors and lawyers

1995: London, BMA, p. 66

To be considered to have capacity to undergo a medical treatment a patient should:

- Understand, in simple language, what the medical treatment is, its purpose and why it is being proposed
- Understand its principal benefits, risks, and alternatives
- Understand in broad terms what the consequences would be of not receiving the proposed treatment
- Retain the information long enough to make an effective decision
- Make a free choice.

Mental Capacity Act 2005 (England and Wales)

This came into effect in October 2007 and is a new framework for decision-making on behalf of adults aged 16 and over.

Basic principles include:

- A presumption of capacity in all
- Maximizing decision-making capacity (e.g. using 'total communication strategies' with a speech and language therapist to determine capacity in an aphasic patient)
- The freedom to make unwise decisions
- Best interests—incorporating the person's past and present wishes (including any advance life directives) and their beliefs or values
- The least restrictive alternative.

The test of capacity should include a patient's ability to demonstrate four things:

- To understand information relevant to the decision
- To retain information relevant to the decision
- To use or weigh the information
- To communicate the decision (by any means).

In practice, it is this test that we routinely use when assessing capacity in the NHS.

- The Act also changed the role of the holder of 'Power of Attorney', formerly known as *Enduring Power of Attorney* (EPA) and now known as *Lasting* Power of Attorney (LPA). Power of Attorney is drawn up by an adult with capacity in anticipation of a future point in time when they may be unable to make decisions for themselves (i.e. lack capacity). The person making the Power of Attorney (the donor) appoints another to act on their behalf (the receiver) and registers this with the Office of the Public Guardian. The Power of Attorney only becomes activated when the donor is deemed to have lost capacity
- Prior to 2007, the holder of Power of Attorney only had control over the donor's financial affairs and estate. Now, the receiver in England, Wales and Scotland is also the voice of the donor with regard to medical decision-making
- The Act has also introduced a new process for adults who lack capacity, have neither an appointed Power of Attorney nor appropriate next of kin. In such a scenario, an Independent Mental Capacity Advocate (IMCA) is legally required to ensure the patient's best interests are being followed. IMCAs are trained advocates, independent of Health and Social services
- Where an adult lacks both capacity and an appointed Power of Attorney, but has an appropriate next of kin, the next of kin can still apply for receivership to manage the person's affairs via the Court of Protection. Like LPAs, deputies appointed by the Court of Protection will be able to take decisions on welfare, healthcare, and financial matters but will not be able to refuse consent to life-sustaining treatment

- Finally, the Act introduces a new criminal offence of ill treatment or neglect of a person who lacks capacity—punishable by imprisonment for up to 5 years
- Full details of the Act are at: http://www.opsi.gov.uk/ACTS/acts2005/ukpga_20050009_en_1

Consent

Informed consent for clinical procedures

- Without valid consent, a healthcare professional may not lawfully examine or treat a competent adult
- Proceeding to physical examination without consent (or valid refusal) risks committing battery (unconsented touching) or assault
- The principle of respect for autonomy grants patients a right to decline investigations or treatment, even if in doing so they risk ill health or death
- UK Department of Health guidelines can be downloaded from the following address: www.doh.gov.uk/consent.

Some key points on consent: the law in England

- The consent process has two possible outcomes—acceptance or refusal
- Issues of consent are principally about acceptance of medical treatment and social care
- Consent can be written, verbal or implied by actions
- A signature on a consent form is *evidence* that a patient has given consent, but is not *proof* of valid consent
- For consent to be valid, the patient must:
  - Be competent to take the particular decision
  - Have received adequate information to take it
  - Not be acting under duress (voluntary).

The last point is interesting in the context of gaining informed consent for stroke thrombolysis. In our experience, whilst in the midst of an acute ischaemic brain injury patients are often incapable of giving informed consent. In such cases it is our practice to gain only *assent* whilst informing the next of kin about the treatment decision.

What is adequate information?

In 1985 The House of Lords adopted the Bolam test (named after a patient who claimed he had not been given adequate information before receiving electroconvulsant therapy in 1954).

This legal standard when deciding whether adequate information has been given to a patient should be the same as that used when judging whether a doctor has been negligent in their treatment or care of a patient (i.e. they would not be considered negligent if their practice conformed to that of a responsible body of medical opinion).

This can still be open to the courts to decide.

Example: consenting for carotid endarterectomy

- Patient must be able to demonstrate capacity around the decision to accept or refuse the operation, i.e.
  - Be able to understand the information relevant to the decision (understand that the cause of the stroke episode is a narrowed carotid artery which, if left untreated, leaves them at higher risk of recurrent stroke than if they accept the operation)
  - To retain the information relevant to the decision
  - To use or weigh the information (risks of surgery against risks of medical treatment)
  - To communicate the decision (verbally, in writing or by gesture)
- Patient must be given sufficient information around the procedure, including risk of stroke, death, other typical complications of surgery (scar, wound healing issues, possible local cranial nerve damage), and any alternative treatments (e.g. stenting if appropriate)
- It is well within a patient's remit to ask an individual surgeon their personal rates of success and complication.

Consent for research trials and other studies

Consenting to enter a research trial involves knowing about:

- The research purpose, questions, aims, and methods
- Relevant terms like 'randomize'
- The treatment, if any, which the research investigates
- Benefits, risks, harms or costs to research subjects
- Hoped-for benefits to other groups such as future patients
- Confidentiality, indemnity, sponsors, and ethical approval
- The research team and a named contact.

Research in adults who lack capacity

- Currently no legislation available
- In the UK, GMC guidelines suggest research into conditions with adults with incapacity should not be undertaken if it could equally well be done with other adults
- Guidance is available in the UK from '*GMC: Research: The role and responsibilities of doctors*', which suggests that if research involves subjects with incapacity, you must demonstrate that:
  - It could be of direct benefit to their health, or
  - It is of special benefit to the health of people in the same age group with the same state of health, or
  - That it will significantly improve the scientific understanding of the adult's incapacity, leading to a direct benefit to them or others with the same incapacity
  - The research is ethical and will not cause the participants emotional, physical or psychological harm
  - The person does not express objections physically or verbally
- The GMC guidelines can be downloaded from the following address: http://www.gmc-uk.org/guidance/ethical_guidance/consent_guidance/index.asp

Withholding treatment and withdrawing medical treatment

This is an extremely emotive and potentially upsetting scenario in stroke care but one which not infrequently arises—especially where the stroke is associated with a bleak prognosis.

It always requires careful attention, a multidisciplinary team approach, and sensitive communication with family, carers, and friends.

Withdrawing artificial nutrition and hydration

- There is considerable variation in what constitutes 'basic care' and what constitutes 'medical treatment' across Europe
- Currently, artificial nutrition and hydration (ANH) is not 'basic care' but medical treatment in English Law
- The intention of withholding or withdrawing life-prolonging treatment is to refrain from providing treatment that is not benefiting the patient. This should not involve making judgements on the value of a patient's life
- The British Medical Association recommends clinical review by a second specialist not involved in the care team, respecting advance life directives if available, and, if not, seeking information from family members and close friends as to what the patient may have considered to be beneficial.

Advanced life directives (ALDs)

Also known as 'Living Wills' or 'Advanced Refusals'.

- Developed in USA after recognition of persistent vegetative state cases
- Now topical in the setting of dementia
- Must be drawn up by competent patients
- Three main types:
  1. Instructive (legally binding); e.g. If I had a stroke and was unable to walk again I would not want any life-prolonging treatment, including tube feeding
  2. Values; e.g. If I had a stroke which meant I was no longer able to complete my favourite newspaper cryptic crossword I would not want any life-prolonging treatment
  3. Proxy; e.g. If as a result of a disabling stroke I am unable to make my own decisions regarding medical treatment I would want my son to do so on my behalf
- Should be respected where appropriate and patient now *lacks* mental capacity *(legally binding)*
- If doubt exists whether ALD applies to current circumstances, then a court declaration should be sought
- The British Medical Association has developed guidelines *(http://www.bma.org.uk/ap.nsf/Content/advancestatements)*
- An example of a living will is available from http://www.dignityindying.org.uk

Further reading

British Medical Association (2007) *Withholding and withdrawing life prolonging treatment (LPT): guidance for decision making*, 3rd edn. London, BMA.
http://www.gmcuk.org/guidance/current/library/witholding_lifeprolonging_guidance.asp.

Persistent vegetative state (PVS)

- First described by Jennett and Plum in 1972 as 'the absence of any adaptive response to the external environment, the absence of any evidence of a functioning mind which is either receiving or projecting information, in a patient who has long periods of wakefulness'
- Clinically, patients are able to breathe without mechanical support and cardiovascular, gastrointestinal, and renal function must be stable. The patient may be aroused by painful stimuli (eye opening or grimacing). Patients also show spontaneous movements such as chewing, teeth grinding, smiling, crying, grunting or screaming
- PVS due to stroke is rare and is most often seen where stroke is complicated by a prolonged hypoxic brain injury caused by a secondary complication
- Differential diagnosis:
  - Coma—state of unconsciousness in which eyes are closed and sleep–wake cycles are absent (usually transient but may lead to vegetative state)
  - Locked-in syndrome—results from brainstem lesions which disrupt voluntary control of movement without abolishing either arousal or content of awareness, e.g. extensive pontine infarction due to basilar artery thrombosis. Patients can typically communicate via eye movements
  - Brain death—loss of brainstem function
- Prognosis—recovery to a state of severe disability is seen in up to 1.6% of patients with PVS at 1 year. Overriding outlook is miserable.

Further reading

Jennett B, Plum F (1972). Persistent vegetative state after brain damage. A syndrome in search of a name. *Lancet* **1**, 734-7.

Wade DT, Johnston C (1999) The permanent vegetative state: practical guidance on diagnosis and management. *BMJ* **319**, 841–4.

Zeman A (1997) Persistent vegetative state. *Lancet* **350**, 795–9.

Brainstem death

- Must be independently confirmed by two medically qualified doctors
- Must wait at least 6 hours after onset of coma or, if anoxia or cardiac arrest was cause of coma, until 24 hours after circulation has been restored
- The two tests must be performed at least 2 hours apart
- No legal requirements for special tests to confirm diagnosis in the UK
- Criteria of brainstem death:
  1. Patient is comatose and apnoeic
  2. There is irremediable structural brain damage due to head injury or intracranial haemorrhage (and be >6 hours after onset of coma), or prolonged anoxia or cardiac arrest (and be >24 hours after circulation restored)
  3. The following have been excluded:
     - Hypothermia
     - Drug or alcohol intoxification
     - Metabolic or endocrine derangement
     - Neuromuscular blockade (no such drugs for 12 hours)
  4. There are no brainstem reflexes
  5. The patient remains apnoeic on disconnection from the ventilator.

Resuscitation (CPR) decisions

- Cardiopulmonary resuscitation (CPR) was first described in 1960 and devised to treat cardiorespiratory arrest consequent upon anaesthesia or surgery
- Cardiac arrest always renders a patient legally incompetent. In England and Wales, up until recently families have had no rights in law over CPR decisions of adults, and doctors have acted as the patient's advocate 'in partnership with those people close to the patient'. Excluding relatives of an incompetent patient from participating in making decisions may be seen to breach Human Rights Act Article 8 (*right to respect private and family life*). However, recent changes outlined in the Mental Capacity Act have now given those with Lasting Power of Attorney the right to make decisions over medical treatment issues, including CPR
- Recent changes in the UK have seen that, as well as doctors, nurses with appropriate training can also make valid resuscitation orders (including Do Not Attempt Resuscitation or DNAR)
- 'Futility' as a rationale for making CPR decisions has now been rejected, although in practice it is still often cited. Instead 'consideration of the prospect for restoration of pulse and respiration initially and then to consider if this will benefit the patient' should be the guide
- Outcome from in-hospital CPR is poor; studies have shown 14–66% (mean 39%) immediate recovery, 0–28% (mean 15%) discharged, and 5–17% alive at 6 months
- Competent patients' attitudes and participation should always be taken into account (unless they indicate they do not want to), especially with decisions regarding DNAR orders. Valid advanced refusals of CPR must be respected
- If a competent patient does not want a DNAR order, then one cannot be written—but at the same time 'doctors cannot be required to give treatment contrary to their clinical judgement, but should, whenever possible, respect patients' wishes to receive treatment which carries only a very small chance of success or benefit'
- Published guidelines regarding good practice in the UK were revised in 2007 (http://www.resus.org.uk/pages/dnar.pdf).

Palliative care

- Stroke is a common cause of death, and most stroke deaths occur in hospital
- Mortality is greatest in the first 28 days of admission
- Where the diagnosis is one of 'end of life' or 'dying', palliation or symptom control will be the most appropriate form of medical and multidisciplinary treatment
- Palliation is alleviating without curing
- Predictors of mortality in stroke include:
  - Deep coma
  - Stroke severity, e.g. NIHSS >25
  - Brain imaging evidence of diffuse intracerebral bleeding, including intraventricular blood, massive hemispheric infarction with mass effect, brainstem stroke
  - Multiorgan failure
  - Great age
  - Depression
- In principle, all interventions should be aimed at relieving symptoms of suffering, distress, and pain. This includes psychological symptoms such as severe anxiety
- There needs to be clear communication between the members of the treating team and family/carers/friends
- The religious and cultural needs of the patient should be addressed
- Involvement of a palliative care specialist may be appropriate.

Deaths reportable to the UK Coroner

This is only applicable to the UK. Under regulation 51 of Registration of Births, Deaths and Marriages Regulations 1968 the following deaths should be reported:

- Element of suspicious death or history of violence
- Death linked to an accident
- Death due to occupation or industrial disease
- Death linked to abortion
- Death during operation or before full anaesthetic recovery
- Death related to medical procedure or treatment
- Actions of deceased may have contributed to their own death (self-neglect, drug or solvent abuse)
- Death occurred in police custody or prison
- Death within 24 hours of admission
- Deceased was detained under the Mental Health Act.

In practice it is only those patients that die within the first 24 hours of admission to hospital that are reported to the Coroner, but it is well to be aware of the other criteria; e.g. death following stroke caused by carotid dissection is likely to need to be discussed with the Coroner owing to the association of such injury with trauma.

Glossary

Name	Description
Activities of daily living (ADLs)	Tasks performed in the daily routine (e.g. washing, dressing)
Advocate	Someone who acts on the patient's behalf
Agnosia	Impairment of ability to understand the meaning of various sensory stimuli
Agraphia	Inability to write
Alexia	Inability to read
Aneurysm	Weak section of an artery wall that balloons out and may rupture
Angiography	Contrast-enhanced X-ray of the blood vessels
Angioplasty	Insertion of a catheter into a narrow artery and dilatation of the artery; inflation of a balloon on the end of the catheter
Anosognosia	Lack of awareness or denial of disease (e.g. the patient denies anything being wrong with the stroke side)
Anticoagulant	A drug (e.g. warfarin) used to prevent blood clots by inhibiting the blood coagulation protein thrombin
Anticonvulsants	Antiepileptic drugs
Antihypertensives	Blood pressure lowering drugs
Antiphospholipid syndrome	A condition that results from antibodies that form against the body's phospholipids, producing thrombosis
Antiplatelet therapy	Drugs used to stop platelets in the blood sticking to one another and forming clots. Aspirin is the most widely used. Others include clopidogrel (Plavix) and dipyridamole (Persantin)
Antithrombotics	Drugs that are used to prevent blood clots
Aphasia	The inability to use language. It can either be a problem understanding language (receptive) or speaking it (expressive)
Apoptosis	Programmed, genetically triggered cell death
Apraxia	Loss of abililty to do well practised tasks (e.g. dressing)
Arrhythmia	Irregular heart beat
Arteriography	X-ray of arteries after the injection of a radio-opaque contrast material
Arteriovenous malformation (AVM)	Disorder characterized by a complex tangle of arteries and veins

Name	Description
Aspiration pneumonia	Chest infection (pneumonia) resulting from the inhalation of foreign material
Asteriognosis	Inability to identify an object by touch
Ataxia	Lack of coordination, unsteadiness
Atheroma	Fatty cholesterol deposits inside of artery walls (*synonym* plaque)
Atherosclerosis	A disease of arteries characterized by deposits of lipid material which make the artery hard, thick (narrow) and brittle
Atrial fibrillation	Where the heart is beating irregularly. There is an increased risk of a blood clot forming inside the heart, which can break off, travel to the brain and cause a stroke
Blood pressure	The pressure inside the arteries, pushing blood through the circulation. Pressure is highest when the ventricles in the heart contract (systole) and lowest when they relax (diastole). The normal BP is about 120/80 mmHg
Blood–brain barrier	The walls of blood vessels and capillaries in the brain regulate which elements of the blood can pass through to the neurons
Brainstem	The stem-like, lower part of the brain that connects the brain's right and left hemispheres to the spinal cord
Bruit	The noise that can be heard when listening over a narrowed artery
Capillaries	Tiny blood vessels whose wall consists of endothelium and basement membrane
Cardiac	Relating to the heart
Cardioembolic stroke	Stroke due to a clot that formed in the heart and travelled to the brain
Cardiovascular	Relating to the heart and blood vessels
Carotid artery	There are two carotid arteries located on either side of the neck that supply the front half of the brain with blood. Disease of a carotid artery is a common cause of stroke
Carotid endarterectomy	The operation to remove atheroma from the narrowed internal carotid artery
Carotid stenosis	Narrowing of the carotid artery
Catheter (urine)	A medical device (tube) used to control urinary incontinence using a receptacle bag

Name	Description
Catheterization	The insertion of a tube inside the body—most commonly this is into the bladder to drain the urine directly into a bag
Central pain	Pain caused by damage and altered pain perception in the brain (often the thalamus)
Cerebellum	The part of the brain at the back which is responsible for coordinating voluntary muscle movements
Cerebral	Relating to the brain
Cerebral blood flow (CBF)	The flow of blood through the arteries in the brain
Cerebral cortex	The outer layer of the brain consisting of grey matter
Cerebral haemorrhage	Bleeding into the brain tissue (intracerebral haemorrhage) or into surrounding areas (subarachnoid haemorrhage)
Cerebral hemisphere	One of the two halves of the brain
Cerebral infarct	An area where brain cells have died
Cerebral oedema	Swelling of the brain
Cerebrovascular accident (CVA)	An old term used for stroke (the term is falling into disuse because stroke is no longer viewed as an accident)
Cerebrovascular disease (CVD)	Encompasses all abnormalities in the brain resulting from pathologies of its blood vessels (narrowing, blockage)
Cerebrum	The largest part of the brain, made up of the left and right hemispheres (sides)
Cholesterol	A fatty substance that, if present in excess, can be deposited in the wall of the artery to produce atherosclerosis
Cognition	Higher intellectual (mental) functioning associated with thinking, learning, perception, and memory
Cognitive impairment	A deficiency in a person's short- or long-term memory, orientation as to place, person and time, thinking and judgement
Coma	A state of deep unconsciousness when the person is not responsive or able to be aroused
Computed tomography (CT) scan	A series of cross-sectional X-rays of the brain and head; also called computerized axial tomography (CAT)

Name	Description
Confabulation	Filling gaps in memory with imagined events
Continence	The ability to control urinary bladder and bowel functions
Contracture	Static muscle shortening so that the muscle cannot be lengthened and loss of motion of the adjacent joint occurs
Contralateral	The opposite side of the body
Coordination	The control of several muscle groups in the execution of complex movements
CVA	The abbreviation for cerebrovascular accident. Not recommended as the concept of stroke being an accident is not helpful
Deep venous thrombosis (DVT)	A clot of blood usually in the leg veins
Delirium	A temporary state of confusion, often linked with other illnesses such as infection (taken from the Latin *de lire*, meaning 'out of furrow')
Dementia	Progressive and irreversible loss of intellectual ability (speech, abstract thinking, judgement, memory loss, physical coordination) that interfere with daily activities (e.g. Alzheimer's disease)
Depression	A reversible psychiatric disorder characterized by an inability to concentrate, difficulty sleeping, feeling of hopelessness, fatigue, the 'blues', and guilt
Diplopia	Double vision
District nurse	A nurse who provides skilled, flexible nursing care to people within the community and at home
Diuretics	Drugs given to make you pass more urine. They are used to control heart failure and high blood pressure
Duplex carotid scan (also termed carotid Doppler)	An ultrasound scan of the carotid arteries in the neck
Dysarthria	A motor disorder of the tongue, mouth, jaw or voicebox resulting in slurred speech
Dyslexia	Difficulty reading
Dyslipidaemia	Abnormality in blood lipids
Dysphagia	Difficulty swallowing

Name	Description
Dysphasia or aphasia	Difficulty in using language owing to problems understanding language (receptive) and speaking it (expressive)
Dysphonia	Impairment of the voice
Dyspraxia	Difficulty with performing skilled or purposeful voluntary movement even though the person is physically able to do it
Echocardiogram	Ultrasound scan of the heart
Electrocardiogram (ECG)	A test that measures electrical activity and rhythm of the heart
Electroencephalogram (EEG)	A test used to record electrical activity in the brain by placing electrodes on the scalp
Embolic stroke	A stroke caused by an embolus
Embolism	Blockage of a blood vessel by an embolus
Embolus	A clot or piece of other material which travels distally in the bloodstream, eventually lodging in the blood vessels at a distant site
Emotional lability	A condition in which the mood of the person swings rapidly (unreasonably) from one state to another (such as laughing, crying or anger)
Endarterectomy	Surgical operation to remove obstructions (usually fatty tissue or blood clot) from inside an artery
Enteral feeding	Feeding using a tube connecting with the stomach
Epidemiology	The study of factors that influence the frequency and distribution of a disease in a population
Epilepsy	Seizures or fits
Extracranial–intracranial (EC–IC) bypass	A type of surgery that restores blood flow to a blood-deprived area of brain tissue by rerouting a healthy artery in the scalp to the area of brain tissue affected by a blocked/narrowed artery
Field of vision	The area that you can see without moving your eyes (or head)
Flaccid	Absence of muscle tone, producing floppy muscles
Gait	Manner of walking
Geriatrician	A doctor who specializes in the care of older people, primarily those who are frail and have complex medical and social problems
Glia	Supportive cells of the nervous system that also play an important role in brain functioning; also called neuroglia

Name	Description
Goal setting	The process whereby the professionals and the patient decide on the main objectives for rehabilitation
Haematoma	A collection of blood forming a definite swelling which compresses and damages the brain around it
Haemorrhagic infarct	An infarct that has had secondary bleeding in it
Haemorrhagic stroke	Bleeding into the brain (intracerebral haemorrhage) or into surrounding areas (subarachnoid haemorrhage)
Handicap	The social consequence of disability for the patient
Hemianaesthesia	Loss of sensation down one side of the body
Hemianopia	Loss of the half field of vision in each eye
Hemi-inattention	Ignoring space on the side of the body; sometimes called unilateral neglect
Hemiparesis	Weakness of one-half of the body
Hemiplegia	Complete paralysis of half of the body
Hemisphere	One half of the brain
Heparin	A type of anticoagulant
High-density lipoprotein cholesterol (HDL-C)	A compound consisting of a lipid and a protein that carries cholesterol in the blood and deposits it in the liver; also known as 'good' cholesterol
Homeostasis	A state of equilibrium or balance in the body with respect to various functions and to the chemical compositions of the fluids and tissues
Homonymous hemianopia	Loss of the same half field of vision in each eye
Hughes' syndrome	See antiphospholipid syndrome
Hydrocephalus	Raised pressure within the skull caused by excess fluid on the brain
Hypercholesterolaemia	A high level of cholesterol in the blood
Hyperlipidaemia	A high level of fats in the blood
Hypertension	High blood pressure
Hypotension	Low blood pressure
Impairment	Loss of function (e.g. weakness, loss of sensation, loss of speech)
Impotence	Inability to obtain or maintain penile erection

Name	Description
Incidence	Frequency with which cases of a disease occur during a certain period of time in a population
Incontinence	Inability to control urinary bladder (urinary incontinence) or bowel functions (bowel incontinence), or both
Infarct or infarction	Area of dead or dying brain tissue
Intermediate care	Services working together to help people recover from illness and stop them going into hospital if it is not necessary or staying in hospital longer than they need to
Intracerebral haemorrhage	Bleeding into the brain substance
Involuntary	Without being willed or intended
Ischaemia	A loss or reduction of blood flow to tissue resulting in reduce nutrients, oxygen, and removal of waste products (such as lactic acid)
Ischaemic penumbra	Area of damaged, but still living, brain cells arranged in a patchwork pattern around areas of dead brain cells
Ischaemic stroke	An area where brain cells have died (*synonyms* cerebral infarct, cerebral infarction)
Key worker	The member of the team who is responsible for making sure that health and social care professionals involved in patient treatment and care know what plans and decisions are being made. The key worker is also responsible for keeping the patient and family informed
Lacunar stroke/infarct	A small stroke less than 1.5 cm in diameter when measured on the brain scan (from the French word 'lacune' meaning a lake)
Large artery disease	Stenosis or occlusion of the carotid arteries, often due to atherosclerosis
Lipoprotein	Small globules of cholesterol covered by a layer of protein
Long-term care	This is provided for people who are unable to live independently and who move into residential or nursing homes
Low-density lipoprotein cholesterol (LDL-C)	A compound consisting of a lipid and a protein that carries cholesterol in the blood and deposits the excess along the inside of arterial walls; also known as 'bad' cholesterol
Lumbar puncture	A procedure whereby some of the spinal fluid is removed by the insertion of a needle into the spine

Name	Description
Magnetic resonance angiography (MRA)	An imaging technique involving injection of radio-opaque contrast material into a blood vessel and using magnetic resonance techniques to create an image of brain arteries and veins
Magnetic resonance imaging (MRI)	A type of scan that, instead of X-rays, uses a large, powerful magnet to create an image (picture) of part of the body
Middle cerebral artery	The artery that most frequently becomes blocked, to cause stroke
Monoparesis, monoplegia	Weakness, paralysis of one limb only
Mortality	Describes the number of persons who die during a certain period of time
Nasogastric tube	Tube put down the nose into the stomach
Neglect, one-sided	A term sometimes used for lack of awareness of one side of the body
Neurologist	A doctor specializing in diseases of the nervous system
Neurology	The study of the structure, functioning, and diseases of the nervous system
Neuron	The main functional cell of the brain and nervous system, consisting of a cell body, an axon, and dendrites
Neuroplasticity	After stroke, dead brain cannot regrow. Unaffected brain tissue that surrounds the dead area takes over part of the lost function. This process is called neuroplasticity
Neuroprotective agents	Medications that protect the brain from secondary injury
Nursing home	A generic term for a skilled nursing facility
Nystagmus	Involuntary jerking of the eyes normally caused by damage to the cerebellum or brainstem
Obesity	Being more than 20% over your recommended weight
Occupational therapist (OT)	A therapist who specializes in helping people to reach their maximum level of function and independence in all aspects of daily life
Oedema	Swelling owing to excess water in the tissue
Ophthalmologist	A doctor who specializes in the investigation and treatment of diseases of the eyes

Name	Description
Orthosis	An external orthopaedic appliance, as a brace or splint, that prevents or assists movement of the spine or the limbs
Papilloedema	Swelling of the optic discs in the eyes
Paraesthesia	An abnormal sensation, such as of burning, pricking, tickling, or tingling
Paralysis	Complete weakness and loss of movement
Paraparesis, paraplegia	Weakness, paralysis of both legs (can happen with bilateral strokes or spinal cord problems)
Paraphrasia	Producing unintended phrases, words or syllables during speech
Paresis	Muscle weakness
Patent foramen ovale (PFO)	A small 'hole' in the heart that may allow blood clots to travel from the right side to the left side without going through the lungs
Peer support	Getting support from people in the same situation as you
PEG tube	Percutaneous endoscopic gastrostomy feeding tube inserted through the abdominal wall into the stomach
Perception	The ability to receive, interpret, and use information
Percutaneous endoscopic gastrostomy (PEG)	Insertion of a tube through the wall of the abdomen into the stomach for the purposes of feeding with a fibreoptic instrument called a gastroscope
Pharmacist	A person who is qualified in pharmacy and authorized to dispense drugs
Phlebotomist	Someone who is trained to take blood specimens from people's veins
Physician	A qualified doctor who specializes in the diagnosis and treatment of disease by other than surgical means
Physiotherapist	A therapist who specializes in physical methods of treatment to promote functional recovery of movement
Plaque	A mixture of fatty substances, including cholesterol and other lipids, deposited inside of artery walls
Plasticity of the brain	See neuroplasticity
Platelets	Blood cells that are known for their role in blood coagulation

Name	Description
Positron emission tomography (PET)	A nuclear medicine scanning technique that uses radioactive isotopes to assess the metabolic function of the brain
Power of Attorney	The legal right to manage financial and other affairs on behalf of another
Prevalence	The number of cases of a disease in a population at any given point in time
Primary care	Care delivered by the GP or healthcare professionals within the community
Prognosis	Expected outcome
Psychiatrist	A specialist in the study and treatment of mental disorders
Psychologist	A person qualified in the scientific study of the mind. A clinical psychologist is trained in the assessment and treatment of people with illness
Pulmonary embolism	A blood clot in the lungs
Randomized controlled trial	A clinical study in which persons are assigned to the experimental or control group by a random selection procedure
Recombinant tissue plasminogen activator (rtPA)	A genetically engineered form of t-PA, a thrombolytic anticlotting substance made naturally by the body
Rehabilitation	The process of regaining function through active treatment
Rehabilitation unit	A place where skilled and experienced staff work to help the stroke patient adjust to the effects of stroke
Respite care	Care given to someone for a short period, usually away from their own home so their family can have a rest from the burdens of caring for them
Rest home	A generic term for a group home, specialized apartment complex or other institution which provides care services where individuals live; sometimes referred to as a private hospital, residential care facility or a care home
Risk factors	The possible underlying causes (for the stroke) such as smoking, high blood pressure, ethnic group, family history of stroke
Small-vessel disease	A disease of small arteries in the brain, often due to hypertension

Name	Description
Social security	A state department which works through the Department of Work and Pensions (DWP) to organize financial aid and assistance in the form of State benefits
Social services	The body run by the local authority or council which provides a number of services for those living at home, including personal care, day centres, equipment and adaptations
Social worker	Someone from the social services department who gives advice and practical help with social problems
Spasm	Involuntary contraction of a muscle
Spastic paralysis	Paralysis with increased muscle tone and spasmodic contraction of the muscles
Spasticity	Abnormally increased tone in a muscle
Speech and language therapist (SALT)	A therapist who specializes in the rehabilitation of people with speech and language difficulties, helping them to improve their speech and language, and/or to find alternative ways of communicating. They also help with problems with swallowing
Spinal cord	The long elliptical part of the central nervous system joining the brain to the peripheral nerves. It runs in the vertebral canal
Stenosis	A narrowing normally in an artery
Stroke	An acute vascular injury of the brain
Stroke unit	The ward for multidisciplinary team management of patients with acute stroke
Subarachnoid haemorrhage	Bleeding between the brain pial surface and the covering membranes, often caused by a ruptured aneurysm
Thalamus (thalamic)	A part of the brain where the nerves carrying information about sensation from the body join with other nerves
Thromboembolic	A blood clot which has embolized
Thrombolysis	The use of drugs to break up a blood clot
Thrombosis	The formation of a blood clot
Thrombotic stroke	A stroke caused by thrombosis
Thrombus	A blood clot
Tone	A slight constant tension in muscles at rest

Name	Description
Total serum cholesterol	A combined measurement of high-density lipoprotein cholesterol (HDL-C) and low-density lipoprotein cholesterol (LDL-C)
Transcranial magnetic stimulation (TMS)	A small magnetic current delivered to stimulate an area of the brain
Transient ischaemic attack (TIA)	A short-lived mini stroke that lasts from a few minutes up to 24 hours
Vascular	Relating to the blood vessels
Vasospasm	Spasm of a blood vessel
Vein	A blood vessel that carries blood back to the heart
Vertebral arteries	The two arteries on either side of the back of the neck that travel to the brain. They supply the posterior part of the brain
Vertigo	An abnormal sensation of movement
Videofluoroscopy	A video X-ray of the swallowing mechanism
Visuospatial disorder	Inability to interpret special problems correctly
Warfarin	The most frequently used oral anticoagulant

Appendix

Useful stroke scales

NIH Stroke Scale

N I H
STROKE
SCALE

Patient Identification. ___ ___-___ ___ ___-___ ___ ___

Pt. Date of Birth ___ ___/___ ___/___ ___

Hospital ______________________(___ ___-___ ___)

Date of Exam ___ ___/___ ___/___ ___

Interval: [ ] Baseline [ ] 2 hours post treatment [ ] 24 hours post onset of symptoms ±20 minutes [ ] 7-10 days
[ ] 3 months [ ] Other ______________________________(___ ___)

Time: ___ ___:___ ___ [ ]am [ ]pm

Person Administering Scale ______________________________

Administer stroke scale items in the order listed. Record performance in each category after each subscale exam. Do not go back and change scores. Follow directions provided for each exam technique. Scores should reflect what the patient does, not what the clinician thinks the patient can do. The clinician should record answers while administering the exam and work quickly. Except where indicated, the patient should not be coached (i.e., repeated requests to patient to make a special effort).

Instructions	Scale Definition	Score
1a. Level of Consciousness: The investigator must choose a response if a full evaluation is prevented by such obstacles as an endotracheal tube, language barrier, orotracheal trauma/bandages. A 3 is scored only if the patient makes no movement (other than reflexive posturing) in response to noxious stimulation.	0 = **Alert**; keenly responsive. 1 = **Not alert**; but arousable by minor stimulation to obey, answer, or respond. 2 = **Not alert**; requires repeated stimulation to attend, or is obtunded and requires strong or painful stimulation to make movements (not stereotyped). 3 = Responds only with reflex motor or autonomic effects or totally unresponsive, flaccid, and areflexic.	___
1b. LOC Questions: The patient is asked the month and his/her age. The answer must be correct - there is no partial credit for being close. Aphasic and stuporous patients who do not comprehend the questions will score 2. Patients unable to speak because of endotracheal intubation, orotracheal trauma, severe dysarthria from any cause, language barrier, or any other problem not secondary to aphasia are given a 1. It is important that only the initial answer be graded and that the examiner not "help" the patient with verbal or non-verbal cues.	0 = **Answers** both questions correctly. 1 = **Answers** one question correctly. 2 = **Answers** neither question correctly.	___
1c. LOC Commands: The patient is asked to open and close the eyes and then to grip and release the non-paretic hand. Substitute another one step command if the hands cannot be used. Credit is given if an unequivocal attempt is made but not completed due to weakness. If the patient does not respond to command, the task should be demonstrated to him or her (pantomime), and the result scored (i.e., follows none, one or two commands). Patients with trauma, amputation, or other physical impediments should be given suitable one-step commands. Only the first attempt is scored.	0 = **Performs** both tasks correctly. 1 = **Performs** one task correctly. 2 = **Performs** neither task correctly.	___
2. Best Gaze: Only horizontal eye movements will be tested. Voluntary or reflexive (oculocephalic) eye movements will be scored, but caloric testing is not done. If the patient has a conjugate deviation of the eyes that can be overcome by voluntary or reflexive activity, the score will be 1. If a patient has an isolated peripheral nerve paresis (CN III, IV or VI), score a 1. Gaze is testable in all aphasic patients. Patients with ocular trauma, bandages, pre-existing blindness, or other disorder of visual acuity or fields should be tested with reflexive movements, and a choice made by the investigator. Establishing eye contact and then moving about the patient from side to side will occasionally clarify the presence of a partial gaze palsy.	0 = **Normal.** 1 = **Partial gaze palsy;** gaze is abnormal in one or both eyes, but forced deviation or total gaze paresis is not present. 2 = **Forced deviation,** or total gaze paresis not overcome by the oculocephalic maneuver.	___
3. Visual: Visual fields (upper and lower quadrants) are tested by confrontation, using finger counting or visual threat, as appropriate. Patients may be encouraged, but if they look at the side of the moving fingers appropriately, this can be scored as normal. If there is unilateral blindness or enucleation, visual fields in the remaining eye are scored. Score 1 only if a clear-cut asymmetry, including quadrantanopia, is found. If patient is blind from any cause, score 3. Double simultaneous stimulation is performed at this point. If there is extinction, patient receives a 1, and the results are used to respond to item 11.	0 = **No visual loss.** 1 = **Partial hemianopia.** 2 = **Complete hemianopia.** 3 = **Bilateral hemianopia** (blind including cortical blindness).	___
4. Facial Palsy: Ask – or use pantomime to encourage – the patient to show teeth or raise eyebrows and close eyes. Score symmetry of grimace in response to noxious stimuli in the poorly responsive or non-comprehending patient. If facial trauma/bandages, orotracheal tube, tape or other physical barriers obscure the face, these should be removed to the extent possible.	0 = **Normal** symmetrical movements. 1 = **Minor paralysis** (flattened nasolabial fold, asymmetry on smiling). 2 = **Partial paralysis** (total or near-total paralysis of lower face). 3 = **Complete paralysis** of one or both sides (absence of facial movement in the upper and lower face).	___
5. Motor Arm: The limb is placed in the appropriate position: extend the arms (palms down) 90 degrees (if sitting) or 45 degrees (if supine). Drift is scored if the arm falls before 10 seconds. The aphasic patient is encouraged using urgency in the voice and pantomime, but not noxious stimulation. Each limb is tested in turn, beginning with the non-paretic arm. Only in the case of amputation or joint fusion at the shoulder, the examiner should record the score as untestable (UN), and clearly write the explanation for this choice.	0 = **No drift;** limb holds 90 (or 45) degrees for full 10 seconds. 1 = **Drift;** limb holds 90 (or 45) degrees, but drifts down before full 10 seconds; does not hit bed or other support. 2 = **Some effort against gravity;** limb cannot get to or maintain (if cued) 90 (or 45) degrees, drifts down to bed, but has some effort against gravity. 3 = **No effort against gravity;** limb falls. 4 = **No movement.** UN = **Amputation** or joint fusion, explain: ________________ **5a. Left Arm** **5b. Right Arm**	 ___ ___

6. Motor Leg: The limb is placed in the appropriate position: hold the leg at 30 degrees (always tested supine). Drift is scored if the leg falls before 5 seconds. The aphasic patient is encouraged using urgency in the voice and pantomime, but not noxious stimulation. Each limb is tested in turn, beginning with the non-paretic leg. Only in the case of amputation or joint fusion at the hip, the examiner should record the score as untestable (UN), and clearly write the explanation for this choice.	0 = **No drift;** leg holds 30-degree position for full 5 seconds. 1 = **Drift;** leg falls by the end of the 5-second period but does not hit bed. 2 = **Some effort against gravity;** leg falls to bed by 5 seconds, but has some effort against gravity. 3 = **No effort against gravity;** leg falls to bed immediately. 4 = **No movement.** UN = **Amputation** or joint fusion, explain: ______ **6a. Left Leg** **6b. Right Leg**	____
7. Limb Ataxia: This item is aimed at finding evidence of a unilateral cerebellar lesion. Test with eyes open. In case of visual defect, ensure testing is done in intact visual field. The finger-nose-finger and heel-shin tests are performed on both sides, and ataxia is scored only if present out of proportion to weakness. Ataxia is absent in the patient who cannot understand or is paralyzed. Only in the case of amputation or joint fusion, the examiner should record the score as untestable (UN), and clearly write the explanation for this choice. In case of blindness, test by having the patient touch nose from extended arm position.	0 = **Absent.** 1 = **Present in one limb.** 2 = **Present in two limbs.** UN = **Amputation** or joint fusion, explain: ______	____
8. Sensory: Sensation or grimace to pinprick when tested, or withdrawal from noxious stimulus in the obtunded or aphasic patient. Only sensory loss attributed to stroke is scored as abnormal and the examiner should test as many body areas (arms [not hands], legs, trunk, face) as needed to accurately check for hemisensory loss. A score of 2, "severe or total sensory loss," should only be given when a severe or total loss of sensation can be clearly demonstrated. Stuporous and aphasic patients will, therefore, probably score 1 or 0. The patient with brainstem stroke who has bilateral loss of sensation is scored 2. If the patient does not respond and is quadriplegic, score 2. Patients in a coma (item 1a=3) are automatically given a 2 on this item.	0 = **Normal;** no sensory loss. 1 = **Mild-to-moderate sensory loss;** patient feels pinprick is less sharp or is dull on the affected side; or there is a loss of superficial pain with pinprick, but patient is aware of being touched. 2 = **Severe to total sensory loss;** patient is not aware of being touched in the face, arm, and leg.	____
9. Best Language: A great deal of information about comprehension will be obtained during the preceding sections of the examination. For this scale item, the patient is asked to describe what is happening in the attached picture, to name the items on the attached naming sheet and to read from the attached list of sentences. Comprehension is judged from responses here, as well as to all of the commands in the preceding general neurological exam. If visual loss interferes with the tests, ask the patient to identify objects placed in the hand, repeat, and produce speech. The intubated patient should be asked to write. The patient in a coma (item 1a=3) will automatically score 3 on this item. The examiner must choose a score for the patient with stupor or limited cooperation, but a score of 3 should be used only if the patient is mute and follows no one-step commands.	0 = **No aphasia;** normal. 1 = **Mild-to-moderate aphasia;** some obvious loss of fluency or facility of comprehension, without significant limitation on ideas expressed or form of expression. Reduction of speech and/or comprehension, however, makes conversation about provided materials difficult or impossible. For example, in conversation about provided materials, examiner can identify picture or naming card content from patient's response. 2 = **Severe aphasia;** all communication is through fragmentary expression; great need for inference, questioning, and guessing by the listener. Range of information that can be exchanged is limited; listener carries burden of communication. Examiner cannot identify materials provided from patient response. 3 = **Mute, global aphasia;** no usable speech or auditory comprehension.	____
10. Dysarthria: If patient is thought to be normal, an adequate sample of speech must be obtained by asking patient to read or repeat words from the attached list. If the patient has severe aphasia, the clarity of articulation of spontaneous speech can be rated. Only if the patient is intubated or has other physical barriers to producing speech, the examiner should record the score as untestable (UN), and clearly write an explanation for this choice. Do not tell the patient why he or she is being tested.	0 = **Normal.** 1 = **Mild-to-moderate dysarthria;** patient slurs at least some words and, at worst, can be understood with some difficulty. 2 = **Severe dysarthria;** patient's speech is so slurred as to be unintelligible in the absence of or out of proportion to any dysphasia, or is mute/anarthric. UN = **Intubated** or other physical barrier, explain: ______	____
11. Extinction and Inattention (formerly Neglect): Sufficient information to identify neglect may be obtained during the prior testing. If the patient has a severe visual loss preventing visual double simultaneous stimulation, and the cutaneous stimuli are normal, the score is normal. If the patient has aphasia but does appear to attend to both sides, the score is normal. The presence of visual spatial neglect or anosagnosia may also be taken as evidence of abnormality. Since the abnormality is scored only if present, the item is never untestable.	0 = **No abnormality.** 1 = **Visual, tactile, auditory, spatial, or personal inattention** or extinction to bilateral simultaneous stimulation in one of the sensory modalities. 2 = **Profound hemi-inattention or extinction to more than one modality;** does not recognize own hand or orients to only one side of space.	____

Scandinavian Stroke Scale

From *Stroke* 1985: 885–90

Initial Prognostic and Long-term Functional Scores

From Stroke 1985: 166: 885–90

	Score	Prognostic score	Long-term score
Consciousness			
fully conscious	6		
somnolent, can be awakened to full consciousness	4	□	
reacts to verbal command, but is not fully conscious	2		
Eye movements			
no gaze plasy	4		
gaze plasy present	2	□	
conjugate eye deviation	0		
Arm, motor power*			
raises arm with normal strength	6		
raises arm with reduced strength	5		
raises arm with flexion in elbow	4	□	□
can move, but not against gravity	2		
paralysis	0		
Hand, motor power*			
normal strength	6		
reduced strength in full range	4		□
some movement, fingertips do not reach palm	2		
paralysis	0		
Leg, motor power			
normal strength	6		
raises straight leg with reduced strength	5		
raises leg with flexion of knee	4	□	□
can move, but not against gravity	2		
paralysis	0		
Orientation			
correct for time, place and person	6		
2 of these	4		□
1 of these	2		
completely disorientated	0		
Speech			
no aphasia	10		
limited vocabulary or incoherent speech	6		□
more than yes/no, but not longer sentences	3		
only yes/no or less	0		
Facial palsy			
none/dubious	2		□
Gait			
walks 5 m without aids	12		
walks with aids	9		
walks with help of another person	6		□
sites without support	3		
bedridden/wheelchair	0		
Maximal score		22	48

*Motor power is assessed only on the affected side.

Barthel Index

	With Help	Independent
1. Feeding (if food needs to be cut up = help)	5	10
2. Moving from wheelchair to bed and return (includes sitting up in bed)	5–10	15
3. Personal toilet (wash face, comb hair, shave, clean teeth)	0	5
4. Getting on and off toilet (handling clothes, wipe, flush)	5	10
5. Bathing self	0	5
6. Walking on level surface (or if unable to walk, propel wheelchair) *score only if unable to walk	0*	5*
7. Ascend and descend stairs	5	10
8. Dressing (includes tying shoes, fastening fasteners)	5	10
9. Controlling bowels	5	10
10. Controlling bladder	5	10

A patient scoring 100 BI is continent, feeds himself, dresses himself, gets up out of bed and chairs, bathes himself, walks at least a block, and can ascend and descend stairs. This does not mean that he is able to live alone: he may not be able to cook, keep house, and meet the public, but he is able to get along without attendant care.

From Mahoney FI, Barthel D (1965) Functional evaluation: the Barthel Index. *Maryland State Medical Journal* **14**, 61–65. Used with permission.

Definition and discussion of scoring

1. Feeding

10 = Independent. The patient can feed himself a meal from a tray or table when someone puts the food within his reach. He must put on an assistive device if this is needed, cut up the food, use salt and pepper, spread butter, etc. He must accomplish this in a reasonable time.

5 = Some help is necessary (with cutting up food, etc., as listed above).

2. Moving from wheelchair to bed and return

15 = Independent in all phases of this activity. Patient can safely approach the bed in his wheelchair, lock brakes, lift footrests, move safely to bed, lie down, come to a sitting position on the side of the bed, change the position of the wheelchair, if necessary, to transfer back into it safely, and return to the wheelchair.

10 = Either some minimal help is needed in some step of this activity or the patient needs to be reminded or supervised for safety of one or more parts of this activity.

5 = Patient can come to a sitting position without the help of a second person but needs to be lifted out of bed, or if he transfers with a great deal of help.

3. Doing personal toilet

5 = Patient can wash hands and face, comb hair, clean teeth, and shave. He may use any kind of razor but must put in blade or plug in razor without help as well as get it from drawer or cabinet. Female patients must put on own makeup, if used, but need not braid or style hair.

4. Getting on and off toilet

10 = Patient is able to get on and off toilet, fasten and unfasten clothes, prevent soiling of clothes, and use toilet paper without help. He may use a wall bar or other stable object for support if needed. If it is necessary to use a bed pan instead of a toilet, he must be able to place it on a chair, empty it, and clean it. Patient needs help because of imbalance or in handling clothes or in using toilet paper.

5. Bathing self

5 = Patient may use a bath tub, a shower, or take a complete sponge bath. He must be able to do all the steps involved in whichever method is employed without another person being present.

6. Walking on a level surface

15 = Patient can walk at least 50 yards without help or supervision. He may wear braces or prostheses and use crutches, canes, or a walk-erette but not a rolling walker. He must be able to lock and unlock braces if used, assume the standing position and sit down, get the necessary mechanical aides into position for use, and dispose of them when he sits. (Putting on and taking off braces is scored under dressing.)

10 = Patient needs help or supervision in any of the above but can walk at least 50 yards with a little help.

6a. Propelling a wheelchair

5 = If a patient cannot walk but can propel a wheelchair independently. He must be able to go around corners, turn around, manoeuver the chair to a table, bed, toilet, etc. He must be able to push a chair at least 50 yards. Do not score this item if the patient gets score for walking.

7. Ascending and descending stairs

10 = Patient is able to go up and down a flight of stairs safely without help or supervision. He may and should use handrails, canes, or crutches when needed. He must be able to carry canes or crutches as he ascends or descends stairs.

5 = Patient needs help with or supervision of any one of the above items.

8. Dressing and undressing

10 = Patient is able to put on and remove and fasten all clothing, and tie shoe laces (unless it is necessary to use adaptations for this). The activity includes putting on and removing and fastening corset or braces when these are prescribed. Such special clothing as suspenders, loafer shoes, dresses that open down the front may be used when necessary.

5 = Patient needs help in putting on and removing or fastening any clothing. He must do at least half the work himself.

He must accomplish this in a reasonable time.

Women need not be scored on use of a brassiere or girdle unless these are prescribed garments.

9. Continence of bowels

10 = Patient is able to control his bowels and have no accidents. He can use a suppository or take an enema when necessary (as for spinal cord injury patients who have had bowel training).

5 = Patient needs help in using a suppository or taking an enema or has occasional accidents.

10. Controlling bladder

10 = Patient is able to control his bladder day and night. Spinal cord injury patients who wear an external device and leg bag must put them on independently, clean and empty bag, and stay dry day and night.

5 = Patient has occasional accidents or can not wait for the bed pan or get to the toilet in time or needs help with an external device.

A score of 0 is given in all of the above activities when the patient cannot meet the criteria as defined above.

The advantage of the BI is its simplicity. It is useful in evaluating a patient's state of independence before treatment, his progress as he undergoes treatment, and his status when he reaches maximum benefit. It can easily be understood by all who work with a patient and can accurately and quickly be scored by anyone who adheres to the definitions of items listed above. The total score is not as significant or meaningful as the breakdown into individual items, since these indicate where the deficiencies are.

Any applicant to a chronic hospital who scores 100 BI should be evaluated carefully before admission to see whether such hospitalization is indicated. Discharged patients with 100 BI should not require further physical therapy but may benefit from a home visit to see whether any environmental adjustments are indicated. Encouragement by family and others may be necessary for a patient to maintain his degree of independence.

Rivermead Mobility Index

http://www.medicine.mcgill.ca/strokengine-assess/PDF/RMA.pdf

RIVERMEAD MOBILITY INDEX

PATIENT'S NAME:

HOSPITAL NUMBER:

Score 0 = No 1 = Yes

	DATE				
1. Do you turn over from your back to your side without help?					
2. From lying in bed, are you able to get up to sit on the edge of the bed on your own?					
3. Could you sit on the edge of the bed without holding on for 10 seconds?					
4. Can you (using hands and an aid if necessary) stand up from a chair in less than 15 seconds, and stand there for 15 seconds,					
5. Observe patient standing for 10 seconds without any aid.					
6. Are you able to move from bed to chair and back without any help?					
7. Can you walk 10 metres with an aid if necessary but with no standby help?					
8. Can you manage a flight of steps alone, without help?					
9. Do you walk around outside alone, on pavements?					
10. Can you walk 10 metres inside with no caliper, splint or aid and no standby help?					
11. If you drop something on the floor, can you manage to walk 5 metres to pick it up and walk back?					
12. Can you walk over uneven ground (grass, gravel, dirt, snow or ice) without help?					
13. Can you get in and out of a shower or bath unsupervised, and wash yourself?					
14. Are you able to climb up and down four steps with no rail but using an aid if necessary?					
15. Could you run 10 metres in 4 seconds without limping? (A fast walk is acceptable.)					
TOTAL					

Modified Ashworth Spasticity Scale

0	No increase in tone
1	Slight increase in muscle tone, manifested by a catch and release or minimal resistance at the end of the ROM when the affected part(s) is moved in flexion or extension
1+	Slight increase in muscle tone, manifested by a catch, followed by minimal resistance throughout the remainder (less than half) of the ROM
2	More marked increase in muscle tone through most of the ROM, but affected part(s) easily moved
3	Considerable increase in muscle tone, passive movement difficult
4	Affected part(s) rigid in flexion or extension

From Katz RT (1997) Spasticity. In: O'Young B, Young MA, Stiens SA (eds) *PM&R Secrets*. Philadelphia; Hanley & Belfus, p. 487, with permission of Elsevier.

Tardieu Scale

From Tardieu G, Shentoub S, Delarue R (1954) A la recherché d'une technique de measure de la spasticite. *Revue Neurologie* **91**, 143–4.

The Tardieu Scale explicitly compares the occurrence of a catch at low and high speeds, and is effective in measuring the velocity-dependent component of hypertonia (this unique test item gives the Tardieu greater validity than either the Ashworth or modified Ashworth). It is an ordinal rating of hypertonicity which measures the intensity of the muscle reaction at specified velocities (slowest to as fast as possible). The angle at which the catch is first felt is also noted as a clinical estimate similar to the threshold angle. The three variables are considered simultaneously when assessing spasticity.

Procedure

- A constant position of the body must be established, and remain constant from one test to another
- Other joints, in particular the neck, must remain in a constant position throughout the assessment
- The quality of muscle reaction and the angle of muscle reaction must be rated at each of the stretch velocities
    - Step 1—subject seated in a chair, elbow flexed by 90°
    - Step 2—move the wrist as slowly as possible through pain-free available range into extension (slower than the rate of the natural drop of the wrist under gravity). Rate the quality of muscle reaction (see below) and measure angle of muscle reaction (angle of a catch) as appropriate
    - Step 3—move the wrist as fast as possible through pain-free available range into extension (faster than the rate of the natural drop of the wrist under gravity). Rate the quality of muscle reaction (see below) and measure angle of muscle reaction (angle of a catch) as appropriate.

Score

Quality of muscle reaction: (X)

- 0—No resistance throughout the course of the passive movement
- 1—Slight resistance throughout the course of the passive movement with no clear catch at a precise angle
- 2—Clear catch at a precise angle, interrupting the passive movement, followed by a release
- 3—Fatiguable clonus, less than 10 seconds when maintaining the pressure, appearing at a precise angle
- 4—Unfatiguable clonus, more than 10 seconds when maintaining the pressure, at a precise angle.

Modified Rankin Scale

Score	Description
0	No symptoms at all
1	No significant disability despite symptoms; able to carry out all usual duties and activities
2	Slight disability; unable to carry out all previous activities, but able to look after own affairs without assistance
3	Moderate disability; requiring some help, but able to walk without assistance
4	Moderately severe disability; unable to walk without assistance and unable to attend to own bodily needs without assistance
5	Severe disability; bedridden, incontinent, and requiring constant nursing care and attention
6	Dead

TOTAL (0–6): ____

Reproduced with permission from Van Swieten JC, Koudstaal PJ, Visser MC, Schouten HJ, van Gijn J (1998) Intraobserver agreement for the assessement of handicap in stroke patients. *Stroke* **19(5)**, 604–7.
http://www.RankinScale.org

References

Bonita R, Beaglehole R (1988) Modification of Rankin Scale: recovery of motor function after stroke. *Stroke* **19(12)**, 1497–500.

Rankin J (1957) Cerebral vascular accidents in patients over the age of 60. *Scottish Medical Journal* **2**, 200–15.

Van Swieten JC, Koudstaal PJ, Visser MC, Schouten HJ, van Gijn J (1988) Interobserver agreement for the assessment of handicap in stroke patients. *Stroke* **19(5)**, 604–7.

Patient Health Questionnaire (PHQ-9)

This easy to use patient questionnaire is a self-administered version of the PRIME-MD diagnostic instrument for common mental disorders.[1] The PHQ-9 is the depression module, which scores each of the 9 DSM-IV criteria as "0" (not at all) to "3" (nearly every day). It has been validated for use in Primary Care.[2]

Personal Health Questionnaire Depression Scale (PHQ-9)

Over the **last 2 weeks**, how often have you been bothered by any of the following problems? *(circle **one** number on each line)*

How often during the past 2 weeks were you bothered by...	**Not at all**	**Several days**	**More than half the days**	**Nearly every day**
1. Little interest or pleasure in doing things	0	1	2	3
2. Feeling down, depressed, or hopeless	0	1	2	3
3. Trouble falling or staying asleep, or sleeping too much	0	1	2	3
4. Feeling tired or having little energy	0	1	2	3
5. Poor appetite or overeating	0	1	2	3
6. Feeling bad about yourself, or that you are a failure, or have let yourself or your family down	0	1	2	3
7. Trouble concentrating on things, such as reading the newspaper or watching television	0	1	2	3
8. Moving or speaking so slowly that other people could have noticed. Or the opposite – being so fidgety or restless that you have been moving around a lot more than usual	0	1	2	3
9. Thoughts that you would be better off dead, or of hurting yourself in some way	0	1	2	3

http://patienteducation.stanford.edu/research/phq.pdf
This scale is free to use without permission.

Hamilton Rating Scale for Depression (HAMDS)

http://healthnet.umassmed.edu/mhealth/HAMD.pdf

THE HAMILTON RATING SCALE FOR DEPRESSION

(to be administered by a health care professional)

Patient's Name ______________________

Date of Assessment ______________________

To rate the severity of depression in patients who are already diagnosed as depressed, administer this questionnaire. The higher the score, the more severe the depression.

For each item, write the correct number on the line next to the item. (Only one response per item)

______ 1. **DEPRESSED MOOD** (Sadness, hopeless, helpless, worthless)

0= Absent
1= These feeling states indicated only on questioning
2= These feeling states spontaneously reported verbally
3= Communicates feeling states non-verbally—i.e., through facial expression, posture, voice, and tendency to weep
4= Patient reports VIRTUALLY ONLY these feeling states in his spontaneous verbal and non-verbal communication

______ 2. **FEELINGS OF GUILT**

0= Absent
1= Self reproach, feels he has let people down
2= Ideas of guilt or rumination over past errors or sinful deeds
3= Present illness is a punishment. Delusions of guilt
4= Hears accusatory or denunciatory voices and/or experiences threatening visual hallucinations

______ 3. **SUICIDE**

0= Absent
1= Feels life is not worth living
2= Wishes he were dead or any thoughts of possible death to self
3= Suicidal ideas or gesture
4= Attempts at suicide (any serious attempt rates 4)

______ 4. **INSOMNIA EARLY**

0= No difficulty falling asleep
1= Complains of occasional difficulty falling asleep—i.e., more than 1/2 hour
2= Complains of nightly difficulty falling asleep

______ 5. **INSOMNIA MIDDLE**

0= No difficulty
1= Patient complains of being restless and disturbed during the night
2= Waking during the night—any getting out of bed rates 2 (except for purposes of voiding)

______ 6. **INSOMNIA LATE**

0= No difficulty
1= Waking in early hours of the morning but goes back to sleep
2= Unable to fall asleep again if he gets out of bed

______ 7. **WORK AND ACTIVITIES**

0= No difficulty
1= Thoughts and feelings of incapacity, fatigue or weakness related to activities; work or hobbies
2= Loss of interest in activity; hobbies or work—either directly reported by patient, or indirect in listlessness, indecision and vacillation (feels he has to push self to work or activities)
3= Decrease in actual time spent in activities or decrease in productivity
4= Stopped working because of present illness

______ 8. **RETARDATION: PSYCHOMOTOR** (Slowness of thought and speech; impaired ability to concentrate; decreased motor activity)

0= Normal speech and thought
1= Slight retardation at interview
2= Obvious retardation at interview
3= Interview difficult
4= Complete stupor

______ 9. **AGITATION**

0= None
1= Fidgetiness
2= Playing with hands, hair, etc.
3= Moving about, can't sit still
4= Hand wringing, nail biting, hair-pulling, biting of lips

______ 10. **ANXIETY (PSYCHOLOGICAL)**

0= No difficulty
1= Subjective tension and irritability
2= Worrying about minor matters
3= Apprehensive attitude apparent in face or speech
4= Fears expressed without questioning

11. ANXIETY SOMATIC: Physiological concomitants of anxiety, (i.e., effects of autonomic overactivity, "butterflies," indigestion, stomach cramps, belching, diarrhea, palpitations, hyperventilation, paresthesia, sweating, flushing, tremor, headache, urinary frequency). Avoid asking about possible medication side effects (i.e., dry mouth, constipation)

______ **0**= Absent
1= Mild
2= Moderate
3= Severe
4= Incapacitating

12. SOMATIC SYMPTOMS (GASTROINTESTINAL)

______ **0**= None
1= Loss of appetite but eating without encouragement from others. Food intake about normal
2= Difficulty eating without urging from others. Marked reduction of appetite and food intake

13. SOMATIC SYMPTOMS GENERAL

______ **0**= None
1= Heaviness in limbs, back or head. Backaches, headache, muscle aches. Loss of energy and fatigability
2= Any clear-cut symptom rates 2

14. GENITAL SYMPTOMS (Symptoms such as: loss of libido; impaired sexual performance; menstrual disturbances)

______ **0**= Absent
1= Mild
2= Severe

15. HYPOCHONDRIASIS

______ **0**= Not present
1= Self-absorption (bodily)
2= Preoccupation with health
3= Frequent complaints, requests for help, etc.
4= Hypochondriacal delusions

16. LOSS OF WEIGHT

______ **A.** When rating by history:
0= No weight loss
1= Probably weight loss associated with present illness
2= Definite (according to patient) weight loss
3= Not assessed

17. INSIGHT

______ **0**= Acknowledges being depressed and ill
1= Acknowledges illness but attributes cause to bad food, climate, overwork, virus, need for rest, etc.
2= Denies being ill at all

18. DIURNAL VARIATION

______ **A.** Note whether symptoms are worse in morning or evening. If NO diurnal variation, mark none
0= No variation
1= Worse in A.M.
2= Worse in P.M.

______ **B.** When present, mark the severity of the variation. Mark "None" if NO variation
0= None
1= Mild
2= Severe

19. DEPERSONALIZATION AND DEREALIZATION (Such as: Feelings of unreality; Nihilistic ideas)

______ **0**= Absent
1= Mild
2= Moderate
3= Severe
4= Incapacitating

20. PARANOID SYMPTOMS

______ **0**= None
1= Suspicious
2= Ideas of reference
3= Delusions of reference and persecution

21. OBSESSIONAL AND COMPULSIVE SYMPTOMS

______ **0**= Absent
1= Mild
2= Severe

Total Score ______

Geriatric Depression Scale (GDS)

The Geriatric Depression Scale (GDS) is in the public domain and not protected by copyright. For more information, go to http://www.stanford.edu/~yesavage/GDS.html.

Choose the best answer for how you have felt over the past week:

1. Are you basically satisfied with your life? YES / **NO**
2. Have you dropped many of your activities and interests? **YES** / NO
3. Do you feel that your life is empty? **YES** / NO
4. Do you often get bored? **YES** / NO
5. Are you in good spirits most of the time? YES / **NO**
6. Are you afraid that something bad is going to happen to you? **YES** / NO
7. Do you feel happy most of the time? YES / **NO**
8. Do you often feel helpless? **YES** / NO
9. Do you prefer to stay at home, rather than going out and doing new things? **YES** / NO
10. Do you feel you have more problems with memory than most? **YES** / NO
11. Do you think it is wonderful to be alive now? YES / **NO**
12. Do you feel pretty worthless the way you are now? **YES** / NO
13. Do you feel full of energy? YES / **NO**
14. Do you feel that your situation is hopeless? **YES** / NO
15. Do you think that most people are better off than you are? **YES** / NO

Answers in **bold** indicate depression. Although differing sensitivities and specificities have been obtained across studies, for clinical purposes a score >5 points is suggestive of depression and should warrent a follow-up interview. Scores >10 are almost always depression.

Useful websites

http://www.strokecenter.org/
Website of Washington University St Louis, USA—an excellent resource for ongoing clinical trials.

http://www.stroke-site.org/
The Brain Attack Coalition is a group of American professional, voluntary, and governmental entities dedicated to reducing the occurrence, disabilities, and death associated with stroke. The site is a good resource of guidelines for stroke treatment.

http://www.medicine.mcgill.ca/strokengine/
Canadian site with up-to-date evidence base of stroke rehabilitation.

http://www.strokeassociation.org/presenter.jhtml?identifier=3030388
Official website of American Stroke Association.

http://www.basp.ac.uk/
Official website of British Stroke Physicians.

http://www.stroke.org.uk/
British Stroke Association is a charity for stroke survivors. The site has a lot of useful background facts around stroke and a wealth of patient information.

http://www.world-stroke.org/
The World Stroke Organization (WSO) was established in October 2006 from the merger of the International Stroke Society (ISS) and the World Stroke Federation (WSF), the two lead organizations representing stroke globally. The website has details of presentations from annual meetings and is a window into global stroke care.

http://www.eso-stroke.org/
European stroke website with European guidelines and virtual stroke university with compendium of previous European Stroke Conference lectures and symposia.

http://www.strokecare.co.uk/
The official website of the authors' local stroke service. Has many useful links and generic patient information.

http://wfnr.co.uk/index.html
The World Federation for NeuroRehabilitation (WFNR) is a multidisciplinary organization open to any professional with an interest in neurological rehabilitation. The organization exists to act as a forum of communication between those with an interest in the subject.

http://clinicaltrials.gov/ct2/home
Website of all current (recruiting and about to recruit) clinical trials in USA.

http://www.strokeassociation.org/presenter.jhtml?identifier=3023009
Online NIH scale training.

http://www.library.nhs.uk/stroke/
NHS evidence-based resource for stroke. A good source of general information about all aspects of stroke.

Index

D

E

T

W

X